Surgical Robotics and Computer-Assisted Surgery

Fundamentals and Advances

Editors:

Kapil Joshi

Department of Computer Science & Engineering
Uttaranchal Institute of Technology (UIT)
Uttaranchal University, Dehradun, India

Kiruthigha R

Assistant Professor, Department of Information Technology
SRM Institute of Science and Technology, Chennai, India

Gopal Krishna

Department of Computer Science & Engineering
Uttaranchal Institute of Technology (UIT)
Uttaranchal University, Dehradun, India

Prabhishek Singh

School of Computer Science Engineering and Technology
Bennett University, Greater Noida, India

Manoj Diwakar

Department of Computer Science and Engineering
Graphic Era Deemed to be University, Dehradun, India

CRC Press
Taylor & Francis Group
Boca Raton London New York

CRC Press is an imprint of the
Taylor & Francis Group, an **informa** business
A SCIENCE PUBLISHERS BOOK

First edition published 2027
by CRC Press
2385 NW Executive Center Drive, Suite 320, Boca Raton FL 33431

and by CRC Press
4 Park Square, Milton Park, Abingdon, Oxon, OX14 4RN

CRC Press is an imprint of Taylor & Francis Group, LLC

Library of Congress Cataloging-in-Publication Data (applied for)

ISBN: 978-1-041-08738-0 (hbk)
ISBN: 978-1-041-10453-7 (pbk)
ISBN: 978-1-003-65512-1 (ebk)

DOI: 10.1201/9781003655121

Typeset in Times New Roman
by Prime Publishing Services

Preface

The rapid convergence of artificial intelligence, machine learning, and robotic technologies is transforming modern healthcare at an unprecedented pace. From intelligent diagnosis and predictive analytics to autonomous surgical assistance and immersive medical training, these innovations are redefining how clinicians deliver care and how patients experience recovery. This book has been conceived to present a comprehensive, critical, and forward-looking view of these technological advances, with a particular emphasis on their clinical relevance, ethical implications, and real-world deployment challenges.

The chapters in this volume collectively explore the expanding ecosystem of AI-enabled healthcare. Early chapters establish the foundations by examining the role of machine learning and deep learning in key diagnostic domains such as neuroimaging, fetal health assessment, bone imaging, cancer detection, and dermatology. These contributions highlight how data-driven models are improving accuracy, enabling early diagnosis, and supporting clinical decision-making, while also addressing persistent issues such as data imbalance, limited annotations, domain adaptation, and the need for trustworthy and explainable systems.

A central theme of the book is the transformative impact of intelligent surgical technologies. Multiple chapters investigate the evolution of surgical robotics—from smart sensing instruments and haptic-enabled tools to AI-integrated robotic platforms capable of real-time navigation, intraoperative decision support, and personalised therapy. The discussion extends to specialised domains such as neurosurgery, cardiac surgery, minimally invasive procedures, and robotic-assisted plastic surgery, demonstrating measurable improvements in precision, ergonomics, functional recovery, and patient safety. At the same time, the authors offer a balanced and critical perspective on cost, training requirements, regulatory frameworks, accountability, and global accessibility.

The volume also looks beyond the operating room. It explores augmented and virtual reality for surgical education, intelligent rehabilitation models, brain–computer interfaces, tele-surgery enabled by 5G, and data-governance frameworks required for responsible AI integration. These topics reflect a paradigm shift toward connected, adaptive, and patient-centric healthcare systems.

By bringing together methodological advances, clinical applications, technological innovations, and ethical considerations, this book aims to serve as a valuable resource for researchers, clinicians, engineers, policymakers, and students. It not only documents the current state of the art but also identifies open challenges and future research directions needed to build safe, affordable, and globally deployable intelligent healthcare solutions.

We hope this volume will stimulate interdisciplinary collaboration and inspire the next generation of innovations in AI-driven and robot-assisted medicine.

Contents

Preface *iii*

List of Contributors *vii*

1. Artificial Intelligence and Autonomous Technologies in Revolutionalizing Neurosurgical Precision and Postoperative Recovery 1
2. Advancing Fetal Health Prediction
   A Review of CTG-Based Classification, MRI, Segmentation, and Abnormality Detection 23
3. Fracture Detection in X-Ray Images Using Deep Supervised Learning 44
4. Transforming Healthcare with AI
   An Introduction to Machine Learning and Deep Learning Techniques 65
5. Semi-Supervised Image Segmentation Techniques for Medical Image Analysis 84
6. Challenges Issues on Low-Quality Images in Cancer Detection within Medical Imaging System and Image Enhancement Using Multifocus Image Fusion Techniques 102
7. Future Challenges and Opportunities in Surgical Robotics 118
8. Artificial intelligence Cardiac Surgery and Medicine Practice
   Hope for the Future 131
9. The Role of AI and Robotic Aided Plastic Surgery in Skin Cancer Management 140
10. Enhancing Medical Competence using AR and VR Techniques 152
11. Smart Surgical Tools
    Sensor-Integrated Instruments in Robotic Surgery 168
12. Surgical Robots
    Principles, Technologies and Clinical Application 191
13. Integrating Robotics into Neurosurgery
    Techniques, Benefits, and Challenges 214
14. Robotics in Minimally Invasive Surgery 235

15. Artificial Intelligence and Machine Learning in Robotic Surgery 250

16. The Role of Artificial Intelligence in Next-Generation Surgical Robotics 271

17. Kinematics, Workflow Integration, and Clinical Applications 296

Index 305

About the Editors 307

List of Contributors

Aakash Sharma
School of Computer Science Engineering and Technology, Bennett University, Greater Noida, UP, India.

Amrendra Tripathi
School of Computing, UPES, Dehradun, India.

Ananta Narayana
Bennett University, Greater Noida, Uttar Pradesh.

Animesh Raturi
Department of Computer Science, Uttaranchal Institute of Technology, Uttaranchal University, Dehradun, India.

Anshika Arora
Department of Computer Science and Engineering, Delhi Technological University, New Delhi, India.

Anuradha Brijwal
Uttaranchal Institute of Technology, Uttaranchal University, Dehradun (INDIA).

Archika Jain
Swami Keshvanand Institute of Technology, Management and Gramothan (SKIT) Jaipur, India.

Arpit Goel
Uttaranchal Institute of Technology, Uttaranchal University, Dehradun (INDIA).

Arvind Mewada
Bennett University, Greater Noida, Uttar Pradesh.

Bhavika Mittal
School of Computer Science Engineering and Technology, Bennett University, Greater Noida, 201310, Uttar Pradesh, India.

Bhowmick, Sangita
Director, Bangladesh University, Bangladesh.

Chugh, Pinki
Department of Computer Science, Uttaranchal Institute of Technology, Uttaranchal University, Dehradun, India.

D. Jayarajan
Program of Medical Laboratory Sciences, Faculty of Paramedical Sciences, Assam Down Town University, Gauwahati, Assam-781026.

Deepika Pantola
School of Computer Science Engineering and Technology, Bennett University, Greater Noida, 201310, Uttar Pradesh, India.

Deepika Vatsa
School of Computer Science Engineering and Technology, Bennett University, Greater Noida, UP, India.

Dipika Rawat
Uttaranchal College of Health Sciences, Uttaranchal University, Dehradun-248007, Uttarakhand, India.

Dr. Akanksha Chauhan (PT)
Uttaranchal College of Health Sciences, Uttaranchal University Dehradun.

Dr. Tripti Choudhary
Department of Computer Science and Engineering, Hi-Tech Institute of Engineering and Technology, Ghaziabad.

Garima Jaiswal
Bennett University, Greater Noida, Uttar Pradesh.

Gaurav Kumar Rajput
College of Computing Sciences & Information Technology, Teerthanker Mahaveer University, Moradabad (INDIA).

Gaurav Mittal
Uttaranchal College of Health Sciences, Uttaranchal University, India.

Gopal Krishna
Uttaranchal Institute of Technology, Uttaranchal University, Dehradun, 248007, India.

Hardik Bhardwaj
School of Computer Science Engineering and Technology, Bennett University, Greater Noida, UP, India.

Harishchander Anandaram
Assistant Professor (Senior Grade), Amrita School of Artificial Intelligence, Coimbatore, Amrita Vishwa Vidyapeetham, India.

Ikshit Mangal
Bennett University, Greater Noida, Uttar Pradesh.

Jai Singhal
Bennett University, Greater Noida, Uttar Pradesh.

Jayant Singh
Bennett University, Greater Noida, Uttar Pradesh.

Jitender Gairolla
Department of Paramedical & Allied Sciences, Sparsh Himalaya University, Dehradun, Uttarakhand, India.

Kangan Saraswati
Chandigarh Group of Colleges, Jhanjeri, Mohali, Punjab, 140307, Chandigarh School of Business, Department of Sciences.

Kapil Joshi
Department of Computer Science, Uttaranchal Institute of Technology, Uttaranchal University, Dehradun, India.

Kapil Kumar Sharma
Department of Computer Science and Engineering, Accurate Institute of Engineering and Technology, Greater Noida.

Kapil Sharma
Department of Computer Science and Engineering, Accurate Institute of Engineering and Technology, Greater Noida, India.

Kartikey
School of Liberal Arts, Uttaranchal University, Dehradun, Uttarakhand, India.

Madhuri Gupta
School of Computer Science Engineering and Technology, Bennett University, Greater Noida, 201310, Uttar Pradesh, India.

Mahima Pant
Uttaranchal College of Health Sciences, Uttaranchal University, Dehradun.

Minakshi
College of Computer Science, King Khalid University, Saudi Arabia.

Mohd. Aquib Ansari
Bennett University, Greater Noida, Uttar Pradesh.

Nidal Al Said
College of Mass Communication, Ajman University, Ajman, UAE.

Nidhi Sharma
Uttaranchal College of Health Sciences, Uttaranchal University, Dehradun, Uttarakhand, India.

Nidhi Sharma
Department of Computer Science and Engineering & Hi-Tech Institute of Engineering and Technology, Ghaziabad.

Niyati Goyal
School of Computer Science Engineering and Technology, Bennett University, Greater Noida, 201310, Uttar Pradesh, India.

Prachi Singh
School of Computer Science Engineering and Technology, Bennett University, Greater Noida, UP, India.

Pratham Jaiswal
School of Computer Science Engineering and Technology, Bennett University, Greater Noida, UP, India.

Quazi Taif Sadat
Director, Bangladesh University, Bangladesh.

Rajkumar Teotia
Bennett University, Greater Noida, Uttar Pradesh.

Ranjay Kumar Chaudhary
Department of Medical Laboratory Sciences, College of applied and Health Sciences, A'Sharqiyah University, P.O. Box-42, Ibra, Sultanate of Oman-400

Reshabh Saini
Pharmacology & Clinical Research. University Institute of Pharma Sciences and Research., Chandigarh University, Mohali Punjab, India.

Richa Srivastava
Bennett University, Greater Noida, Uttar Pradesh.

Rohit Ranjan
Uttaranchal College of Health Sciences, Uttaranchal University, Dehradun-248007, Uttarakhand, India.

Sakshi Koli
Uttaranchal Institute of Technology, Uttaranchal University, Dehradun, 248007, India.

Sameer Ahmad Sheikh
Department of Dialysis Therapy Technology, (USAHS), Rayat-Bahra University, Mohali. India 140104.

Sapna
Allied Health Sciences: Saraswati Group of Pharmacy, SGC Group, Gharuan-140413, Mohali, Punjab, India.

Shruti Goel
Staff Software Engineer, Turo Inc, San Francisco, CA, USA 94104.

Sinha, Rahul
Uttaranchal Institute of Technology, Dehradun, India.

Stuti Bhatt
Assistant Professor, Department of Computer Science, Graphic Era Hill University, Dehradun, India.

Suresh Babu Kondaveeti
Department of Biochemistry, Symbiosis Medical College for Women, Symbiosis International (Deemed University), Pune, India.

Utkarsh Kumar Verma
Bennett University, Greater Noida, Uttar Pradesh.

Utkarsh Singh
Bennett University, Greater Noida, Uttar Pradesh.

Vandna Sharma
School of Computer Science Engineering and Technology, Bennett University, Greater Noida, 201310, Uttar Pradesh, India.

Vineeta Singh
Department of Computer Science and Engineering, School of Engineering and Technology (Formerly known as UIET Kanpur), Chhatrapati Shahu Ji Maharaj University, Kalyanpur, Kanpur, Uttar Pradesh 208024 U.P. India.

Vivek Chandra Sunori
School of Allied Health sciences, ARNI University, (Kathgarh), Tehsil Indora, Distt. Kangra, Himachal Pradesh–176401, India.

Vivek Kumar Garg
Department of Medical Lab Sciences (USAHS), Rayat-Bahra University, Mohali, Punjab, India.

1 Artificial Intelligence and Autonomous Technologies in Revolutionalizing Neurosurgical Precision and Postoperative Recovery

Nidhi Sharma[1*], Kartikey[2] and Nidal Al Said[3]

Robotic-assisted neurosurgery is transforming surgical treatment involving the brain and spine through improved accuracy, reduced invasiveness, and better outcomes. Rapid advances in artificial intelligence (AI), Machine Learning (ML), and real-time imaging have enabled unprecedented levels of accuracy and safety in neurosurgery. AI-driven neurorehabilitation, and early intervention tactics to maximize functional restoration and life experience. This chapter reviews recent literature, technological advances, clinical applications, and integration into educational paradigms in robotic-assisted neurosurgery and AI-enabled rehabilitation, providing an overview of important neurosurgical innovations such as Neuroimaging based on AI, Intraoperative Neuromonitoring, and minimally invasive robotic techniques as well as AI or AI-powered rehabilitation strategies, brain-computer interfaces (BCI), robotic exoskeleton, virtual reality (VR), and neurostimulation underscoring the potential of AI and robotic-assisted techniques in enhancing the precision of surgical procedures, minimizing intraoperative risks, and shortening recovery timelines. Neurofunctional assessment tools powered by AI help continuously monitor neural functions in real-time, facilitating immediate detection of complications and timely intervention, transforming neural rehabilitation with robotic rehabilitation programs that harness neuroplasticity for functional recovery. Tele-rehabilitation platforms ensure ongoing patient assistance, and predictive AI models fine-tune individualized therapy schedules. AI and robotics developments work closely together to connect neurosurgery and rehabilitation experiences for individual patients in uninterrupted ways. But many challenges remain—data privacy, ethical concerns, and clinical workflow integration, which must be overcome to ensure that AI realizes its full potential. However, this convergence of AI, robotics, and real-time monitoring fosters greater precision in surgery, tailored rehabilitation, and optimized long-term outcomes,

[1] Uttaranchal College of Health Sciences, Uttaranchal University, Dehradun, Uttarakhand, India.
[2] School of Liberal Arts, Uttaranchal University, Dehradun, Uttarakhand, India.
[3] College of Mass Communication, Ajman University, Ajman, UAE.
* Corresponding author: sharmanidhi1411@gmail.com

DOI: 10.1201/9781003655121-1

ushering in the next era of neurobiologically-informed, patient-centered, and autonomy-focused surgical excellence.

1. Introduction

Robotics, Artificial Intelligence (AI), and advanced imaging technologies have enabled neurosurgeons to perform complex operative procedures with increased precision. Such advancements, in the past 20 years, have greatly decreased the risks associated with surgery, enabled effective and safe neurosurgical procedures and promoted early recovery. The evolution of robotic-assisted neurosurgery began with the inception of stereotactic frames in the 1950s in the mid-20th century, which enabled accurate localization of Central Nervous System structures (Kazemzadeh et al., 2023). The introduction and emergence of robotic assistance in surgical procedures brought a change in the neurosurgical approach, enabling stabilized and systematized assistance to neurosurgeons. Some key milestones have been NeuroMate (1997), the first FDA-approved robotic system for stereotactic neurosurgery, and NeuroArm (2008), the first MRI-compatible robotic system, which was designed for microsurgical precision and the ability to perform tumor resections. Subsequent advancements like ROSA Brain (2014), Renaissance from Mazor Robotics, and ExcelsiusGPS introduced enhanced neurosurgical accuracy and intraoperative navigation, as well as real-time adjustments during procedures (Shaikh et al., 2024). Figure 1 illustrates Evolution of Robotic Neurosurgery Systems.

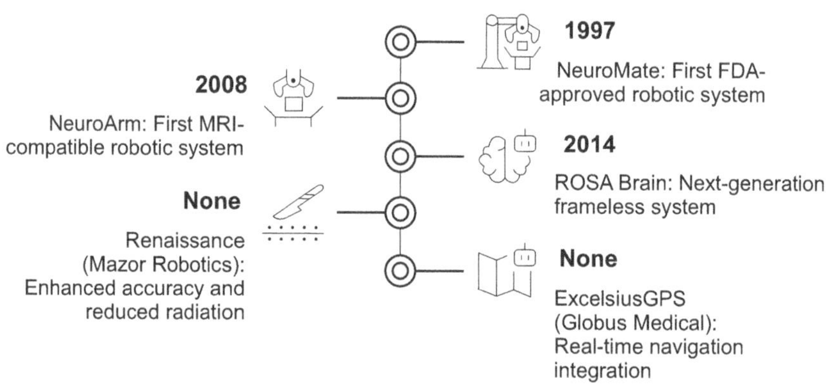

Fig. 1 Evolution of Robotic Neurosurgery Systems.

Some key developments in robotic-assisted neurosurgery are AI-enhanced precision and automation, advanced intraoperative imaging and navigation, minimally invasive robotic surgery, and invasive or automated robotic surgery. AI-powered image analysis and surgical planning tools help neurosurgeons determine the safest, most effective surgical trajectories, and automated robotic arms offer enhanced dexterity. Predictive analytics enables administrators to see the potential for complications before they happen and improve patient safety. Moreover, real-time Magnetic Resonance Imaging (MRI), Computerized Tomography (CT), and functional MRI (fMRI) visualization and integration into robotic systems provide continuous visualization of the interaction of neural structures during surgery (Abdalla Osman et al., 2025). On the other hand, using augmented reality (AR) and virtual reality (VR) in surgical navigation further improves surgical navigation and has been used to decrease the risks of tumor resection as well as the operation of deep brain stimulation (DBS). Minimally invasive robotic modalities such as keyhole and endoscopic surgeries spare the surrounding brain tissue, while laser interstitial thermal therapy (LITT) achieves non-invasive tumor ablation via robotic platforms. And fewer, smaller incisions are associated with less blood loss, reduced infection risk and quicker recovery times. In addition, telesurgery technologies allow neurosurgeons to conduct surgery via robotic-assisted platforms from a distance, and AI-powered microsurgery instruments execute adjustments on their own to decrease human error and reduce fatigue (Khor et al., 2016). Figure 2 depicts key AI applications in Neurosurgical Interventions.

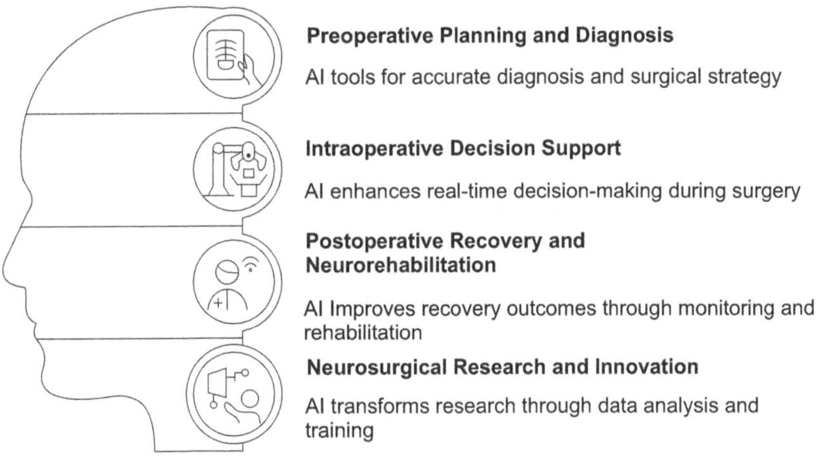
Preoperative Planning and Diagnosis
AI tools for accurate diagnosis and surgical strategy
Intraoperative Decision Support
AI enhances real-time decision-making during surgery
Postoperative Recovery and Neurorehabilitation
AI Improves recovery outcomes through monitoring and rehabilitation
Neurosurgical Research and Innovation
AI transforms research through data analysis and training

Fig. 2 Key AI Applications in Neurosurgical Interventions.

Neurosurgeons routinely use robotic technology for several neurosurgical procedures, including DBS for Parkinsonian palsy, the treatment of essential tremor, and dystonic movement disorders. It also improves stereo-electroencephalography (SEEG) electrode placement for epilepsy surgery and provides microsurgical precision for tumor resections. A similar trend appears in spinal neurosurgery as robotic-assisted spinal fusion and decompression surgeries offer improved surgical accuracy and outcomes. As AI (artificial intelligence), ML (machine learning), and real-time imaging evolve, the future of robotics in the operating theatre is likely to involve increased automation, remote surgical applications, and targeted AI-enabled therapies. This technological evolution is not only redefining neurosurgical excellence, but also bridging the careful transition between surgery and post operative neurorehabilitation, which is essential for the most favorable recovery for our patients (Larson, 2014).

2. The Evolving Role of Artificial Intelligence (AI) in Neurosurgical Interventions

Neurosurgical interventions are being revolutionized by the use of AI in improving diagnostic precisions, surgical planning, intra operative assistance and post operative management. The use of ML, deep learning (DL), and computer vision within the hospital environment is improving precision and reducing human error within neurosurgical procedures, improving patient safety. AI-based tools help with preoperative planning and diagnosis by analyzing MRI, CT, and Positron Emission Tomography (PET) scans to identify tumors, aneurysms, and vascular abnormalities. AI is helping in the segmentation of the brain, enabling proper identification of all the brain structures without damaging healthy tissues, and utilizing radiomics as AI biomarkers helps to predict tumor growth patterns and treatment planning (Tangsrivimol, et al., 2023). AI models analyze patient-specific data to evaluate preoperative risks, enabling predictions of post-surgical complications and facilitating timely interventions. In the operating room, AI improves real-time decision-making by fusing data from robotic, imaging, and neural monitoring devices. 3-D visualization of the surgical area using AI-supported AR and VR also assists in making optimal surgical choices, and intraoperative mapping ensures precision in tumor resection while protecting viable functional zones. Robotic arms are handled by AI algorithms for consistent and accurate movements, which has broadened the trajectory planning in DBS and limited hand shaking with laparoscopic and microsurgery. Intraoperative electroencephalography (EEG), magnetoencephalography (MEG), and neurophysiological signals are being interpreted by real-time AI-driven neurophysiological monitoring to mitigate the risk of neuronal damage and prevent stroke, ischemia, and cognitive deficits. AI also overlaps with postoperative recovery and neurorehabilitation by analyzing patient vitals and brain activity through the use of wearable sensors (Nam et al., 2025).

AI-based chatbots and virtual assistants help users evaluate symptoms in real-time and plan rehabilitation instructions, while ML algorithms tailor rehabilitation exercises based on users' improvement. Low-end BCI (brain-computer interface) would restore movement in patients with limb impairments, while AI-driven neurofeedback would enable effective restoration of motor and cognitive functions by using VR systems. AI-based predictions help uncover drug compounds for neurological disorders like Parkinson's or Alzheimer's disease, by detecting potential drug candidates and predicting treatment or drug responses (Rasa, 2024). AI examines metrics of practice to assess a trainee's skill and provide feedback instantaneously with haptic feedback systems in a VR-based neurosurgical simulator that allows for the creation of new immersive environments that showcase the pathology and structures of bodies. AI-assisted neurosurgical technologies are poised to revolutionize the clinical landscape, as they evolve towards fully autonomous robotic interventions, integrated AI-driven neuro-prosthesis, and advanced real-time brain mapping techniques that will prove to be faster, more precise, and personalized. From diagnosis to intra operative and postoperative management, AI has the potential to make neurosurgery safer, more efficient, and individualized in unprecedented ways (Abedi et al., 2024).

3. The Importance of a Comprehensive Approach from Surgery to Rehabilitation

Neurosurgical management, especially for brain and spinal cord pathologies, involves a comprehensive approach that goes beyond surgical intervention. Although robotic-assisted neurosurgery and AI will most certainly help improve surgical accuracy, achieving long-term functional recovery relies on an integrated care involving postoperative surveillance, early intervention strategies, and AI-based neurorehabilitation. Ensuring the best patient outcomes with minimal complications and improved quality of life requires a coordinated approach from surgery through rehabilitation. Success or failure of a neurosurgical intervention often depends on the subsequent rehabilitation phase, as neurological surgeries involving the brain and spine can result in motor, cognitive, sensory, or speech deficits, as well as the need for a recovery period to follow (Karas et al., 2007). These can be well coordinated by performing precise surgery to minimize trauma to adjacent neural tissues, AI-guided monitoring systems to detect potential post operative complications at the earliest, and the use of personalized rehabilitation approaches utilizing AI-directed and robotics-enabled neurorehabilitation programs based on need. This includes predictive AI models for estimating patient-specific risks, collaborative efforts between the neurosurgical team and rehabilitation team during pre operative planning to devise an appropriate early intervention strategy, and patient education for enhancing compliance in rehabilitation regimens. Beneficial intraoperative measures that optimize recovery consist of minimally invasive robotic-assisted methods to minimize tissue insult, AI-assisted transcendental mapping and neuromonitoring to preserve critical functional sites, and intraoperative data integration that enables surgeons to better tailor surgical maneuvers to achieve the best results for every patient (Hassan et al., 2023).

For postoperative monitoring and early rehabilitation, it includes distributed neural-computer interface (NCI) powered wearable sensors and imaging tools for tracking rapid neural recovery, an automated rehabilitation protocol capable of adapting treatment intensity, and neuroplasticity-promoting domains, such as transcranial magnetic stimulation and DBS. Robotics and AI-based neurorehabilitation are crucial to recovery, while BCI supports restoration of motor and cognitive function, robotic-based exoskeletons assist in recovery in paralyzed subjects, and the combination of VR and gamified AI-based therapy holistically enhances participation and neuroplasticity. The rehabilitation exercises are made more personal through the use of AI algorithms that identify the data points that require iteration based on patient performance and changes in neural response (Young et al., 2021). Tele-rehabilitation platforms enable long-term follow-up and integration into daily life with access to therapy, AI-based predictive analytics to assess long-term risk and motivate lifestyle changes, and social and psychological support systems to enhance patient adherence and mental well-being. By integrating accurate surgical interventions with AI-integrated rehabilitation approaches, practitioners can deliver comprehensive care trajectories that focus on patient health and autonomy (Calabrò et al., 2025).

4. Precision and Innovation in Robotic Neurosurgery

Robotic systems in neurosurgery have transformed the field by introducing greater precision, safety, and outcome improvements through enhanced technologies such as real-time navigation and AI. Robotic systems have evolved from NeuroMate, the first FDA-approved stereotactic robot for DBS, since 1997. The NeuroArm, which was first launched in 2008, was the first MRI-compatible robotic system allowing for sub-millimeter precision microsurgical tumor resections. Mazor Robotics' Renaissance improved spinal and cranial surgeries with image-guided tracking and greater precision, and ROSA Brain provided multi tasking, AI-supported options for brain epilepsy and DBS procedures (Shaikh et al., 2024). ExcelsiusGPS combines ML with intraoperative imaging to create the best possible platform for spinal navigation. As a result of these advancements, minimally invasive techniques have become possible, complications have been reduced, and patient outcomes have been significantly improved. The evolution of robotic platforms will enable autonomous neurosurgery, remote surgical intervention, and tailored, AI-based surgical planning, paving the way for a new era of neurosurgical care (Rivero-Moreno et al., 2023).

5. Role of ML and AI in Real-Time Intraoperative Decision-Making

AI-based systems process intraoperative images (MRI, CT, ultrasound) for automatic segmentation and dynamic image fusion during surgery, improving tumor resections and allowing for preservation of healthy brain structures. AI-guided path planning aids robotics navigation platforms, ensuring optimal trajectories of instruments and reducing invasiveness. ML algorithms track neurophysiological signals and patient vitals in real- time, enabling dynamic decision-making during surgery as well as the immediate detection of arising complications. This data-driven intelligence and adaptive precision are reshaping neurosurgical care by tailoring surgical procedures through AI-based insights and accurately predicting patient outcomes in the long run (Nitsch et al., 2019).

6. AI-Powered Intraoperative Decision Support Systems

AI-based intraoperative imaging and navigation technology incorporation of AI into intraoperative imaging and navigation modalities has considerably improved the specificity, safety, and adaptability of neurosurgical procedures. AI-driven image reconstruction and real-time updating improve intraoperative MRI, and the integration of AI with fMRI enables accurate mapping of motor and language areas before tumor excisions, thus reducing cognitive or motor deficits afterwards. Moreover, AI-augmented DTI enhances tractography and fiber tracking, enabling preservation of crucial white matter pathways in resection. AI facilitates holistic and adaptive navigation through interweaving data from several imaging sources into interactive 3-D maps, which support real-time adjustment during surgery and improve prediction of outcomes. Integrating AI with various imaging modalities enables patient-specific, data-driven approaches that support safe, efficient, optimal short- and long-term patient outcomes through cross-validated surgical communication (Upreti, 2024).

7. Predictive Analytics in Neurosurgery

AI and ML-based predictive analytics tools are revolutionizing contemporary neurosurgery by providing real-time, data-driven decision-making that improves surgical accuracy and safety. This progress aids neurosurgeons in every phase of surgery—preoperative planning, intraoperative monitoring, and postoperative outcome prediction—through patient-specific risk assessment and dynamic strategy optimization (Tangsrivimol et al., 2023). Key highlights include:

- AI-driven risk stratification analyzes patient data (age, comorbidities, vitals, imaging) to predict complications (bleeding, neurovascular injury), allowing timely management.
- MRI, fMRI, and DTI data-based, personalized surgical planning creates individualized maps of the brain in 3-D, allowing neurosurgeons to keep out of harm's way of important areas of the organ.
- Predictive models assist surgeons in deciding incision locations and resection size—particularly important with tumor surgeries—maximizing excision while sparing function.
- ML-based systems adjust their surgical strategies in real- time to intraoperative variations (e.g., brain shift/swelling) during the surgeries.
- AI aids in predicting tumor growth, identifying neural targets, and the placement of DBS electrodes for optimal outcomes in intricate procedures such as tumor resections, epilepsy surgery whereas in spinal neurosurgery,

predictive analytics contributes by modeling spinal biomechanics to support precise fusion or decompression strategies.

7.1 Real-Time Neurophysiological Monitoring with AI for Better Surgical Outcomes

AI and ML are revolutionizing real-time intraoperative neurophysiological monitoring (IONM) by increasing precision, decreasing risk, and improving patient outcomes in neurosurgery (Parduzi et al., 2025). Figure 3 represents the role of AI in enhancing neurosurgical outcomes. Techniques of IONM provide real-time evaluation of peripheral, spinal, and cortical neural function during surgical interventions, and the application of AI-enhancements of monitoring data amplification is the key to their successful application by:

- AI-enabled IONM has improved the accuracy of monitoring processes, allowing filtering of undesirable noise and artifacts, separating actual neural signals from surgical interference, thereby allowing for more effective intraoperative decisions.
- AI-powered real-time anomaly detection enables detection of minimally invasive changes (e.g., early signs of ischemia or nerve degeneration) before irreversible damage, allowing for early intervention.
- Forecasting intraoperative trends plays a valuable role in reducing neurological deficits through predictive modeling, particularly within challenging surgical procedures such as brain tumor resections and spinal cord surgeries.
- Individualized monitoring adjusts to the patient's architecture of neural structures, continuously adjusting sensitivity in real time, and directly interfacing with robotic systems and imaging (M.RI, fMRI, DTI) to protect critical structures.

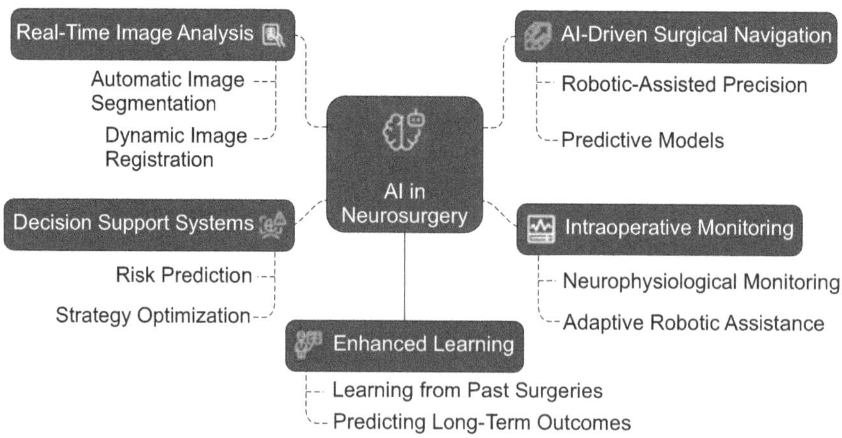

Fig. 3 Role of AI in enhancing neurosurgical outcomes.

- AI-assisted systems additionally offer decision support for complex neurosurgical procedures, including spinal fusions, DBS, and epilepsy surgery, through optimization of electrode placement and identification of high-risk areas.

7.2 Post-Surgical Challenges in Neurosurgical Patients

Neurologic complications are frequent and may be devastating resulting in incurable neurological deficits or death especially in neurosurgical procedures involving the brain or spinal cord. These complications mainly arise from the complex structure of the nervous system, the complexity of neural connections, and the sensitivity of the surgical field. Despite the use of robotics and AI that has considerably improved the precision of surgical procedures, post-surgical complications like motor deficits, cognitive impairment, and speech problems continue to be common and severely impact rehabilitation and recovery. Motor deficits are a common postoperative complication resulting either from the primary disease pathology, (e.g., during tumor resection or stroke surgery), or from surgical injury itself (e.g., spinal surgery), where the intrinsic physiology is not yet well understood and is unique to each patient. These may also be due to brain edema that temporarily or permanently interrupts motor signaling. Important motor complications are hemiparesis/hemiplegia (weakness/paralysis on one side of the body), ataxia (coordinative impairment), spasticity (increased muscle tone secondary to upper motor neuron injury) and peripheral neuropathy (numbness/weakness due to nerve injury) (Chaudhary et al., 2024). Management Strategies involving robotic-assisted neurorehabilitation using AI-Powered exoskeletons, and BCIs assist in movement through neural-controlled prosthesis.

Cognitive dysfunction is another common complication after neurosurgery, often resulting from direct injury to frontal or temporal lobes, ischemic injuries, or postoperative delirium associated with anesthesia and metabolic disturbances. Cognitive deficits arise as forgetfulness (especially if the hippocampus is involved), executive dysfunction (difficulties in decisions and planning), and attention deficits, which disrupt one's capabilities to function (sedentary life), among others. Rehabilitation includes cognitive therapy to strengthen memory and reasoning, incorporating techniques for AI-assisted neurostimulation, including transcranial magnetic stimulation (TMS) by which the number of neuronal action potentials could be improved. Moreover, impaired verbal communication is a frequent consequence in neurosurgical patients with invasions near language networks or cranial nerves (Deiner et al., 2009). These difficulties can stem from damage to Broca's or Wernicke's areas, involvement of the cerebellum or injury to the facial and vocal nerves. Other speech-related complications are aphasia (loss of the ability to use or comprehend language), dysarthria (a speech disorder resulting from muscle weakness, causing slurred or imprecise speech) and apraxia of speech (inability to coordinate speech movements). Speech recognition tools incorporating AI-based technology assist non-verbal patients, and enable neural plasticity-based training to identify and rehabilitate language ability (Daiello et al., 2019).

7.3 *Role of AI in Predicting Post-Surgical Complications and Recovery Trajectories*

The integration of big data, continuous patient monitoring, and predictive analytics within the scope of AI is changing the postoperative landscape of neurosurgical practice, allowing identification of at-risk individuals for neurological deficits and systemic complications. By harnessing the power of advanced algorithms and intelligent systems, AI enables early detection, personalized interventions, and enhanced patient outcomes, positioning it as an indispensable component of contemporary neurosurgical practice. AI models that predict complications utilize DLNs trained on large-scale neurosurgical datasets, which are powerful models. Such models identify relationships across electronic health records (EHRs), imaging findings, and intraoperative factors to predict postoperative risks such as stroke, infection, or cognitive decline (Senadheera et al., 2024). Furthermore, Natural Language Processing (NLP) allows AI to process clinical notes and uncover hidden risk factors, and Explainable AI (XAI) promotes transparency by offering clinicians clear rationales for the risk predictions, building trust, and enabling informed decision-making. Through smart wearable devices and sensors, AI can also play a large role in helping to conduct real-time monitoring of post-surgical recovery. AI-controlled exoskeletons adapt flexible motor rehabilitation programs in real-time, and brainwave-monitoring tools (e.g., EEG-based) automatically report even subtle changes in CNS (central nervous system) functioning characteristic of early neurodegeneration. AI-enabled telemedicine platforms also provide continuous monitoring remotely, which reduces the chances of hospital readmission while also allowing timely interventions (Dixon et al., 2024). Figure 4 illustrates the role of AI in predicting post-surgical complications.

Characteristic	Motor Deficits	Cognitive Impairment	Speech Difficulties	Surgical Site Infections	Brain Swelling & Hemorrhage
AI Approach	Analyzes fMRI, IONM, EMG	Assesses EEG, biomarkers, connectivity	Integrates speech analysis, neural networks	Detects biomarkers, temperature, immune response	Analyzes post-op CT/MRI scans

Fig. 4 Predicting post-surgical complications using AI models.

In addition, predictive analytics models analyze post operative recovery patterns to predict the likelihood of hospital readmission, and chatbots monitor patient-reported outcomes, identifying issues such as postoperative depression or cognitive dysfunction. The robotic rehabilitation systems powered by AI enhance therapy by adapting the stress applied by the patient in real- time based on the predicted trajectory of recovery. AI also paves the way for personalized recovery trajectories, guiding the transition towards precision medicine in neurorehabilitation. Through genetic profiles, brain plasticity, and individual neural recovery potential, AI adjusts the intensity and length of rehabilitation to the patient's progress. Predictive models provide information related to the likelihood of complete functional recovery, which can help guide clinicians in establishing realistic goals that are grounded in underlying data (Lee et al., 2021).

8. Importance of Early Intervention Strategies in Neurorehabilitation

Owing to functional and cognitive deficits associated with neurosurgical procedures, especially for the brain and spinal cord, rehabilitative measures incorporating strategies for early intervention are required. These counteract the associated deficits and increase chances of recovery. Neuroplasticity is an emerging approach targeting on building new neuronal connections in the brain using the brain's natural capacity to engage neuronal networks in post-surgical and traumatic conditions. Early incorporation of rehabilitative measures is associated with enhanced recovery, decreased disability, improvement in long term functional ability. Nerve-growth factor (NGF)-mediated facilitation of neuroplasticity is preferentially enabled directly following surgical augmentation, when a high level of neuronal excitability permits rapid rates of synaptic remodeling and functional reorganization (Dailah et al., 2024). Early rehabilitation allows for recovery of motor and cognitive function before malformation compensatory pathways are established. Moreover, early rehabilitation is necessary to avoid other complications, including muscle wasting, joint contractures, and spasms, as well as cognitive decline. Additionally, these keep the brain engaged and emotionally happy, lowering the chances of post-surgery depression. Clinical studies have demonstrated that early mobilization and therapy, as part of a structured care program, greatly reduces the risk for long-term disability, thereby not only increasing functional independence, but also returning to normal daily life (Zotey et al., 2023).

Motor rehabilitation, cognitive and speech therapy, as well as neurophysiological stimulation are among the main modalities of an effective early neurorehabilitation. Motor rehabilitation should, if possible, start within 24–48 hours post-surgery with the intention to preserve muscle function and initiate motor relearning. During this critical stage, robotic-assisted rehabilitation, especially with AI-guided exoskeletons, improves the accuracy and safety of movement. In terms of cognition, early interventions targeting memory, problem-solving, and attention help diminish the severity of long-term cognitive deficits AI-powered speech therapy tools are even more beneficial in focusing communication rehabilitation for patients with aphasia or dysarthria. In patients with severe neurological impairment, BCIs assist with early motor training, and neuromodulation techniques—such as TMS (track management system) and AI-enhanced biofeedback—facilitate accelerated and pronounced neuroplastic responses and improved functionality (Shahid et al.,

2023). AI and robotics applied in early neurorehabilitation provide significant improvement in the personalization and efficiency of the therapy. ML algorithms evaluate patient data—genetic markers, surgical results, recovery patterns—to create tailored treatment plans that adjust in real-time. These predictive models help clinicians by guiding the patient onto the best path towards recovery while making sure that rehabilitation is goal-driven and cost-effective. Robotic-assisted, neuroprosthetic, and VR rehabilitation tools provide interactive environments that can support the retraining of motor and cognitive abilities. AI-assisted telemedicine solutions may enable home rehabilitation and follow-up in days instead of weeks post-discharge. Biosensors worn on the body quantify physiological and functional endpoints and adjust treatment parameters according to individual recovery, ensuring continuous care (Pollock et al., 2014).

8.1 AI-Driven Neurorehabilitation Post Neurosurgery: Wearable Sensors and Brain-Computer Interfaces (BCI) for Tracking Recovery

Neurorehabilitation is essential once the patient has undergone neurosurgical intervention in order to regain motor skills, cognitive function, and brain function. AI has made the industry transformative by paving the way to solutions that improve the recovery quality. Wearable sensors and BCIs are among the two prominent breakthroughs in this domain. Wearable sensors, with integrated AI, enable real-time tracking of biomechanical and physiological parameters, including gait, muscle activity, and joint motion. They employ real-time data analytics and predictive models to identify complications early such as motor delays or fatigue, and provide timely feedback to maximize rehabilitation exercises, minimize improper movements, and facilitate remote care through telemedicine. AI-driven feedback loop guarantees efficient and tailored rehabilitation programs. BCIs also provide innovative assistance for patients with major motor or communication disabilities. Non-invasive methods such as EEG are used for BCIs to detect brain signals corresponding to motor intent. ML algorithms decode these signals and can convert them into digital outputs for controlling a range of assistive technologies ranging from robotic limbs and VR-based therapy systems to neuroprosthetics (Calderone et al., 2024).

8.2 AI-Driven Personalized Rehabilitation Protocols Based on Real-Time Patient Data

Standard recommendations dominate in traditional rehabilitation, disregarding potential complications or differences between individual recovery profiles. In comparison, AI-driven rehabilitation leverages real-time, patient-specific data from multiple modalities—including sensors, imaging, and clinical assessments—to individualize treatment. Based on the day-to-day developments in the clinic, AI systems adapt treatment into the right intensity/ type/duration to ensure maximum practical outcomes. These AI-enhanced systems collate real-time neurological, physiological, and biomechanical data for timing and targeting of precise, responsive interventions. Investigations of EEG and EMG are deployed to monitor brain and skeletal muscle activity, respectively, while imaging techniques, including fMRI (magnetic resonance imaging) and DTI (diffusion tensor imaging), assess changes in functional connectivity and neuroplastic alterations within the brain (Yen et al., 2023). Wearable technologies like smart exoskeletons and inertial measurement units (IMUs) of the body record gait and postural anomalies to assist robotic and VR-rehabilitative therapies. AI also analyzes vital signs, which include heart rate variability and oxygen saturation, as well as patient-reported outcomes like fatigue and emotional state, to adjust therapy. Continuous *in situ* optimization maintains therapeutic commitment within the patient's ability. AI-assisted robotics and VR also adjust task difficulty in response to patient performance for motor recovery, and cognitive and speech recovery is aided by tailored neurofeedback and micro-stimulation regimens with AI-demarcated parameters (McDevitt et al., 2022).

9. Robotic Exoskeletons and Neurostimulation for Motor Recovery

Motor deficits, weakness, and impaired coordination are common among patients who have undergone neurosurgery due to damage to the brain or spinal cord. Physical rehabilitation is traditionally reliant on intensive physiotherapy that can be slow and strenuous for both patients and therapists. On the other hand, AI-based robotic exoskeletons and neurostimulation technologies have shown great potential to promote the restoration of motor function, increase neuroplasticity, and facilitate functional independence. The precision, adaptiveness, and intensive nature of motor rehabilitation with these technologies in the form of real-time feedback and individualized recovery strategies pave the way for expedited and optimized patient rehabilitation (Aldhahi et al., 2025). Table 1 depicts applications of AI-powered wearable devices and neurostimulation techniques in optimizing recovery post-neurosurgical interventions.

***Robotic Exoskeletons in Enhancing Mobility and Strength*:** AI algorithms help analyze neuromuscular signals and adapt levels of robotic assistance according to patient progress. The rehab machine modifies different elements like force, speed, and resistance based on recovery levels and provides feedback in real-time, enabling early mobilization of severely weak patients, providing repetitive training for neuroplasticity, offering patient-specific adjustments according to strength and endurance, and ameliorating gait and postural stability to correct asymmetrical walking patterns and reduce fall risk.

***Activating Neural Pathways for Faster Recovery*:** AI actively adjusts stimulation parameters in real-time through EEG/EMG monitoring according to brain muscle connectivity, and ML algorithms predict optimal stimulation sites to facilitate recovery. AI-based neurofeedback goes a step further, tailoring treatment intensity to the specific level at which a patient responds.

Table 1 Applications of AI-powered wearable devices and neurostimulation techniques in optimizing recovery post-neurosurgical interventions.

AI-Powered Robotic Exoskeletons		
Exoskeleton Type	*Function*	*Application in Post-Neurosurgery Recovery*
Lower-Limb Exoskeletons (e.g., EksoGT, ReWalk)	Assist with standing, walking, and weight shifting	Gait training for patients with spinal cord injury or stroke
Upper-Limb Exoskeletons (e.g., Armeo, Myomo)	Restore arm and hand movements	Helps stroke and brain injury patients regain fine motor control
Full-Body Exoskeletons (e.g., HAL by Cyberdyne)	Enhance mobility and core stability	Beneficial for severe neuromuscular impairments
AI-Driven Neurostimulation Techniques		
Neurostimulation Type	**Function**	**Clinical Application**
Transcranial Magnetic Stimulation (TMS)	Non-invasive magnetic pulses stimulate the motor cortex	Enhances neuroplasticity for motor and speech recovery
Transcranial Direct Current Stimulation (tDCS)	Low-intensity electrical currents modulate brain activity	Improves motor learning and cognitive recovery
Functional Electrical Stimulation (FES)	Activates paralyzed muscles via electrical impulses	Assists limb movement for gait and hand function restoration
Epidural Spinal Cord Stimulation (SCS)	Stimulates spinal cord circuits	Restores voluntary movement in spinal cord injury patients

***Combining Robotics and Neurostimulation for Optimal Recovery*:** By encouraging active neuroplasticity and muscular reactivation, these two potent technological features work in concert to speed up motor recovery. Synergistic applications such as TMS (transcranial magnetic stimulation) and exoskeletons that overlay TMS to modulate both cortical excitability and functional recovery by priming the motor cortex during rehabilitation in robotic gait devices to improve walking recovery.

***Virtual Reality* (*VR*) in *Neurorehabilitation*:** Computer-generated environments that can offer multiple sensory inputs to support motor and cognitive rehabilitation are used in VR-based neurorehabilitation to deliver realistic sensory stimulation. By closely analyzing a patient's performance, AI enhances the VR experience by assisting in real-time therapy adjustments and recovery trajectory prediction.

***Gamified Rehabilitation in Enhancing Engagement and Recovery*:** In order to make therapy exercises interesting, inspiring, and goal-oriented, gamification integrates game-like elements such as challenges, rewards, and real-time feedback. This approach increases patient motivation, encourages the repetition of movements that are essential for neuroplasticity, and provides real-time AI feedback that modifies game difficulty based on emotional reaction, motor control, and cognitive function. The use of AI-based virtual reality systems in post-neurosurgical rehabilitation is shown in Figure 5.

Characteristic	Immersive VR	Non-Immersive VR	Augmented Reality	AI-VR Neurofeedback
Environment	360-degree virtual environment	Simulated interactive environments	Overlays virtual objects	Adjusts therapy based on brain activity
Application	Gait training cognitive exercises	Hand-eye coordination, executive function	Motor skill retraining, spatial awareness	Brain injury recovery, neuroplasticity

Fig. 5 Application of AI-based VR systems in post-neurosurgical rehabilitation.

9.1 Robotics in Post-Surgical Neurorehabilitation

In the postoperative phase of neurological rehabilitation, rehabilitation robotic devices are crucial because they offer high-accuracy interventions in a controlled, repeatable, and patient-specific manner, improving recovery by maximizing therapeutic outcomes and reducing dependency on therapists for effective and efficient rehabilitation. They support neuroplasticity by enhancing therapy, boosting patient involvement, giving prompt feedback, and reinforcing repetitive, task-oriented behaviors. Because the field is always changing, robotic rehabilitation will probably be combined with other modalities like remote rehabilitation, BCIs, and co-therapy with other interventions like VR and neurostimulation to target more neurobiological systems and improve recovery outcomes (Vaida et al., 2025).

9.2 AI-Enhanced Telerehabilitation Platforms for Remote Patient Monitoring

Platforms for AI-enhanced telerehabilitation have emerged as a promising option for services that allow for remote monitoring, personalized feedback, and real-time therapy protocol adjustments. Together with wearable sensors and robotic equipment, these platforms enable patients to receive excellent rehabilitation treatment at home under the constant supervision of therapists. Incorporating AI allows for tailored therapy, predictive analytics, and real-time feedback, providing individualized and patient-centric pathways to recovery. As a result, this process improves access to care, increases independence, enhances efficiency of rehabilitation, and lowers costs (Dobkin B. H., 2009).

10. AI-Powered Prosthetics for Neuroplasticity Enhancement

An innovative approach in post-surgical neurorehabilitation is the implementation of the neural implants along with the AI-based prosthetics to improve the functional outcomes and to promote the recovery rate. Neural implants are devices, such as deep brain stimulators and spinal cord stimulators (SCS), that physically engage the nervous system to restore or amplify neural functions. These devices modulate specific brain or spinal cord areas with electrical stimulation to enhance neuroplasticity, reduce neuropathic pain, or drive motor recovery. Through incorporation of advanced AI technologies, these devices incorporate AI systems and sensors that help them track joint movements and adjust the design to suit the user. These assistive devices help restore mobility or use of limbs after neurosurgery, personalized rehabilitation using real-time adjustments based on neurological feedback (Hidler et al., 2011). Neural Implants Support Neuroplasticity via:

***Precision Electrical Stimulation*:** Through the formation of new synaptic connections and enhanced neural communication, neural implants promote neuroplasticity by delivering precise electrical impulses to particular regions of the brain or spinal cord.

***Relearning and Neural Activation*:** These devices have the ability to reactivate dormant or weak neurons, which enables the central nervous system to retarget neural pathways that are essential for movement or sensory reception following a neurological injury.

***Enhancing Motor Function*:** By focusing on the areas that are in charge of voluntary movement, DBS techniques facilitate motor recovery and are being used more and more to treat movement disorders following surgery.

***Neuropathic Pain Relief*:** Spinal cord stimulators are used for the treatment of chronic neuropathic pain, modifying pain processing pathways and evoking a state of decreased pain perception via long-term neuroplasticity.

***Support for Neuroplasticity after Surgery*:** Neural implants play a key role in functional restoration by enabling the brain to use its natural plasticity mechanism, through which healthy areas of the brain reorganize and compensate for a damaged region due to stroke, trauma or surgery.

10.1 AI-Powered Prosthetics in Enhancing Neuroplasticity

AI-enhanced prosthetics are crucial for personalized rehabilitation as they integrate with the user's neurophysiology. These devices employ real-time adjustments in response to user feedback, which fosters adaptive recovery through ongoing learning via:

***Real-Time Learning and Adaptation*:** AI algorithms integrated into prosthetic devices enable continuous learning from user movements, dynamically adjusting the prosthetic's functionality according to neurological feedback. This adaptation strengthens the brain-device connections, similar to how the brain learns.

***Personalized Movement Support*:** Rather than purely mechanical Appliances, prosthetics works as Individual Bodies, utilizing Real-Time Data that the Neuro-

Receptor Receives to Build and Reshape its Individual Neural Pathways System, thus making it similar to the Natural & Biological Movement of Humans & Circulating a motor control-System.

***Feedback Loops*:** Sensory feedback received from prosthetics can stimulate the somatosensory cortex, facilitating neuroplasticity and functional recovery.

10.2 Key Clinical Applications of Neural Implants and AI-Powered Prosthetics in Neurosurgical Rehabilitation

***Neural Implants and AI- Powered Prosthetics*:** Two up and coming technologies that have the potential of drastically changing rehabilitation practices, through promoting motor recovery, cognitive enhancement, and neuroplasticity, following neurosurgical interventions.

***Stroke Rehabilitation*:** DBS can be used to stimulate the motor cortex for motor recovery, while AI-enhanced prosthetics can assist with limb movement and manipulation.

***Spinal Cord Injury Recovery*:** Spinal cord stimulators enable functional recovery and pain relief, while AI-based exoskeletons assist patients in relearning to walk by allowing controlled limb movement.

***CNS Rehabilitation*:** Neural implants and prosthetics activate lesions of the brain to promote neural organization and increase patient independence.

10.3 Challenges in AI and Robotic Integration

Challenges in AI and robotic integration in neurosurgery and rehabilitation are outlined in Table 2.

10.4 Ethical Implications

Integration of AI and Robotics in Neurosurgery and Neurorehabilitation have multiple ethical considerations—specifically regarding data confidentiality, algorithmic biases, and AI cognition. Some of the key ethical issues include protecting sensitive health data, addressing algorithmic bias, ensuring transparency in AI systems, and ensuring that there is human oversight in clinical decision-making. Particularly, data security is very important because AI systems need large quantities of patient data, so they are at risk for being hacked. Moreover, biased AI models can lead to inequitable healthcare outcomes if the data used to train the algorithms are not diverse or representative (Calabrò et al., 2025). In addition to that, patient comprehension and AI accountability are critical issues raised by autonomy vs. oversight regarding AI-driven decisions, particularly in high-stakes settings. Predictive analytics will need ethics frameworks to help insulate them from the vagaries of society that would want to control or limit what patients can choose or what can happen to them. In addressing these ethical

Table 2 Challenges in AI and robotic integration in neurosurgery and rehabilitation.

Parameters	*Challenges*	*Ethical Implications*
Patient Safety and Risk Management	**Ensuring Safety in AI-Driven Systems**: Risk of system errors in neurosurgery, leading to complications.	• **Accountability and Liability:** Difficult to assign responsibility for surgical errors. Clear liability frameworks needed. • **Continuous Monitoring:** Need for real-time professional oversight to ensure AI aligns with patient interests.
Informed Consent and Patient Autonomy	**Ensuring Transparent Communication**: Difficulty for patients to fully understand AI-driven interventions.	• **Complexity of AI and Robotic Systems:** Need for clear communication to ensure patients understand risks and benefits. • **Understanding AI's Role:** Healthcare providers must educate patients on AI's decision-making role.
Data Privacy and Security	**Managing Sensitive Patient Data**: AI and robotic systems require large volumes of sensitive patient data.	• **Data Breaches and Misuse:** Concerns about unauthorized access to medical information. • **Data Ownership:** Issues with who owns patient data and how it is used. • **Informed Consent for Data Usage:** Patients must be informed about how their data is used in research and AI model development.
Socioeconomic Impacts and Accessibility	**Ensuring Equitable Access**: Limited access to advanced AI technologies in low-resource settings.	• **Health Disparities:** Inequitable access to AI-driven healthcare technologies. • **Rising Healthcare Costs:** High costs of AI and robotics could widen the gap between rich and poor patients. • **Global Health Inequities:** Risk of developing countries lagging in adopting AI technologies, creating a digital divide.
Ethical Use of AI in Clinical Decision-Making	**Defining AI's Role in Decision-Making**: AI's involvement in clinical decision-making raises concerns about bias and transparency.	• **Bias in Algorithms:** AI systems may reflect biases from non-representative datasets. • **Algorithmic Transparency:** Lack of transparency in AI decision-making processes may undermine trust. • **Physician Autonomy and Responsibility:** Ethical concerns arise when AI overrules physician judgment or is given too much decision-making autonomy.

challenges, several approaches can guide the implementation and development of AI and robotic technologies within neurosurgery and neurorehabilitation including making AI algorithms transparent by explaining their decision-making processes to clinicians and patients, bias mitigation, enhancing data security, creating regulatory frameworks to delineate responsibility and liability when AI systems take part in clinical decisions and implementing AI systems in ways that promote patient autonomy and empowerment.

10.5 Future Directions

AI and robotics in neurosurgery anticipate the advent of completely autonomous operating room procedures as well as the potential to revolutionize healthcare through more accurate, efficient, and customized treatment. These systems require extensive testing in complex applications and high-level verification, especially in situations with greater stakes. Algorithmic bias is still a major worry as well because training datasets may leave out particular populations, which could result in unequal surgical outcomes. The responsible advancement of autonomous neurosurgery will require the development of legal frameworks, ethical principles, and patient-centered protective frameworks that balance our reliance on technology with the necessity of human oversight and compassion in healthcare. Furthermore, AI-based rehabilitation should go beyond the physical domain to address psychological and emotional health in order to meet the comprehensive needs of neurosurgical patients. In order to support long-term monitoring, smart rehabilitation networks, and inclusive, flexible collaborative care models, AI must be incorporated into multidisciplinary care ecosystems in the future. This comprehensive strategy is required to maintain patient-driven, sustainable innovation in the field of neurorehabilitation and to fully realize AI's potential in enhancing neurosurgical recovery.

11. Conclusion

The rapid transformation of the healthcare landscape brought about by the integration of robotics and AI into neurosurgical care is revolutionizing the standards and delivery of surgery and rehabilitation. Neurosurgeons have access to technologies that support accuracy, safety, and real-time decision-making, such as ML to enhance intraoperative guidance and systems like ROSA and NeuroArm that can perform minimally invasive procedures. By utilizing wearable sensors, BCIs, and robotic exoskeletons to track recovery and modify treatment in real-time, AI enables customized and adaptive neurorehabilitation outside of the operating room. This integrated pathway from OR (operating room) to recovery promotes a coordinated approach to a patient-centric continuum of care. Furthermore, the application of AI to neurosurgical care suggests the development of highly advanced, self-governing systems that can optimize surgical and rehabilitation results. The ethical use of these technologies, which includes preserving patient autonomy, safeguarding data privacy, and addressing healthcare disparities, must be addressed by the system we design. AI and robotics must be integrated with the help of the professionals—patients, engineers, and clinicians—to guarantee fair access and care delivery. To sum up, efforts are underway to integrate cutting-edge technology and human interaction to deliver more accurate, customized, consistent, and cost-effective neurosurgical care in the future; this will rethink recovery and enhance patients' quality of life everywhere.

References

Abdalla Osman, E.I., Mubarak Ismail, M.M.E., Hassan Mukhtar, M.A., Babiker Ahmed, A.U., Abd Elfrag Mohamed, N.A. and Alamin Ibrahim, A.A. (2025). Artificial Intelligence and Robotics in Minimally Invasive and Complex Surgical Procedures: A Systematic Review. *Cureus*, *17*(3), e81339. https://doi.org/10.7759/cureus.81339.

Abedi, A., Colella, T.J.F., Pakosh, M. and Khan, S.S. (2024). Artificial intelligence-driven virtual rehabilitation for people living in the community: A scoping review. *NPJ Digital Medicine*, *7*(1), 25. https://doi.org/10.1038/s41746-024-00998-w.

Aldhahi, M.I., Alorainy, A.I., Abuzaid, M.M., Gareeballah, A., Alsubaie, N.F., Alshamary, A.S. and Hamd, Z.Y. (2025). Adoption of Artificial Intelligence in Rehabilitation: Perceptions, Knowledge, and Challenges among Healthcare Providers. *Healthcare* (*Basel, Switzerland*), *13*(4), 350. https://doi.org/10.3390/healthcare13040350.

Calabrò, R.S. and Mojdehdehbaher, S. (2025). AI-Driven Telerehabilitation: Benefits and Challenges of a Transformative Healthcare Approach. *AI*, *6*(3), 62. https://doi.org/10.3390/ai6030062.

Calderone, A., Latella, D., Bonanno, M., Quartarone, A., Mojdehdehbaher, S., Celesti, A. and Calabrò, R.S. (2024). Towards Transforming Neurorehabilitation: The Impact of Artificial Intelligence on Diagnosis and Treatment of Neurological Disorders. *Biomedicines*, *12*(10), 2415. https://doi.org/10.3390/biomedicines12102415.

Chaudhary, F., Ahmed, Z. and Agrawal, D.K. (2024). Critical Assessment of the Neurological Complications during High-Risk Anesthesia Procedures. *Journal of Surgery and Research*, *7*(2), 250–266.

Daiello, L.A., Racine, A.M., Yun Gou, R., Marcantonio, E.R., Xie, Z., Kunze, L.J., Vlassakov, K.V., Inouye, S.K., Jones, R.N., Alsop, D., Travison, T., Arnold, S., Cooper, Z., Dickerson, B., Fong, T., Metzger, E., Pascual-Leone, A., Schmitt, E. M., Shafi, M., Cavallari, M., … SAGES Study Group (2019). Postoperative Delirium and Postoperative Cognitive Dysfunction: Overlap and Divergence. *Anesthesiology*, *131*(3), 477–491. https://doi.org/10.1097/ALN.0000000000002729.

Dailah, H.G., Koriri, M., Sabei, A., Kriry, T. and Zakri, M. (2024). Artificial Intelligence in Nursing: Technological Benefits to Nurse's Mental Health and Patient Care Quality. *Healthcare (Basel, Switzerland)*, *12*(24), 2555. https://doi.org/10.3390/healthcare12242555.

Deiner, S. and Silverstein, J.H. (2009). Postoperative delirium and cognitive dysfunction. *British Journal of Anaesthesia*, *103 Suppl 1*(Suppl 1), i41–i46. https://doi.org/10.1093/bja/aep291.

Dixon, D., Sattar, H., Moros, N., Kesireddy, S.R., Ahsan, H., Lakkimsetti, M., Fatima, M., Doshi, D., Sadhu, K. and Junaid Hassan, M. (2024). Unveiling the Influence of AI Predictive Analytics on Patient Outcomes: A Comprehensive Narrative Review. *Cureus*, *16*(5), e59954. https://doi.org/10.7759/cureus.59954.

Dobkin B.H. (2009). Motor rehabilitation after stroke, traumatic brain, and spinal cord injury: common denominators within recent clinical trials. *Current Opinion in Neurology*, *22*(6), 563–569. https://doi.org/10.1097/WCO.0b013e3283314b11.

Hassan, A.M., Rajesh, A., Asaad, M., Nelson, J.A., Coert, J.H., Mehrara, B.J. and Butler, C.E. (2023). Artificial Intelligence and Machine Learning in Prediction of Surgical Complications: Current State, Applications, and Implications. *The American Surgeon*, *89*(1), 25–30. https://doi.org/10.1177/00031348221101488.

Hidler, J. and Sainburg, R. (2011). Role of Robotics in Neurorehabilitation. *Topics in Spinal Cord Injury Rehabilitation*, *17*(1), 42–49. https://doi.org/10.1310/sci1701-42.

Karas, C.S. and Chiocca, E.A. (2007). Neurosurgical robotics: A review of brain and spine applications. *Journal of Robotic Surgery*, *1*(1), 39–43. https://doi.org/10.1007/s11701-006-0006-6.

Kazemzadeh, K., Akhlaghdoust, M. and Zali, A. (2023). Advances in artificial intelligence, robotics, augmented and virtual reality in neurosurgery. *Frontiers in Surgery*, *10*, 1241923. https://doi.org/10.3389/fsurg.2023.1241923.

Khor, W.S., Baker, B., Amin, K., Chan, A., Patel, K. and Wong, J. (2016). Augmented and virtual reality in surgery-the digital surgical environment: Applications, limitations, and legal pitfalls. *Annals of Translational Medicine*, *4*(23), 454. https://doi.org/10.21037/atm.2016.12.23.

Larson P.S. (2014). Deep brain stimulation for movement disorders. *Neurotherapeutics : The Journal of the American Society for Experimental NeuroTherapeutics*, *11*(3), 465–474. https://doi.org/10.1007/s13311-014-0274-1.

Lee, E. E., Torous, J., De Choudhury, M., Depp, C. A., Graham, S. A., Kim, H. C., Paulus, M. P., Krystal, J. H. and Jeste, D. V. (2021). Artificial Intelligence for Mental Health Care: Clinical Applications, Barriers, Facilitators, and Artificial Wisdom. *Biological Psychiatry. Cognitive Neuroscience and Neuroimaging*, *6*(9), 856–864. https://doi.org/10.1016/j.bpsc.2021.02.001.

McDevitt, S., Hernandez, H., Hicks, J., Lowell, R., Bentahaikt, H., Burch, R., Ball, J., Chander, H., Freeman, C., Taylor, C. and Anderson, B. (2022). Wearables for Biomechanical Performance Optimization and Risk Assessment in Industrial and Sports Applications. *Bioengineering* (*Basel, Switzerland*), *9*(1), 33. https://doi.org/10.3390/bioengineering9010033.

Nam, S.M., Byun, Y.H., Dho, Y.S. and Park, C.K. (2025). Envisioning the Future of the Neurosurgical Operating Room with the Concept of the Medical Metaverse. *Journal of Korean Neurosurgical Society*, *68*(2), 137–149. https://doi.org/10.3340/jkns.2024.0160.

Nitsch, J., Klein, J., Dammann, P., Wrede, K., Gembruch, O., Moltz, J.H., Meine, H., Sure, U., Kikinis, R. and Miller, D. (2019). Automatic and efficient MRI-US segmentations for improving intraoperative image fusion in image-guided neurosurgery. *NeuroImage Clinical*, *22*, 101766. https://doi.org/10.1016/j.nicl.2019.101766.

Parduzi, Q., Wermelinger, J., Koller, S.D., Sariyar, M., Schneider, U., Raabe, A. and Seidel, K. (2025). Explainable AI for Intraoperative Motor-Evoked Potential Muscle Classification in Neurosurgery: Bicentric Retrospective Study. *Journal of Medical Internet Research*, *27*, e63937. https://doi.org/10.2196/63937.

Pollock, A., Farmer, S.E., Brady, M.C., Langhorne, P., Mead, G.E., Mehrholz, J. and van Wijck, F. (2014). Interventions for improving upper limb function after stroke. *The Cochrane Database of Systematic Reviews*, *2014*(11), CD010820. https://doi.org/10.1002/14651858.CD010820.pub2.

Rasa A.R. (2024). Artificial Intelligence and Its Revolutionary Role in Physical and Mental Rehabilitation: A Review of Recent Advancements. *BioMed Research International*, *2024*, 9554590. https://doi.org/10.1155/bmri/9554590.

Rivero-Moreno, Y., Echevarria, S., Vidal-Valderrama, C., Pianetti, L., Cordova-Guilarte, J., Navarro-Gonzalez, J., Acevedo-Rodríguez, J., Dorado-Avila, G., Osorio-Romero, L., Chavez-Campos, C. and Acero-Alvarracín, K. (2023). Robotic Surgery: A Comprehensive Review of the Literature and Current Trends. *Cureus*, *15*(7), e42370. https://doi.org/10.7759/cureus.42370.

Senadheera, I., Hettiarachchi, P., Haslam, B., Nawaratne, R., Sheehan, J., Lockwood, K.J., Alahakoon, D. and Carey, L.M. (2024). AI Applications in Adult Stroke Recovery and Rehabilitation: A Scoping Review Using AI. *Sensors* (*Basel, Switzerland*), *24*(20), 6585. https://doi.org/10.3390/s24206585.

Shahid, J., Kashif, A. and Shahid, M.K. (2023). A Comprehensive Review of Physical Therapy Interventions for Stroke Rehabilitation: Impairment-Based Approaches and Functional Goals. *Brain Sciences*, *13*(5), 717. https://doi.org/10.3390/brainsci13050717.

Shaikh, S.T., Dwarakanath, T.A. and Moiyadi, A.V. (2024). Evolution of Robotics in Neurosurgery. *Asian Journal of Neurosurgery*, *19*(4), 598–609. https://doi.org/10.1055/s-0044-1790606.

Tangsrivimol, J.A., Schonfeld, E., Zhang, M., Veeravagu, A., Smith, T.R., Härtl, R., Lawton, M.T., El-Sherbini, A.H., Prevedello, D.M., Glicksberg, B.S. and Krittanawong, C. (2023). Artificial Intelligence in Neurosurgery: A State-of-the-Art Review from Past to Future. *Diagnostics* (*Basel, Switzerland*), *13*(14), 2429. https://doi.org/10.3390/diagnostics13142429.

Upreti G. (2024). Advancements in Skull Base Surgery: Navigating Complex Challenges with Artificial Intelligence. *Indian Journal of Otolaryngology and Head and Neck Surgery : Official Publication of the Association of Otolaryngologists of India*, *76*(2), 2184–2190. https://doi.org/10.1007/s12070-023-04415-8.

Vaida, C., Rus, G. and Pisla, D. (2025). A Sensor-Based Classification for Neuromotor Robot-Assisted Rehabilitation. *Bioengineering* (*Basel, Switzerland*), *12*(3), 287. https://doi.org/10.3390/bioengineering12030287.

Yen, C., Lin, C.L. and Chiang, M.C. (2023). Exploring the Frontiers of Neuroimaging: A Review of Recent Advances in Understanding Brain Functioning and Disorders. *Life* (*Basel, Switzerland*), *13*(7), 1472. https://doi.org/10.3390/life13071472.

Young, M.J., Lin, D.J. and Hochberg, L.R. (2021). Brain-Computer Interfaces in Neurorecovery and Neurorehabilitation. *Seminars in Neurology*, *41*(2), 206–216. https://doi.org/10.1055/s-0041-1725137.

Zotey, V., Andhale, A., Shegekar, T. and Juganavar, A. (2023). Adaptive Neuroplasticity in Brain Injury Recovery: Strategies and Insights. *Cureus*, *15*(9), e45873. https://doi.org/10.7759/cureus.45873.

2 Advancing Fetal Health Prediction
A Review of CTG-Based Classification, MRI, Segmentation, and Abnormality Detection

Deepika Pantola[1], Madhuri Gupta[2*], Vandna Sharma[3], Bhavika Mittal[4] and Niyati Goyal[5]

The fetal health prediction is a significant area of research which aims to safeguard the maternal and the prenatal well-being during pregnancy. Advances in medical imaging, monitoring technologies, and computational approaches have revolutionized this field, enabling accurate analysis of complex physiological data, thus helping in taking timely actions to reduce risks and improve overall pregnancy outcomes. This paper is designed to review and discuss the pioneering recent innovations and key challenges of using Machine Learning (ML) and Deep Learning (DL) in this domain, emphasizing their applications in areas such as classification using Cardiotocography (CTG) data, segmentation with fetal Magnetic Resonance Imaging (MRI), and anomaly detection for early fetal health diagnosis. This paper covers state-of-the-art research works from 2018 to 2024 with in-depth quantitative and qualitative analysis of the research papers. This study answers several questions such as challenges posed while diagnosing fetal health using various ML/DL techniques; significance of CTG data and MRI data; and identifies the research gaps. This study therefore provides a robust groundwork to impending researchers in the domain of fetal health identification.

1. Introduction

Fetal well-being monitoring is a decisive prospect to observe and guarantee the well-being of both the mother and the fetus. Because, with the progressing pregnancy, multiple complexities can arise due to the occurrence of hormonal and physical changes in the maternal body, wherein the complexities can negatively affect the well-being of the fetus, it becomes vital to monitor the health of the fetus and detect any abnormalities or issue early on (Nandipati, et al., 2020).

Fetal health monitoring can not only help to identify various risks and complications liable to further jeopardize the outcome of pregnancy but can also

[1-5] School of Computer Science Engineering and Technology, Bennett University, Greater Noida, 201310, Uttar Pradesh, India.
email: Deepika.pantola@bennett.edu.in[1]; vandnasharma26304@gmail.com[3]; mittalbhavika094@gmail.com[4]; niygyl167@gmail.com[5]
* Corresponding author: madhuri.gupta@bennett.edu.in

DOI: 10.1201/9781003655121-2

help diagnose incidences such as the distress of a fetus, irregular growth, or lack of proper oxygen supply very early in the gestation period (Bhowmik et al., 2021). Detecting or diagnosing such unwanted conditions early on could help the mothers and doctors to act on a viable treatment timely (Kuzu & Santur, 2023), increasing the chances of reducing, and maybe even avoiding any adverse effects of the conditions of the fetus and mother both.

Machine learning (ML) is required in fetal health because it enhances accuracy and speeds-up monitoring in the diagnosis of pregnancy-related conditions (Mushtaq & Veningston, 2024). It is intended to predict and point out a problem early on so that interventions can be taken and implemented to avoid complications both for the fetus and for the mother (Nagavibha et al. (2024). Recent trends in the research in fetal health have shown much progress in data analysis and imaging techniques that have gained interest in high-speed early diagnosis along with accurate classification of fetal conditions. Researchers use various classification techniques on Cardiotocography (CTG) data for identifying whether the fetal is normal or pathological (Kaliappan et al., 2023 & Mehbodniya et al. (2022)). Deep Learning (DL), a sub field of ML, trains artificial neural networks to behave like the human brain by using layers of interconnected nodes to acquire patterns and features from the data. It has attracted significant attention in Magnetic Resonance Imaging (MRI)-based analysis namely segmentation and anomaly detection. In addition, 3-dimensional (3D) Convolutional Neural Networks (CNNs) are applied for spatial feature extraction more precisely from volumetric MRI data (Kuzu & Santur, 2023). Anomaly detection methods, which include deep residual networks and transfer learning, have found application, such that pathologies in the fetal brain can be identified with highly accurate detection of other anomalies. These

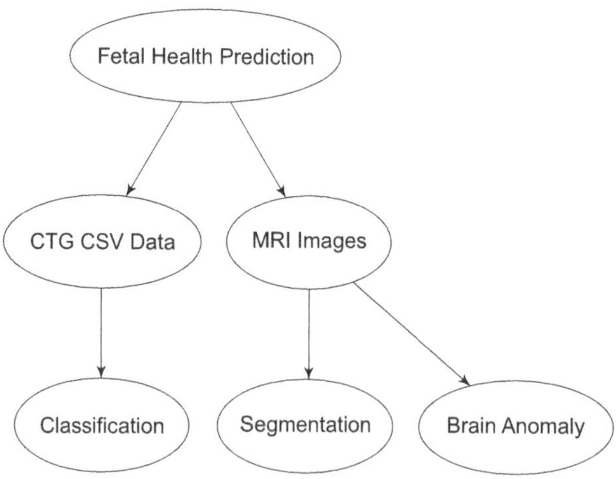

Fig. 1 Categorization of data for fetal health prediction.

advances are extremely helpful for clinical applications, which may happen earlier and accurately detect health issues related to the fetus (Abiyev et al., 2023). Identification of possible complications during gestation in a timely manner along with accurate assessments has been found to play a central role in assuring the fetus's and mother's safety.

This paper presents a detailed analysis of existing methods of ML and DL used for diagnosing the fetal's health. This study includes the research papers published during 2018–2024 and provides a comprehensive evaluation through qualitative and quantitative analysis of published papers. The comparative analysis is conducted broadly using two different types of data used for fetal health prediction, namely, CTG data in Comma-Separated Values (CSV) file format and MRI images. Figure 1 shows the categorization of fetal data. The classification-based ML/DL models use CTG data, whereas MRI images can be used for performing segmentation or detecting brain anomalies. The technique of recognizing and defining particular fetal brain regions or structures from MRI pictures is known as "segmentation of fetal MRI data". In order to comprehend embryonic growth and identify any potential problems early in pregnancy, this step is essential. This study discusses the existing state and prospects of research in fetal well-being prediction. It focuses on the significance of ongoing advancements in this field and emphasizes the potential for further improvements in the prediction ability of ML and DL models.

The paper has been alienated into the following sections: Section 1 is an overview of the existing problem in monitoring fetal well-being; Section 2 is the literature review; Section 3 provides the analysis of CTG data studies; Section 4 discusses the analysis of MRI images data's segmentation as well as anomaly detection; Section 5 discusses the experimental setup outcomes; and Section 6 contains conclusion of the paper.

1.1 Questions to be Answered by this Review

Through this review study, we aim to address key questions in the field of fetal health analysis, such as:

Q1. What are the key challenges in MRI-based fetal brain segmentation?
Q2. What are the contributions of ML and DL to fetal health prediction?
Q3. What is the specific contribution of ensemble methods to analysis in fetal health?
Q4. What is the significance of pathological data in fetal brain analysis?

2. Methodology Adopted in this Study

The approach used to analyse the current research publications for fetal health diagnosis is covered in this section. The process consists of three steps: 1. acquiring research papers; 2. conducting qualitative analysis; and 3. conducting quantitative analysis. The next subsections go over these steps.

2.1 Research Paper Attainment

The research publications are chosen in the first step. The selection of the papers has been done using search engines such as PubMed, Scihub, Google Scholar, and ResearchGate. The subsequent are the exploration keywords; fetal health classification, fetal hypoxia, cardiotocography, fetal anomaly detection, fetal MRI scan, pregnancy complications, etc. The search query has been restricted to journal papers and conference papers in the database from January 2018– November 2024.

2.2 Conducting Qualitative Investigation

Qualitative investigation is conducted in two phases. In the first phase, the overall research articles considered was 55 based on the exploration pattern defined in the research paper acquisition sub section. Nevertheless, in the second reconsideration, the elimination and addition of research articles for qualitative investigation using different dimensions is steered. In this, we have disqualified those research papers which were only related to the health of mothers and incorporated those research articles that explore ML/DL based techniques for diagnosing the health and development of the fetal. The total number of ML/DL based fetal health related research papers incorporated in this qualitative investigation study is 42 (forty-two).

2.3 Conducting Quantitative Investigation

This sub section presents the quantitative investigation of the research articles related to DNNs (dense neural networks). The questions driving this analysis as given below:

Q1. What is the count of research articles disseminated year-wise and also based on the sub-categories of fetal health diagnosis such as CTG data classification, MRI segmentation, and anomaly detection?

Q2. What is the count of ML/DL based research articles for fetal health prediction throughout numerous journals and conferences?

Q3. What are the various ML models utilized in research articles for identifying the health of the fetus?

The preceding research questions are addressed below.

Answer 1: Figure 2 displays the bar chart for visualizing the current trend of research activities in the fetal well-being prediction domain from 2018–2024. After 2019, there is a huge spike in the usage of ML/DL models in diagnosing fetal well-being. In Figure 3, the bar chart presents the research papers broadly categorized into three categories such as CTG classification, MRI segmentation, and brain anomaly.

From the bar chart in Figure 3, we can identify most of the research work is majorly focused on segmentation of MRI to understand fetal development.

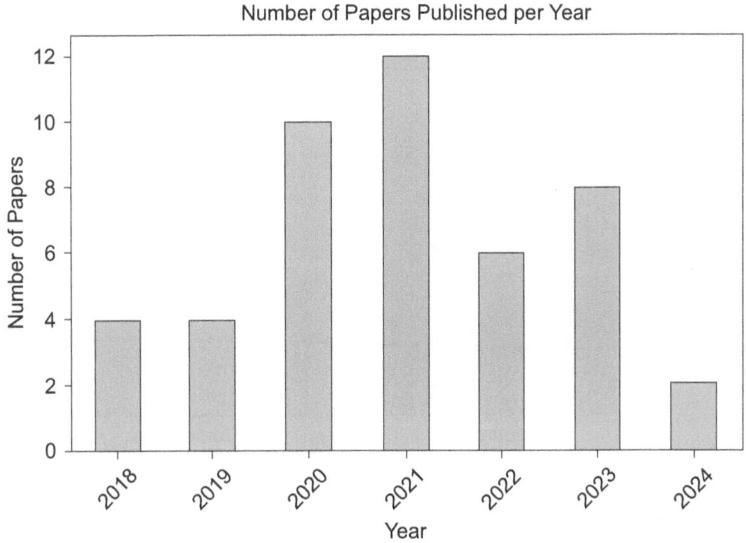

Fig. 2 Publication trend from 2018 to 2024.

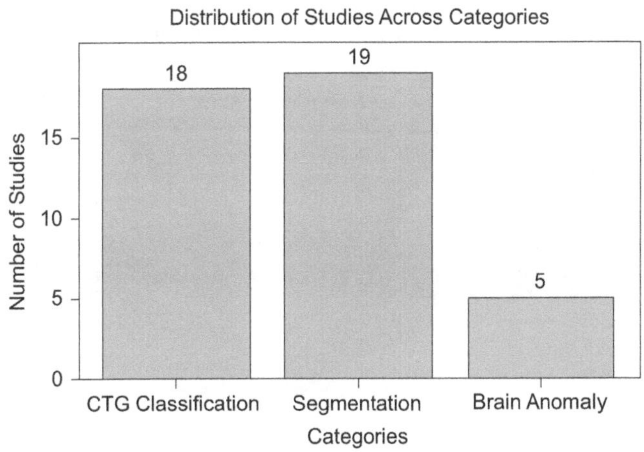

Fig. 3 Summary of fetal well-being prediction studies based on CTG classification, segmentation, and brain anomaly.

Another commonly explored area as can be seen in the bar chart, is CTG data-based classification of fetal as normal, suspected, or pathological.

Answer 2: Figure 4 represents the number of research articles published in international conferences and various journals. In this survey most of the research articles are considered from reputed journals.

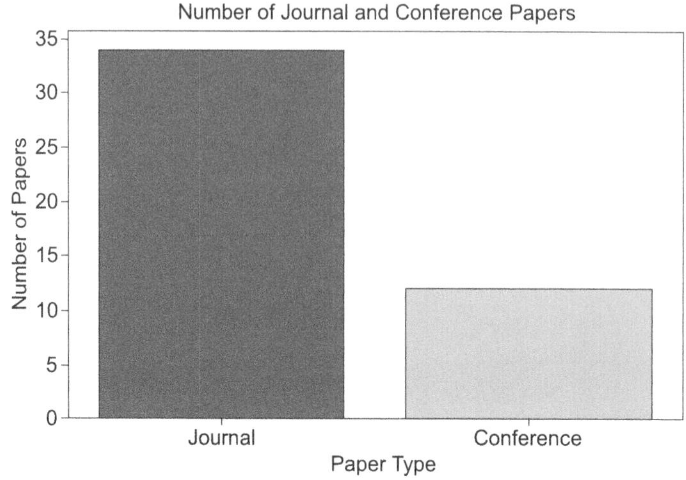

Fig. 4 Ratio of journal to conference papers in the literature review.

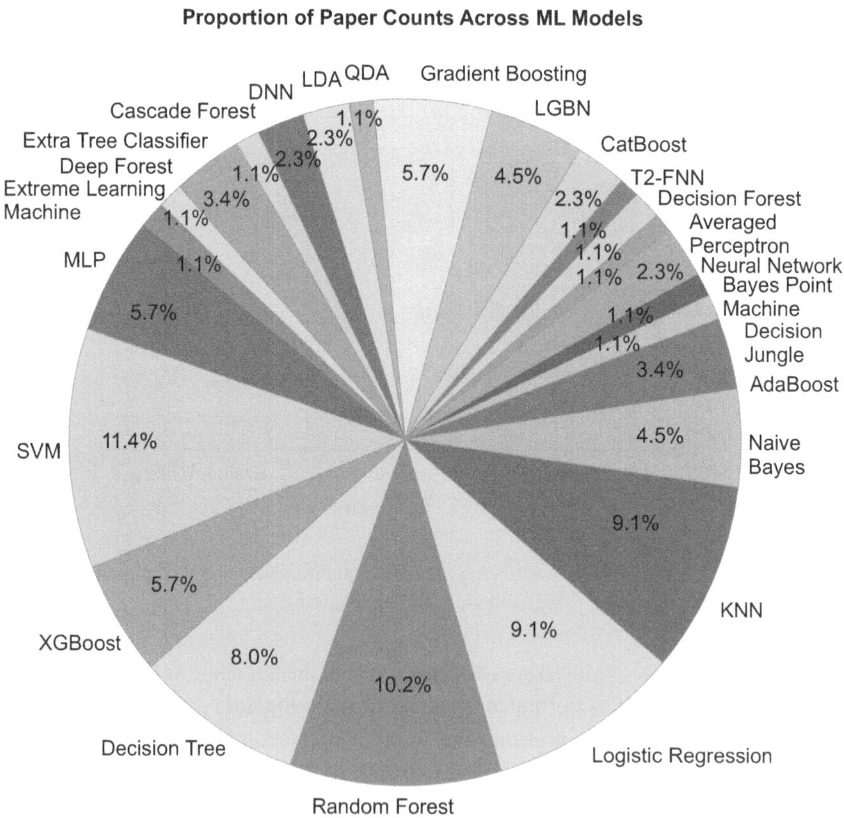

Fig. 5 Different ML/DL models used in fetal health predictions.

Answer 3: The different ML/DL models used by various researchers are shown through the pie-chart in Figure 5. It can be noticed from this pie-chart that SVM (support vector machine) and random forest models are highly used by the researchers for diagnosing the health of the fetus.

3. State-of-the-Art Research Study

This section provides the literature review which is broadly categorized into two subsections based on dataset type such as CTG dataset and MRI dataset. The research papers using MRI dataset are further sub-categorized based on the application such as segmentation or anomaly detection for the fetus.

3.1 CTG Dataset

This sub section presents the analysis of the CTG data used in the state-of-the-art research articles. This section also discusses the methods used to pre process and analyze the CTG data. The CTG dataset comprises 2,126 records obtained from the CTG scans categorized into three classes of fetal well-being: normal, suspect, and pathological. It is composed of 1,655 normal examples, 295 suspect, and 176 pathological examples. The normal class label indicates that the fetal heart rate and uterine contraction patterns are within normal ranges, suggesting no signs of distress, whereas suspect class label suggests that there may be a potential abnormality in the patterns, but it is not definitive for fetal distress. The pathological class represents a strong indication of fetal distress, such as oxygen deprivation, which could necessitate immediate medical intervention (Al Duhayyim et al., 2023). There are 21 features in the CTG dataset and one fetal health class feature. Table 1 describes all the features of this dataset.

3.2 Data Preprocessing and Feature Engineering

Various fetal health classification studies on CTG datasets have employed different pre processing techniques to improve model performance. This sub section provides an overview of different pre processing techniques used in state-of-the-art processes to improve the prediction ability of the trained models.

Normalization has been performed by (Nandipati, et al., 2020; Bhowmik et al., 2021; Mushtaq & Veningston, 2024; Nagavibha et al., 2024; Kaliappan et al., 2023; Kuzu & Santur, 2023; Abiyev et al., 2023; AL Duhayyim et al., 2023). Bhowmik et al. (2021) specifically used Min-Max Scaling, while Mushtaq & Veningston (2024) utilized the StandardScaler. The CTG dataset is highly imbalanced dataset where the suspect and pathological class instances are very few in contrast to the normal class label. Therefore, to tackle the class imbalance problem a technique, named as Synthetic Minority Oversampling Technique (SMOTE), has been applied (Nagavibha et al., 2024; Kapila et al., 2023; Kaliappan et al., 2023; Hoodbhoy et al., 2019), generating synthetic data to balance the class distributions.

Table 1 Description of the CTG dataset features.

Feature	*Description*
Baseline value	Baseline fetal heart rate
Accelerations	Frequency of fetal heart rate accelerations
Fetal movement	Fetal movement occurrences
Uterine contractions	Uterine contraction occurrences
Light decelerations	Light fetal heart rate decelerations
Severe decelerations	Severe fetal heart rate decelerations
Prolonged decelerations	Prolonged fetal heart rate decelerations
Abnormal short-term variability	Abnormal short-term heart rate variability
Mean value of short-term variability	Average short-term heart rate variability
Percentage of time with abnormal long-term variability	Percentage time with abnormal long-term variability
Mean value of long-term variability	Average long-term heart rate variability
Histogram width	Width of the histogram
Histogram min	Minimum value of the histogram
Histogram max	Maximum value of the histogram
Histogram number of peaks	Number of peaks in the histogram
Histogram number of zeroes	Number of zeroes in the histogram
Histogram mode	Mode value in the histogram
Histogram mean	Mean value of the histogram
Histogram median	Median value of the histogram
Histogram variance	Variance in the histogram
Histogram tendency	Tendency in the histogram
Fetal health (class)	Class label (Normal, Suspect, Pathological)

Random Oversampling, which duplicates minority class samples to balance class distributions, was applied by some researchers (Dixit, 2022; Al Duhayyim et al., 2023; Yin & Bingi, 2023). Additionally, Kuzu and Santur (2023) used class weighting to tackle class imbalance problems. The class weighting technique regulates the significance of each class throughout the training process, allocating higher weights to underrepresented classes so the model pays more attention to them, thereby reducing bias towards the majority class. Outlier detection has been utilized by Al Duhayyim et al. (2023) for removing outliers. To handle categorical variables, One-Hot Encoding has been employed by Mushtaq and Veningston (2024), converting these variables into ML-friendly formats.

Additionally, several feature selection techniques have been applied in several studies. Feature selection helps in reducing overfitting, computational cost, and enhances model interpretability. Bhowmik et al. (2021) used the Chi-Square method, while Dixit (2022) applied Univariate Feature Selection with SelectKBest method. Kapila and Saleti*(2023) combined Analysis of Variance (ANOVA) and Chi-Square with dimensionality reduction techniques like PCA (Principal Component Analysis), which identifies key features by transforming data into fewer dimensions, and ICA (Independent Component Analysis), which separates statistically independent components from the data. Kuzu and Santur (2023) employed feature extraction through polynomial expansion, which generates new features by introducing polynomial combinations of the existing ones. These methods collectively help extract the most significant features for improved model performance. To view the summary of various pre processing techniques used in different studies on CTG dataset refer to Table 2.

Table 2 Pre processing techniques used in fetal health classifications studies.

Authors	*Pre processing Used*
Nandipati et al., 2020	Normalization
Bhowmik et al., 2021	Normalization (Min-Max Scaling), Feature Selection: Chi-Square Method
Mushtaq & Veningston, 2024	StandardScaler and One-hot Encoding on target column
Dixit , 2024	Univariate Feature Selection (SelectKBest), RandomOverSampler
Nagavibha et al., 2024	Data Balancing (SMOTE), Data Scaling
Kaliappan et al., 2023	Data Balancing (Over Sampling), Standardization
Kapila & Saleti, 2023	SMOTE, Feature Selection: ANOVA and Chi-Square, Feature Extraction: PCA and ICA
Hoodbhoy et al., 2019	SMOTE
Kuzu & Santur, 2023	Normalization, Feature Extraction (Polynomial Expansion), Class Weighting
Abiyev et al., 2023	Normalization
Al Duhayyim et al., 2023	RandomOverSampler, Outlier Removal
Yin & Bingi, 2023	OverSampling

3.3 Comparative Analysis of ML/DL Techniques for CTG Dataset

The research on the prediction of fetal health uses different ML techniques, each exhibiting different approaches and results. Different models and data were explored by researchers (Hoodbhoy et al., 2019; Kuzu & Santur, 2023; Akbulut et al., 2018), and others that reveal the superiority of a particular algorithm, such as XGBoost, random forest, and decision forest. Hoodbhoy et al. (2019) managed an accuracy of up to 93% when using the XGBoost approach, whereas Kuzu and Santur (2023) hybrid model with Random Forest and XGBoost executed with over 99.5% accuracy. Contrarily, Akbulut et al. (2018) deduced that Decision Forest worked the best with an accuracy of 89.5%. However, each of these studies poses a dependence of the datasets as well as the model being used.

Several studies employed ensemble methods to improve the predictive capacity of the models Li et al (2021). Al Duhayyim et al. (2023) utilized XGBoost, CatBoost, and Light Gradient Boosting Algorithm (LGBM) in amalgamation within a voting classifier which attained an accuracy as well as AUC of 0.99. In another research work, Yin and Bingi et al. (2023) used SVM with a high accuracy of 99.59% combined with Shapley Additive Explanations (SHAP) and Local Interpretable Model-Agnostic Explanations (LIME) to employ model transparency. Nandipati et al. (2020) focuses on the model environment, where random forest and naive bayes perform best in the R environment. In a similar setup, Bhowmik et al. (2021) used a stacked ensemble approach, which demonstrates that providing the power of base models performs better with higher accuracy. Thus, these results indicated ensemble methods, especially voting and stacking classifiers, to be generally winning models in contrast to individual models.

Model optimization and evaluation strategy was another frequent theme of the studies. In Dixit's (2022) study, feature selection happened to be one of the major indicators in identification whereas Nagavibha et al. (2024) and Kaliappan et al. (2023) focused on hyperparameter tuning and evaluation approaches for optimal performance. Nagavibha et al. (2024) demonstrated that LGBM, random forest, and gradient boosting improved after tuning. Once again, Kaliappan et al. (2023) utilized multiple models where the studies were assessed using K-fold and monte carlo cross-validation methods with increased accuracy of the outcome. Authors (Kapila & Saleti, 2023; Mehbodniya et al., 2022; Li & Liu, 2021) tried different combinations of models to predict fetal health using stacking and soft voting classifiers. In their experiments, Kapila and Saleti (2023) got the highest accuracy rate at 98.79% using a stacking classifier with random forest whereas Mehbodniya et al. (2022) got random forest as the top performer. Li and Liu (2021) combined soft voting with gradient boosting, CatBoost, LightGBM, and XGBoost to achieve an accuracy of 95.9% and an AUC of 98.8%. All these studies have further proved that ensemble of multiple models highly enhances the ability and reliability of the prediction.

The contributions of Abiyev et al. (2023) and Mushtaq and Veningston (2024) established the importance of fetal health classification using neural network-based architecture. Abiyev et al. (2023) used a Type-2 Fuzzy Neural Networks (T2-FNN) system for detecting the fetal well-being. Mushtaq and Veningston (2024) used a deep neural network with batch normalization and dropout layers to prevent overfitting with the objective of optimizing the fetal health into multiple categories' classification. Although being able to classify examples with a very high accuracy, especially for pathological cases, their sensitivity has proven to be one of the main advantages over the other models. In general, the studies discussed here represent various methods and approaches in the prediction of fetal health, each bringing value added to the understanding of the effectiveness of different ML methods. Table 3 provides a summary of the various fetal health predictions studies conducted on CTG dataset.

Table 3 Summary of fetal health prediction studies.

Study	*Dataset*	*Method Used*	*Accuracy*	*Key Findings*
Hoodbhoy et al., 2019	Public	XGBoost	93%	High accuracy
Kuzu & Santur, 2023	Public	Hybrid (random forest, XGBoost)	99.5%	Superior accuracy but struggled with class imbalance.
Akbulut et al., 2018	Private	Decision forest	89.5%	Most effective in the Turkish dataset with high AUC (0.958).
Al Duhayyim et al., 2023	Public	Voting classifier (XGBoost,Cat-Boost, LGBM)	99%	Strong accuracy and AUC (0.99).
Yin & Bingi, 2023	Public	SVM	99.59%	High accuracy, with model transparency using SHAP and LIME.
Nandipati et al., 2020	Public	Random forest, naive bayes (R environment)	97.87%	Performance varied with the programming environment (R).
Bhowmik et al., 2021	Public	Stacked ensemble	High accuracy	Higher accuracy compared to individual models.
Dixit, 2022	Public	Feature Selection	Varied	Identified important indicators for fetal health prediction but limited by dataset size and biases.
Nagavibha et al., 2024	Public	LGBM, random forest, gradient boosting	Highest in LGBM	Outperformed other models after hyper-parameter tuning.
Kaliappan et al., 2023	Public	Decision tree, random forest, SVM	High accuracy	Improved interpretability with SHAP and LIME.
Kapila & Saleti, 2023	Private	Stacking classifier (random forest meta-classifier)	98.79%	Best performance with stacking classifiers using random forest.
Mehbodniya et al., 2022	Private	Random forest	High accuracy	Outperformed SVM, MLP, and KNN across accuracy, precision, recall, and F1-score.
Li & Liu, 2021	Public	Soft voting (gradient boosting, CatBoost, XGBoost, LightGBM)	95.9%	Achieved high accuracy and AUC (98.8%) using a blended model approach.
Abiyev et al., 2023	Public	T2-FNN (gradient descent)	96.6%	Strong performance with precision, recall, F1-score, accuracy.
Mushtaq & Veningston, 2024	Public	Deep neural network (with dropout and batch normalization)	High accuracy	High accuracy, especially for pathological cases, with good sensitivity.

4. MRI Data

MRI is a non-invasive technique for imaging which makes the use of powerful magnetic rays and radio rays for generating complete pictures of internal structures. In fetal health, MRI becomes very necessary for visualizing the fetus under development, the presence of abnormalities, and assessment of organ development, especially when results of ultrasound are indeterminate. It is especially valuable in the evaluation of complex cases, including neurological, musculoskeletal, and cardiovascular abnormalities. MRI helps in early diagnosis; hence it will lead to timely intervention, which is crucial for better fetal outcome and helps guide prenatal care.

4.1 Advancements in Fetal Brain MRI Segmentation

The most important technique in medical diagnostics is the segmentation of MRI images, referring to the division of scanned MRI images into distinguishable regions that focus attention on specific structures, like organs, tissues, or abnormalities. It improves the capability of analyzing complex medical conditions, thus leading to more consistent analyses and treatment planning. The process of segmenting areas of interest helps to provide evaluation of disease intensity and progression as well as the ability to give tailor-made treatment. Fetal brain structure segmentation from MRI images is an important process in the reliable diagnosis and the clinical decision-making task. The task has also been confronted with several challenges; this includes fetal movement, variation in shape of the brains, and interference of maternal tissues. There have been numerous studies lately to address all these challenges in DL techniques that concentrate on enhancing the precision, speed, and robustness of the models developed for segmentations. In this review, we critically discuss and compare ten studies which introduce novel approaches to fetal MRI segmentation.

In their research work, Salehi et al. (2018), describe the application of a DL model based on the U-Net architecture for real-time 2D slices-based fetal brain segmentation with high Dice scores (96.52% for normal cases, 78.83% for challenging cases). This proposed U-Net model is superior to other approaches like voxel-wise CNNs and random forests with SIFT features in terms of speed and precision. Zhao et al. (2022) researched on a deep learning model to be used in the segmentation of fetal images, especially those relating with congenital heart disease. Based on the experimental results, the authors presented that the DL-based model could segment a fetus by an average Dice score of 0.831, with slight degenerations in abnormal cases (7% for specific regions).

Faghihpirayesh et al. (2022) proposed a DL model using multiple branches and skip connections which integrates both high-resolution spatial details and contextual features. This model outperforms state-of-the-art methods with dice scores of 97.99% for normal cases and 84.04% for challenging cases. Liao et al. (2020) presented a multi stage deep learning model which was designed to handle different variable shapes of the brain by using the brain detector for localization and deformable convolution.

Zhang et al. (2021) designed a confidence-aware cascaded framework, a two-stage strategy which uses a slice consistency loss function. It significantly outperformed several existing methods with impressive segmentation accuracy and promising future clinical use in real-time. Dudovitch et al. (2020) introduced a deep learning method for the automatic volumetric segmentation of fetal structures. This framework involves three stages: automatic structure segmentation, estimation of segmentation error, and error correction. It showed high accuracy values for both the fetal brain and body, with low average symmetric surface distances that ensure precision and low observer variability.

In their research, Rampun et al. (2021), presented a new hybrid DL called SIMOU-Net, which integrated U-Net and holistically nested edge detection features with the task of fetal brain segmentation. This approach shows high accuracy in both normal and abnormal cases, including Dice scores of 94.2% for normal cases and 91.2% for abnormal cases. In the research work, Li et al. (2020) introduced a two-branch FCN (fully convolutional network) framework for fetal brain localization and multi scale FCN for the refinement of segmentation within the ROI. This method obtained 100% localization accuracy in the brain and gained very high segmentation performance with a Dice score of 0.958, sensitivity of 0.950, and precision of 0.968, making promising clinical application at a processing time of only 6 seconds per MRI stack. Justin Lo et al. (2021) presented the CASE-Net that combines U-Net with attention mechanisms, and squeeze-and-excitation (SE) blocks to perform better image segmentation. CASE-Net achieved the high Dice score of 87.36% on the dataset of 34 patients, surpassing state-of-the-art methods.

Chen et al. (2021) presented a multi step framework for fetal brain extraction with three networks, including global localization network, a local refinement network, and a fusion network. The results show great improvement in brain extraction from 3D MRI images and present a trustworthy result for fetal brain extraction compared with state-of-the-art DL based methods. In the work (Khalili et al., 2019; Kapila & Saleti, 2023) used DL techniques to segment the fetal brain, placenta, and other intrauterine tissues. De Asis-Cruz et al. (2022 proposed a completely automatic segmentation of complex fetal brain structures by hybrid loss functions and multi view data aggregation. Such a scheme significantly increases the accuracy of cortical plate segmentation, which is important for fetal brain development understanding, while reducing the efforts of human annotation. Researchers (Ebner et al. 2020; De Dumast, et al. (2021); Hong et al. (2020)) considered the application of advanced DL (deep learning) models, particularly CNNs, which were implemented for segmenting crucial fetal brain structures, such as the cortical plate. These works elaborated on the merits of using multiple anatomical views to maximize optimal segmentation of cortical regions, which is essential for tracking the development over time of the fetal brain.

Researchers (Fetit et al. (2020); Gu et al. (2020)) discussed issues and improvements related to segmentation methods developed for various fetal tissues by using MRI and ultrasound imaging. They convincingly established evidence that the inclusion of radiomic features, and ML-based approaches can transcend segmentation hurdles caused by fetal movements and image quality issues. Hong et al. (2020) used a fetal brain MRI cortical plate segmentation method based on hybrid loss function and multi-view aggregation. This study holds promise as an example of potential automatic and reproducible segmentation in clinical settings, likely to overrule issues such as scanner variability and differences in gestational age. Dumast et al. (2021) offered a DL based segmentation method of fetal brain MRI that considered dynamic changes in tissue over the course of development. It used the Contextual Transformer Block (CTB) and Hybrid Dilated Convolution (HDC) to improve segmentation results, particularly on distinguishing gray and white matter differences with varying gestational stages. Ebner et al. (2020) designed a fully automatic segmentation framework based on a coarse-to-fine CNN approach for the segmentation of fetal brain MRI. In the developed strategy, it incorporates robust outlier rejection. Huang et al. (2023) used the advanced network architectures such as CoT-Block and HDC for the enhanced segmentation of fetal brain tissues.

4.2 Comparative Analysis of MRI Image Segmentation

This section covers the analysis of DL techniques used in MRI image segmentation. In (Salehi et al., 2018), a CNN model based on the U-Net architecture was applied to segmentation purposes. However, in studies such as (Dumast et al., 2021; Michael et al., 2018; Huang et al., 2023) hybrid approaches were used along with modules such as CoT-Block and HDC for better performance in dynamic fetal brain tissue contrasts. Studies such as (Liao et al., 2020; Rampun et al., 2021) introduced 3D-CNNs that help in extracting spatial features across volumetric MRI scans. Zhao et al.'s (2022) study was based on a large data set of 100 fetal MRI scans that include a very broad range of age: from 20– 36 weeks. Michael et al. (2018) and Huang et al. (2023) used more focused sets, including pathological cases, such as congenital heart disease.

Most other studies rely on standard metrics, such as DSC, Hausdorff Distance (HD95), and Volume Similarity (VS)) for segmentation. Zhao et al. (2022) led to an excellent DSC score of 0.91. Rampun et al. (2021) provided lesser DSC values (0.85), but balances with innovative techniques for handling dynamic fetal brain development. Researchers (Salehi et al., 2018; Razieh et al., 2022; Zhang et al., 2021) studies presented methods that are strong in the segmentation task, with considerable gains over manual segmentation. Liao et al. (2020) proposed a coarse-to-fine CNN strategy, which was well suited for enhancement in segmentation accuracy. Authors (Michael et al., 2018; Huang et al., 2023) introduced new approaches to tissue contrast adaptation between stages, using CoT-Block and HDC.

Future directions for improvement were also highlighted by the studies. Michael et al. (2018) hinted at including additional fetal pathologies to further train and fine-tune models. Other studies emphasized larger datasets and cross-validation across multiple institutions to be confident that these models generalize well across diverse clinical environments. Figure 6 shows the ratio of 2D vs 3D images used in various research studies considered in this review.

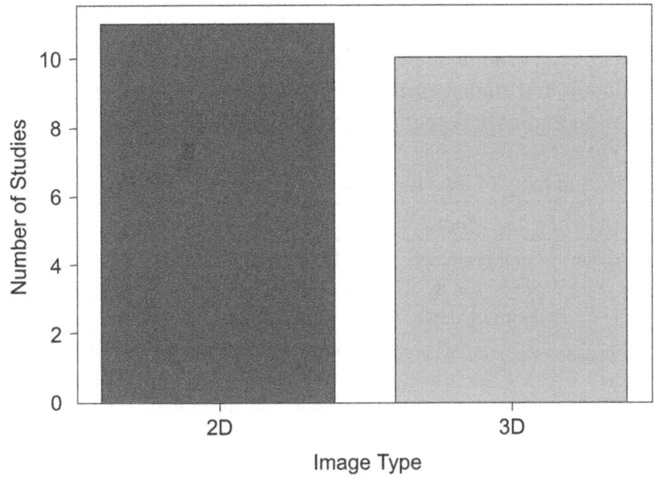

Fig. 6 Ratio of 2D v/s 3D images used.

4.3 Anomaly Detection in MRI Images

The studies by authors (Shi et al., 2020, Attallah et al., 2020) used DL methodology to examine fetal brain abnormalities from MRI. Shi et al. (2020) used deep residual networks with attention and probabilistic mechanisms to predict fetal brain age and detect conditions such as small head size and malformations, which has a strong emphasis on prediction uncertainty. Their approach primarily aimed at enhancing early diagnosis by assessing the likelihood of abnormalities. On the other hand, Attallah et al. (2020) focused on identifying Embryonic Neurodevelopmental Disorders (ENDs) using transfer learning, deep feature extraction, and PCA for feature reduction. They highlighted the importance of multiple CNN architectures for improving classification accuracy.

Conversely, the studies by (Justin Lo et al., 2022; Attallah et al., 2019; Attallah et al., 2018) revolved around detecting fetal brain abnormalities. Lo et al. (2022) proposed a DL model, named FOAC-Net, which is based on squeeze-and-excitation modules and naive inception modules that achieved an anomaly classification accuracy of 85.32% from anomalies within the brain, spinal cord, and heart. In fact, it is unique as it mainly focuses on multi-organ anomaly detection. Moreover, Attallah et al. (2019) classified fetal abnormalities in the brain by applying classifiers like k-NN and Random Forest, attaining an accuracy of 95.6% with k-NN. Furthermore, Attallah et al. (2018) used a four-phase pipeline with image enhancement by using Ensemble Subspace Discriminates (ESD). Justin Lo et al. (2021), designed a versatile model to detect anomalies in multi-fetal organs. Shi et al. (2020) proposed a focused approach that places special emphasis on uncertainties in predictions, a methodology that isn't explored by the other studies. While both sets of studies identify the great capability of DL in prenatal diagnosis, Justin Lo et al.'s (2021) method stands out in detecting multiorgan, while the studies of Attallah et al. (2019) shine in accurately classifying brain abnormalities by using traditional models and enhancement images. Table 4 provides the summary of fetal health studies on anomaly detection in fetus using MRI image data.

Table 4 Summary of fetal health anomaly detection studies using MRI data.

Study	*Dataset*	*Focus*	*Methodology*	*Key Results*
Shi et al., 2020	Private	Fetal brain age prediction & anomaly detection	Deep residual network (ResNet) with attention & probabilistic mechanisms for prediction uncertainty	Emphasized prediction uncertainty; focused on brain age prediction and malformation detection.
Attallah et al., 2020	Public	Embryonic neurodevelopmental disorders (ENDs)	Transfer learning, deep feature extraction, PCA for feature reduction, SVM classification	Used multiple CNN architectures for improved classification accuracy.
Justin Lo et al., 2022	Private	Multi organ fetal anomaly detection	FOAC-Net: combines Squeeze-and-Excitation (SE) and Naive Inception (NI) modules	Achieved 85.32% accuracy in classifying anomalies in brain, spinal cord, and heart.
Attallah et al., 2019	Public	Fetal brain abnormalities detection	Traditional ML approach (KNN, Random Forest, Ensemble models like Bagging and Adaboost)	KNN classifier achieved 95.6% accuracy; ensemble models improved performance in detecting brain abnormalities.
Attallah et al., 2018	Public	Fetal brain abnormalities detection	Four-phase pipeline: segmentation, enhancement, feature extraction, and classification with Ensemble Subspace Discriminates	After image enhancement, achieved 80% accuracy with Ensemble Subspace Discriminates.

4.4 Research Gaps Identified

Most studies on current CTG data studies lack to emphasize the importance of features. Most of the research was focused on the comparison of ML models (Diwakar et al., 2021, 2022; Dhaundiyal et al., 2020) only to identify the most effective algorithm with little attention towards understanding which features most influence the model's performance. Besides, despite the high usage of tree-based models and boosting techniques, advanced neural networks, particularly complex architectures like deep neural networks, are still far from being exploited. Moreover, the datasets used in most of the studies are multi class by nature classifying the fetus as normal, risky, or suspicious but fails to provide specific information about which abnormalities are presently affecting the fetus, which limits the depth of insight available for making clinical decisions. Furthermore, the usage of Explainable Artificial Intelligence (XAI) techniques to deliver more transparency and to build trust on ML/DL models is still not much explored in the domain of identifying the fetus health status.

5. Results

Modern research updates in classification, segmentation, as well as anomaly detection have been extremely impressive. Some research done to classify fetal health using the UCI CTG data presented excellent performance results. Among them, Kuzu et al. (2023) had a hybrid methodology that uses random forest with XGBoost. For the segmentation task, an architecture based on the U-Net was used to effectively segment fetal brain MRI images with great accuracy and attain Dice scores. Concerning anomaly detection, Shi et al. (2020) assessed the age of the fetus's brain using deep residual networks and incorporated attention mechanisms for anomaly identification. These studies focus on the superior ability of ensemble methods, along with DL techniques in predicting and analyzing fetal health. Current explorations of fetal well-being based on CTG and MRI data offer some limitations that do not allow broader improvements. Most explorations of datasets for CTG reports are mainly based on the comparison of algorithms related to the best performing algorithm, and most time is spent identifying which features influence predictions the most. Although tree based as well as boosting models are predominantly used, more complex neural networks have been adopted very seldom; except for simple architectures like MLPs. Most of the work in MRI-based research focuses on fetal brain segmentation, and the remaining organs are relatively under-represented. Secondly, anomaly detection in MRI images is still relatively unexplored regarding issues aside from the brain. In the future, more work needs to be done to expand the scope of segmentation and anomaly detection on even more organs in fetuses as well as conditions, and develop neural networks in the analysis of CTG.

Below are the answers to the questions framed in Section 1.

Answer 1: Challenges of MRI-based fetal brain segmentation include the presence of noisy imaging, resolution not high enough, and overlapping structures with anatomical variations related to gestation. These together make it difficult to accurately delineate the brain tissues. The promising types of advanced hybrid models that include attention mechanisms and 3D CNNs handle these challenges by improving accuracy together with adaptation to complex morphological changes occurring during gestation.

Answer 2: ML models like random forest and XGBoost are utilized with techniques of class imbalance to enhance the accuracy of classification of fetal well-being based on CTG data. DL models, namely U-Net and Hybrid Dilated CNNs, are especially effective for MRI segmentation, given their ability to capture intricate contrasts of tissues and the dynamic nature of changes in fetal development, significantly improving predictive accuracy and segmentation precision.

Answer 3: Ensemble methods, namely stacking and voting classifiers, combine the best features of multiple models to enhance accuracy and robustness. For example, an ensemble model that combines XGBoost, LightGBM, or random forest achieves very good accuracy and minimizes overfitting, hence, ensemble approaches are ideal for analyzing a wide variety of datasets and classifying fetal health with zero or very less error.

Answer 4: Studies have been strengthened by including pathological cases such as those with congenital heart disease. For example, the addition of 41 pathological cases to (Huang et al., 2023) proved that DL methods successfully segmented the tissues of the brain over both normal and abnormal datasets of clinical applications for early diagnosis and intervention.

6. Conclusion

Summarized literature reviews indicate a growing role for ML/DL and provide special focus towards diagnosis accuracy, allowing for the early detection of possible fetal complications. Generally, ML classification models using only CTG data will achieve high accuracy if ensemble models are applied, especially combinations of random forest and XGBoost can handle problems of class imbalance and those of feature selection. Moreover, DL models, particularly the U-Net model, are highly effective (with respect to speed and precision) in comparison to traditional techniques in MRI segmentation and delineation of fetal brain structures. Anomaly detection is another domain where the models that used deep neural networks, attention mechanisms, even transfer learning improved considerably in the prediction of anomalies or abnormalities in fetal development. Despite these innovations, there are many open challenges such as designing more sophisticated feature selection techniques, showing better interpretability of DL models, extending their scope from the fetal brain to other organs and concentrating in the direction of multi-modal data integration models. In a nutshell, further development along these lines of ML/DL promises safer pregnancies, as well as healthier newborns, through more reliable and timely diagnostics.

References

Abiyev, R., Idoko, J.B., Altıparmak, H. and Tüzünkan, M. (2023). Fetal health state detection using interval type-2 fuzzy neural networks. *Diagnostics*, *13*(10), 1690.

Akbulut, A., Ertugrul, E. and Topcu, V. (2018). Fetal health status prediction based on maternal clinical history using machine learning techniques. *Computer Methods and Programs in Biomedicine*, *163*, 87–100.

Al Duhayyim, M., Abbas, S., Al Hejaili, A., Kryvinska, N., Almadhor, A. and Mughal, H. (2023). Ensemble Learning for Fetal Health Classification. *Computer Systems Science and Engineering*, *47*(1).

Attallah, O., Gadelkarim, H. and Sharkas, M.A. (2018, December). Detecting and classifying fetal brain abnormalities using machine learning techniques. In: *2018 17th IEEE International Conference on Machine Learning and Applications* (*ICMLA*) (pp. 1371–1376). IEEE.

Attallah, O., Sharkas, M.A. and Gadelkarim, H. (2019). Fetal brain abnormality classification from MRI images of different gestational age. *Brain Sciences*, *9*(9), 231.

Attallah, O., Sharkas, M.A. and Gadelkarim, H. (2020). Deep learning techniques for automatic detection of embryonic neurodevelopmental disorders. *Diagnostics*, *10*(1), 27.

Bhowmik, P., Bhowmik, P.C., Ali, U.M.E. and Sohrawordi, M. (2021). Cardiotocography data analysis to predict fetal health risks with tree-based ensemble learning. *Inf. Technol. Comput. Sci.*, *5*, 30–40.

Chen, J., Fang, Z., Zhang, G., Ling, L., Li, G., Zhang, H. and Wang, L. (2021). Automatic brain extraction from 3D fetal MR image with deep learning-based multi step framework. *Computerized Medical Imaging and Graphics*, *88*, 101848.

De Asis-Cruz, J., Krishnamurthy, D., Jose, C., Cook, K.M. and Limperopoulos, C. (2022). Fetalgan: automated segmentation of fetal functional brain MRI using deep generative adversarial learning and multi scale 3D u-Net. *Frontiers in Neuroscience*, *16*, 887634.

De Dumast, P., Kebiri, H., Atat, C., Dunet, V., Koob, M. and Cuadra, M.B. (2021, September). Segmentation of the cortical plate in fetal brain MRI with a topological loss. In: *International Workshop on Uncertainty for Safe Utilization of Machine Learning in Medical Imaging* (pp. 200–209). Cham: Springer International Publishing.

Dhaundiyal, R., Tripathi, A., Joshi, K., Diwakar, M. and Singh, P. (2020, April). Clustering based multi-modality medical image fusion. In: *Journal of Physics: Conference Series* (*1478* (1), 012024). IOP Publishing.

Diwakar, M., Singh, P., Shankar, A., Nayak, S.R., Nayak, J., Vimal, S., ... & Sisodia, D. (2022). Directive clustering contrast-based multi-modality medical image fusion for smart healthcare system. *Network Modeling Analysis in Health Informatics and Bioinformatics*, *11*(1), 15.

Diwakar, M., Tripathi, A., Joshi, K., Memoria, M. and Singh, P. (2021). Latest trends on heart disease prediction using machine learning and image fusion. *Materials Today: Proceedings*, *37*, 3213–3218.

Dixit, R. R. (2022). Predicting fetal health using cardiotocograms: A machine learning approach. *Journal of Advanced Analytics in Healthcare Management*, *6*(1), 43–57.

Dudovitch, G., Link-Sourani, D., Ben Sira, L., Miller, E., Ben Bashat, D. and Joskowicz, L. (2020, September). Deep learning automatic fetal structures segmentation in MRI scans with few annotated datasets. In: *International Conference on Medical Image Computing and Computer-assisted Intervention* (pp. 365–374). Cham: Springer International Publishing.

Ebner, M., Wang, G., Li,W., Aertsen, M., Patel, P.A., Aughwane, R., ... & Vercauteren, T. (2020). An automated framework for localization, segmentation, and super-resolution reconstruction of fetal brain MRI. *NeuroImage*, *206*, 116324.

Faghihpirayesh, R., Karimi, D., Erdoğmuş, D. and Gholipour, A. (2022, September). Deep learning framework for real-time fetal brain segmentation in MRI. In: *International Workshop on Preterm, Perinatal, and Paediatric Image Analysis* (pp. 60–70). Cham: Springer Nature Switzerland.

Fetit, A.E., Alansary, A., Cordero-Grande, L., Cupitt, J., Davidson, A.B., Edwards, A.D., ... & Rueckert, D. (2020, September). A deep learning approach to segmentation of the developing cortex in fetal brain MRI with minimal manual labeling. In: *Medical Imaging with Deep Learning* (pp. 241–261). PMLR.

Gu, R., Wang, G., Song, T., Huang, R., Aertsen, M., Deprest, J., ... & Zhang, S. (2020). CA-Net: Comprehensive attention convolutional neural networks for explainable medical image segmentation. *IEEE Transactions on Medical Imaging*, *40*(2), 699–711.

Hong, J., Yun, H.J., Park, G., Kim, S., Laurentys, C.T., Siqueira, L.C., ... & Im, K. (2020). Fetal cortical plate segmentation using fully convolutional networks with multiple plane aggregation. *Frontiers in Neuroscience*, *14*, 591683.

Hoodbhoy, Z., Noman, M., Shafique, A., Nasim, A., Chowdhury, D. and Hasan, B. (2019). Use of machine learning algorithms for prediction of fetal risk using cardiotocographic data. *International Journal of Applied and Basic Medical Research*, *9*(4), 226–230.

Huang, X., Liu, Y., Li, Y., Qi, K., Gao, A., Zheng, B., ... & Long, X. (2023). Deep learning-based multiclass brain tissue segmentation in fetal MRIs. *Sensors*, *23*(2), 655.

Kaliappan, J., Bagepalli, A.R., Almal, S., Mishra, R., Hu, Y. C. and Srinivasan, K. (2023). Impact of cross-validation on machine learning models for early detection of intrauterine fetal demise. *Diagnostics*, *13*(10), 1692.

Kapila, R. and Saleti, S. (2023). Optimizing fetal health prediction: Ensemble modeling with fusion of feature selection and extraction techniques for cardiotocography data. *Computational Biology and Chemistry*, *107*, 107973.

Khalili, N., Lessmann, N., Turk, E., Claessens, N., de Heus, R., Kolk, T., ... & Išgum, I. (2019). Automatic brain tissue segmentation in fetal MRI using convolutional neural networks. *Magnetic Resonance Imaging*, *64*, 77–89.

Kuzu, A. and Santur, Y. (2023). Early diagnosis and classification of fetal health status from a fetal cardiotocography dataset using ensemble learning. *Diagnostics*, *13*(15), 2471.

Li, J. and Liu, X. (2021, March). Fetal health classification based on machine learning. In: *2021 IEEE 2nd International Conference on Big Data, Artificial Intelligence, and Internet of Things Engineering* (*ICBAIE*) (pp. 899–902). IEEE.

Li, J., Luo, Y., Shi, L., Zhang, X., Li, M., Zhang, B. and Wang, D. (2020). Automatic fetal brain extraction from 2D in utero fetal MRI slices using deep neural network. *Neurocomputing*, *378*, 335–349.

Liao, L., Zhang, X., Zhao, F., Zhong, T., Pei, Y., Xu, X., ... & Li, G. (2020, September). Joint image quality assessment and brain extraction of fetal MRI using deep learning. In: *International Conference on Medical Image Computing and Computer-assisted Intervention* (pp. 415–424). Cham: Springer International Publishing.

Lo, J., Lim, A., Wagner, M.W., Ertl-Wagner, B. and Sussman, D. (2022). Fetal organ anomaly classification network for identifying organ anomalies in fetal MRI. *Frontiers in Artificial Intelligence*, *5*, 832485.

Lo, J., Nithiyanantham, S., Cardinell, J., Young, D., Cho, S., Kirubarajan, A., ... & Sussman, D. (2021). Cross attention squeeze excitation network (CASE-Net) for whole body fetal MRI segmentation. *Sensors*, *21*(13), 4490.

Mehbodniya, A., Lazar, A.J.P., Webber, J., Sharma, D.K., Jayagopalan, S., K, K., ... & Sengan, S. (2022). Fetal health classification from cardiotocographic data using machine learning. *Expert Systems*, *39*(6), e12899.

Mushtaq, G. and Veningston, K. (2024). AI driven interpretable deep learning based fetal health classification. *SLAS Technology*, *29*(6), 100206.

Nagavibha, R., Satheesh, M.M., Chandy, M.P. and Prathap, B.R. (2024, March). An empirical and statistical analysis of fetal health classification using different machine learning algorithm. In: *2024 4th International Conference on Data Engineering and Communication Systems (ICDECS)* (pp. 1–7). IEEE.

Nandipati, S.C.R. and XinYing, C. (2020). Classification and feature selection approaches for cardiotocography by machine learning techniques. *Journal of Telecommunication, Electronic and Computer Engineering (JTEC)*, *12*(1), 7–14.

Rampun, A., Jarvis, D., Griffiths, P.D., Zwiggelaar, R., Scotney, B.W. and Armitage, P.A. (2021). Single-input multi-output U-Net for automated 2D foetal brain segmentation of MR images. *Journal of Imaging*, *7*(10), 200.

Rampun, A., Jarvis, D., Griffiths, P. and Armitage, P. (2020, October). Fetal brain segmentation using convolutional neural networks with fusion strategies. In: *International Symposium on Visual Computing* (pp. 113–124). Cham: Springer International Publishing.

Salehi, S.S.M., Hashemi, S.R., Velasco-Annis, C., Ouaalam, A., Estroff, J.A., Erdogmus, D., ... & Gholipour, A. (2018, April). Real-time automatic fetal brain extraction in fetal MRI by deep learning. In: *2018 IEEE 15th International Symposium on Biomedical Imaging (ISBI 2018)* (pp. 720–724). IEEE.

Shi, W., Yan, G., Li, Y., Li, H., Liu, T., Sun, C., ... & Wu, D. (2020). Fetal brain age estimation and anomaly detection using attention-based deep ensembles with uncertainty. *Neuroimage*, *223*, 117316.

Torrents-Barrena, J., Monill, N., Piella, G., Gratacos, E., Eixarch, E., Ceresa, M. and Ballester, M.A. G. (2021). Assessment of radiomics and deep learning for the segmentation of fetal and maternal anatomy in magnetic resonance imaging and ultrasound. *Academic Radiology*, *28*(2), 173–188.

Yin, Y. and Bingi, Y. (2023). Using machine learning to classify human fetal health and analyze feature importance. *BioMedInformatics*, *3*(2), 280–298.

Zhang, X., Cui, Z., Chen, C., Wei, J., Lou, J., Hu, W., ... & Shen, D. (2021, September). Confidence-aware cascaded network for fetal brain segmentation on MR images. In: *International Conference on Medical Image Computing and Computer-assisted Intervention* (pp. 584–593). Cham: Springer International Publishing.

Zhao, L., Asis-Cruz, J.D., Feng, X., Wu, Y., Kapse, K., Largent, A., ... & Limperopoulos, C. (2022). Automated 3D fetal brain segmentation using an optimized deep learning approach. *American Journal of Neuroradiology*, *43*(3), 448–454.

3 Fracture Detection in X-Ray Images Using Deep Supervised Learning

Utkarsh Singh[1], Jayant Singh[2], Jai Singhal[3], Ikshit Mangal[4] and Garima Jaiswal[5*]

Bone issues are prevalent and can lead to various problems with the body's muscles and skeleton. Roughly 1.71 billion individuals worldwide experience musculoskeletal issues. In addition to bone fractures, problems with the femoral neck, knee osteoarthritis, and fractures are very common bone conditions, and the number of cases is expected to double in the next 30 years. Hence, it is crucial to accurately and promptly diagnose and treat a patient with a fracture. On the other hand, overlooked breaks are frequently misidentified in accidents and critical situations. DL can be extensively utilized in the analysis of medical images. Numerous studies on trauma and bone deterioration have shown that deep learning is effective and may be used to detect diseases and fractures from x-rays. This summary gives an outline of how DL is used in bone imaging to assist radiologists in identifying different problems, especially fractures. We also discussed the challenges and problems faced in the DL-based method, and what the future holds for DL in bone imaging.

1. Introduction

In radiology, artificial intelligence (AI) is utilized for a variety of activities, including measurement, segmentation, classification, and automatic sickness diagnosis. According to studies, a particular sort of AI known as deep learning (DL) can occasionally interpret medical images more accurately than medical experts (Roy & Bandyopadhya, 2016). DL applications rely heavily on medical imaging modalities such as computed tomography, X-rays, and magnetic resonance imaging (MRI). Pathologists and clinicians continue to struggle with large datasets, necessitating the use of sophisticated and adaptable DL approaches to interpret specific bone imaging data. There is a strong drive to enhance intelligent radiology systems, as indicated by the growing number of publications in this area. Less than 100 annual publications on AI in radiology were published about ten years

[1-5] Bennett University, Greater Noida, Uttar Pradesh.
email: e22cseu0540@bennett.edu.in[1]; e22cseu0517@bennett.edu.in[2]; e22cseu0536@bennett.edu.in[3]; e22cseu0525@bennett.edu.in[4]
* Corresponding author: garima.jaiswal@bennett.edu.in

DOI: 10.1201/9781003655121-3

ago. Since then, the number has expanded, and there are now between 1,000 and 2,000 publications every year. PubMed contains a huge number of articles on AI in radiology. Figure 1 shows how DL increases the speed and quality of image capture during acquisition and decompression. DL also makes it easy to collect, align, and convert photographs into various formats while reducing costs and image quality degradation.

However, there is a lot of variability among users, within users, and in decision-making and protocols (Gulshan et al., 2016; Roy et al., 2020) because of different experiences and settings. This may result in a loud signal. Hence, the assessment of the picture tag remains effective in DL.

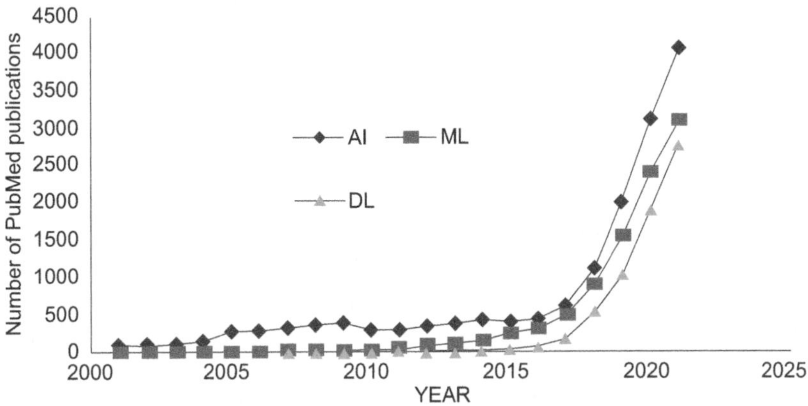

Fig. 1 The number of PubMed publications found when searching for "radiology" and "artificial intelligence," "machine learning," or "deep learning" demonstrates how artificial intelligence is becoming more common in radiography.

At present, numerous AI techniques, particularly DL, are assisting researchers by automating the handling and examination of pictures, including in medical trials, a method known as "computational radiology" (Roy et al., 2022). Understanding medical observations, determining the scope of illness, foreseeing medical results (such as in cancerous and non-cancerous cells), and diverse computerized techniques, may be referred to as a system decision- making aid These are some instances of computer programs that can be created. Because of time limitations and an inability to visualize and measure, these instances are not included in current radiology reports. Figure 2 shows the variations in DL images in bone X-rays.

This article discusses the application of DL g in X-ray imaging and how it can be used to diagnose bone fractures. Fracture detection was thoroughly reviewed using a rigorous approach. This study reviews research data from the past retrospectively. The PubMed, Research gate, and Radiology databases all had relevant materials. The search phrases include "artificial intelligence in fracture analysis", "deep learning or machine learning in fracture analysis", as well as "neural networks in fracture analysis". The quest ended in 2022. This review is to address the following questions:

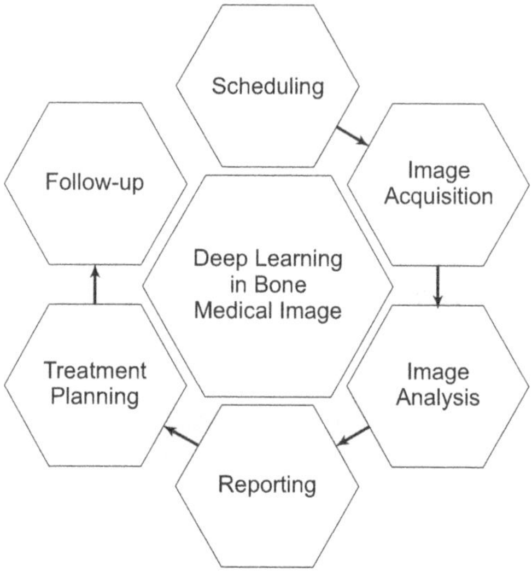

Fig. 2 Examples of machine learning in radiology.

- What are the various types of bone fractures?
- What kinds of deep learning methods are utilized in identifying and categorizing bone fractures?
- How can deep learning in radiology greatly assist doctors?
- What are the existing problems and potential advantages in using computers to detect diseases in bones?
- What are the potential research opportunities in this area?

1.1 Widespread Bone Condition

Orthopaedic specialists and radiologists detect bone diseases using X-rays, MRIs, or CT scans of the affected bone. Recent advances in the discipline have enabled the healthcare sector to efficiently deploy and assess DL models. Musculoskeletal issues, including arthritis, bursitis, tendinitis, and other related disorders, are a prominent concern in orthopedics. These illnesses begin with extreme pain and have the potential to deteriorate over time, resulting in disability. DL is thus essential for speedy and accurate recognition.

With 2.7 million breaks happening every year in six EU countries (Sweden, Germany, Italy, France, Spain, and the United Kingdom), a visibly broken bone in an X-ray is among the most frequent injuries nowadays (Krupinski et al., 2010). Doctors face several challenges while examining X-rays: first, some bone properties may be obscured; second, effectively diagnosing different types of fractures takes a high degree of knowledge; and third, doctors may grow exhausted when working under time constraints. According to research, radiologists become less accurate in detecting fractures on musculoskeletal X-rays as the day progresses (International Osteoporosis Foundation, 2019. Furthermore, it is typical for X-ray examinations to be performed without experienced colleagues present to provide second opinions (Hallas & Ellingsen, 2006). Accurate fracture categorization is required for effective diagnosis and therapy, as per criteria established by the Arbeitsgemeinschaft für Osteosynthesisfragen. A computer-assisted design system for physicians can have a significant impact on patient outcomes. Figure 3 illustrates a proposed DL method for fracture diagnosis.

1.2 Significance of Advanced Learning in Orthopaedic and Radiology

By automating time-consuming processes, mixing DL algorithms with traditional radiology methodologies offers the potential to improve diagnostic efficiency and reduce radiologists' burden. Nonetheless, interpretive variability across observers or even within a single observer may provide challenges for DL algorithms. In academic studies, DL has consistently outperformed humans in identifying and classifying fractures from X-rays. DL has recently gained a lot of attention, and studies have demonstrated that it is capable of making complex assessments comparable to those performed by medical professionals (Lindsey et al., 2018). There has been minimal study on using DL for fracture detection in CT images (Layan et al., 2019), despite the fact that numerous orthopedic trauma studies use DL to diagnose and classify fractures in X-rays (Urukawa et al., 2019; Wang et al., 2022).

Speaking about the customer journey, it is crucial to pay attention to the specifics of the interactions of organizations, providing products and services, and customers, to whom these offers are proposed. This sensitive bond has transformed significantly throughout the years as compared to the early thought that the firms have the power to influence the market into the current thought that the customers have the power. It is true that the world was not an interconnected world as it is today. The customers were buying with local sellers or basing their decisions on external factors like word-of-mouth by friends and family as well as exposure to conventional advertising. The limited choice offered, as it was closely linked to either of the above-mentioned factors, meant that a business that had a good local presence, or spent a lot on advertising, stood a chance to succeed. Nevertheless, with the increased interconnection of the world, the amount of information that customers have access to when making their decisions on the products and services grew exponentially, and it provided customers with a more detailed picture of the possible products and services and the ability to choose the most suitable to meet their needs. In a world like this, consumers started to learn overall in the most varied ways to receive the holistic response to their needs. The period of making passive customers buy marketed products and services is gone, and new opportunities are created to many organizations that were formerly unable to be competitive. In fact, it is not uncommon to see a startup firm grow fast and compete effectively with other bigger and more successful competitors. The reason behind this is that the modern customers are proactively finding solutions to their needs and therefore any organization that can fulfill such needs and wants has a chance of attracting attention. According to Strauss, J., & Frost, R. (2014). E-Marketing (7th ed.). Pearson Education., this phenomenon is known as a Power Shift of Sellers to Purchasers (p. 30) and it is mentioned that individual and company buyers are more than ever demanding because of the tremendous number of alternatives available with just a couple of clicks. In fact, word-of-mouth has been an important component of the decision-making process in the past, yet technology facilitated the ability to share opinions of a new form. Contemporary personal and business customers can utilize various sources (blogs, vlogs, social media content, product, service reviews, influencers, communities, and the likes) on top of the views of their relatives, colleagues and best friends (Frigenti, 2022b). This made the shift of a centralized push (businesses to people) to a decentralized pull with regards to the direction of flow of information (individuals collecting the information through various sources). The relationship between businesses and individuals has undergone changes as shown in Figure 1.

1.3 Historical Perspective

Convolutional neural networks (CNNs) revolutionized image classification by dominating the ImageNet competition in 2012 (Krizhersky et al., 2012), accelerating DL advancements. This sparked discussions on DL applications in medical imaging, particularly addressing data scarcity due to limited labelled datasets.

Transfer learning (TL), introduced in 2015–2016, enabled the application of pre trained models from nonmedical datasets to medical imaging. Studies (Kim et al., 2022; Jaiswal et al., 2022; Anand et al., 2021) demonstrated that ImageNet-trained networks improved accuracy in bone imaging. Data augmentation, emerging around 2017–2018, became crucial for training on small datasets.

Key questions arose on using generative models to synthesize medical data and improve performance. A study (Shah et al., 2022) showed generative adversarial network (GAN)-based image enhancement boosted CNN accuracy for liver lesion detection, producing images indistinguishable from real ones. Advances in GANs, variational encoders, and U-Net architectures have since driven progress in bone disorder analysis and other medical imaging tasks (Sannat et al., 2022).

2. Advanced Learning and Important Methods in Bone Scanning

There are substantial practical benefits to taking high-quality images with less radiation exposure and/or shorter capture times. Whether for display or further diagnostic analysis, improving clinical images includes adjusting pixel brightness to increase image quality.

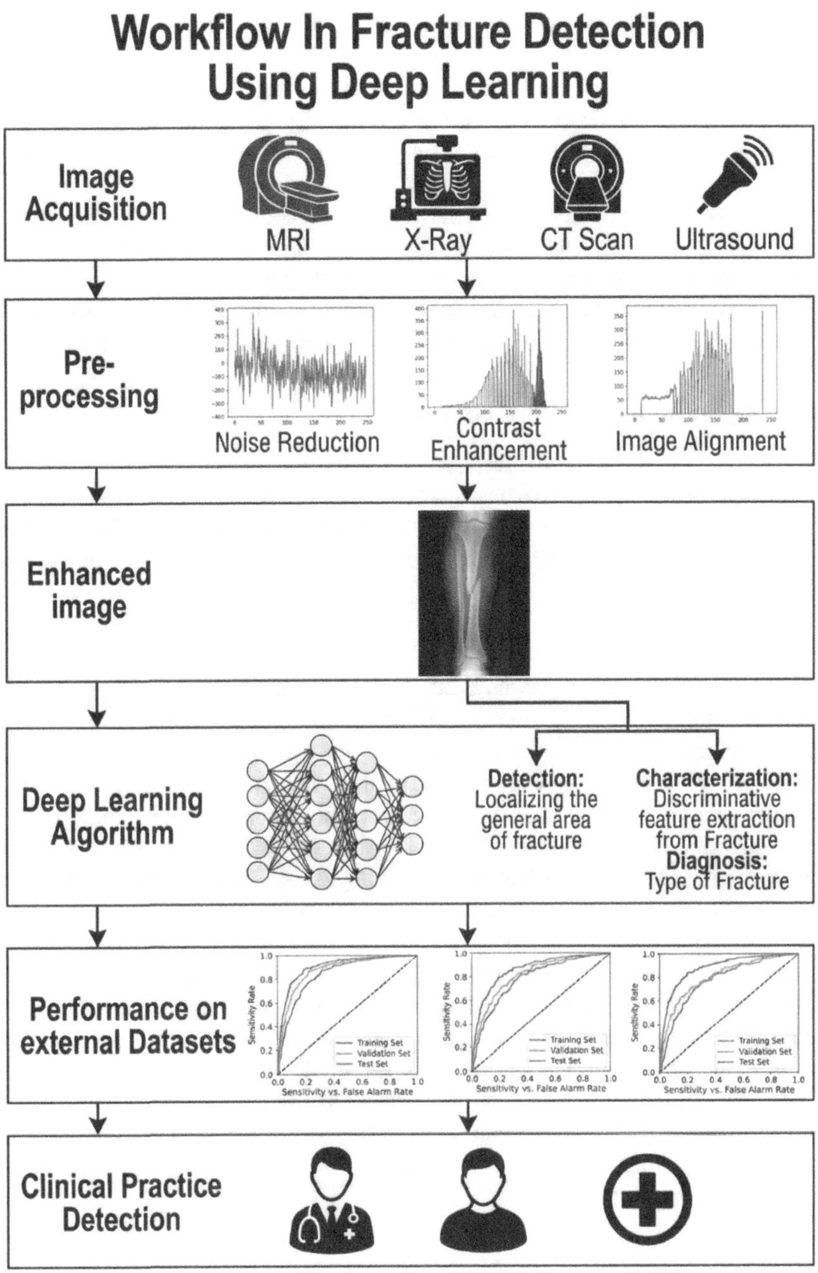

Fig. 3 Process in identifying fractures using advanced learning.

Improvements include adjusting the MR (magnetic resonance) field, eliminating noise, increasing resolution, and synchronizing images. Translation and synthesis, also called image improvement methods, have also been widely studied. DL can assist in diagnosing strokes and in measuring clinical outcomes, as well as in planning treatment and surgeries. DL-based registration is commonly used in combining multiple modes, analyzing populations over time, and transferring labels for image segmentation. Additional DL and pre processing technologies encompass target and reference, display or image recognition, and automatic report creation (Roy et al., 2019; Roy et al., 2017; Al Ghaiti & Al Maskari, 2021).

DL models are stronger and more adaptable than basic neural network models. DL techniques trained on vast amounts of data can yield much better and superior results compared to typical algorithms and capabilities for a specific task.

2.1 Arrangement of Connections

The ResNet, VGGNet, and Inception Net belong to the branch of research that began with the AlexNet (Krizhersky et al., 2012) to develop networks and apply bone marrow images. The case of both denseNet (Marwa et al., 2022; Anand et al., 2021) and U-Net (Papandrianos et al., 2020) demonstrates that a deep network can be improved by including skip connections. U-net was meant to be used in segmentation unlike other networks that were meant to be used in classifying the image. The ability to identify is improved through continuous surveillance (Rahmaniar & Wang, 2019) Bone imaging, the procedure of taking medical images, improving quality of images and image segmentation has wide uses in machine learning. In summarizing the bone-shaped data or in making structured decisions, the focus method is able to automatically identify the where and the what to focus on. The channel can be controlled with the help of pressing and activating. The concentration is used with a GAN in (Zhang et al., 2019) and the focus is used with a U-Net in (Sarvamangala & Kulkarni, 2022). The GAN in question can be illustrated in its simplest form in Figure 4. GANs consist of a discriminator and a generator, and they are adversarial networks. The machine acquires significant characteristics and creates maps of those characteristics through linking them to the concealed region. The discriminator is conditioned to learn the difference between the shape maps generated by the generator and the actual data distribution. The sensitivity gates enable the pipeline to process feature vectors with large dimensions without the need to complicate the computation. The acquired characteristics are in terms of surface vector distributions, which are inputted in the image encoder. This is then passed on to an endpoint layer so as to achieve the required result.

2.2 Annotation Effective Methods

The minimum detectable level in bone imaging should match the image brightness of current models and data for the same job, even if they are from different areas.

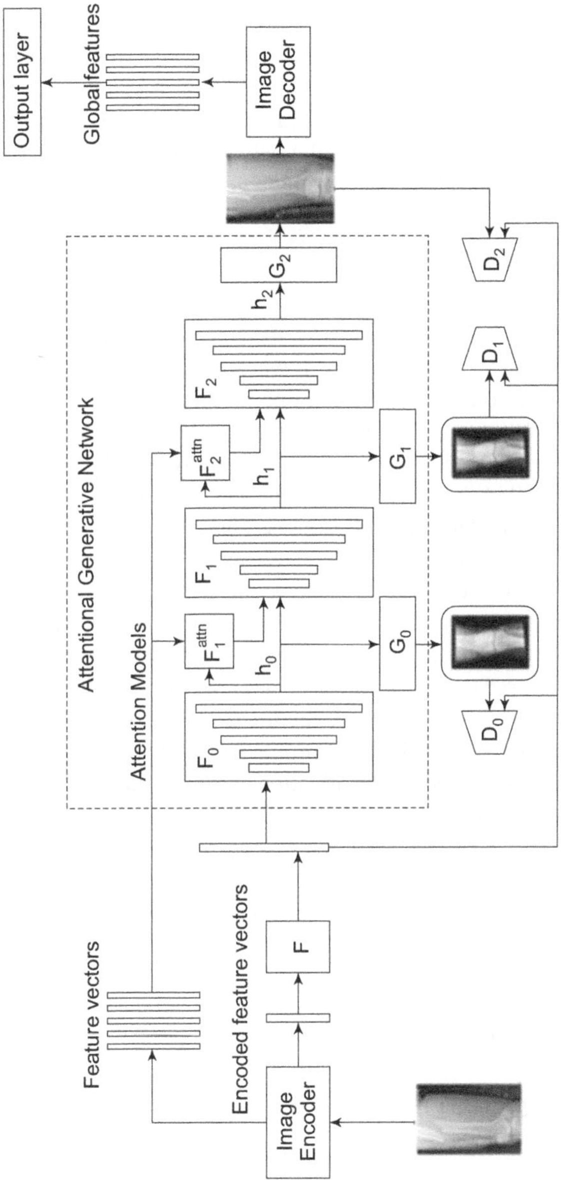

Fig. 4 Basic structure of attention assisted GAN.

This new learning approach enables you to discover various fields and professions for the first time. One way to achieve learning of new features is through supervised learning, as illustrated in Figure 5. Figure 5A uses reference images and an image encoder to help the encoder learn important patterns, increasing the picture to greater clarity. The particular characteristics are moved to the final layer. The last layer could contain a thick layer for grouping or a 1 x 1 layer for recognizing items or areas. Figure 5B is used to apply the obtained features to a modified design to achieve the aim of prototyping. Various learning characteristics are combined into weighted patterns and inputted into the network. This enables the student to complete multiple tasks simultaneously using a version with several tabs.

2.3 Fractures in Upper Limbs

The probability of failing to detect fractures is equal for both the upper and lower limbs. The rate of unidentified fractures in the upper body, including the neck, wrist, hand, and shoulder, was 6%, 5.4%, 4.2%, and 1.9%, in that order (Tyson & Hasan, 2015). Kim and colleagues (2018) trained the model using 1,112 hand x-ray pictures, then added 100 more images (50 fractures and 50 normal images). They reached an 88% accuracy in diagnosis, with a sensitivity of 90% and an area under the curve (AUC) of 0.954. Lindsey and colleagues (2018) utilized 135,409 x-rays to create a CNN model to detect wrist fractures. They stated that doctors' ability to interpret images improved (with and without assistance) from 88% to 94%, leading to a 53% decrease in misinterpretation. Olchak and colleagues created a model for breaks in the lower part of the forearm and evaluated it using x-rays of the hand and wrist. They examined how well the network worked with very skilled bone specialists and discovered that it did well with a sensitivity of 90% and a specificity of 88%. The type and complexity of the fracture diagnosis were not specified.

Chung et al., 2018 developed a CNN model to detect and categorize proximal humerus fractures by using Neer's classification and 1890 shoulder X-ray pictures. In contrast to experts, the example's strength and the average level below the curve are 96% and 1%, while the strength is 99% and the average level is 97%. The primary challenge is determining the kind of fractures. The anticipated accuracy was around 63 to 85%. Rayan and his team introduced a model using a multi-perspective method that allows the radiologist to rotate while examining multiple images of severe pediatric neck fractures. The authors analyzed 21,453 radiology assessments, which involved 58,817 X-rays of the elbow. The model's sensitivity, accuracy, and specificity were 87%, 90%, and 83%, respectively.

2.4 Fractures in Lower Limb

Hip fractures constitute 21% of the patients who are under orthopedic surgery and hidden fractures on x-rays are between 4–9% (Wang et al., 2022). Urakawa et al. (2019) developed a CNN based on the diagnostics of hip intertrochanteric fracture. The number of hip X-rays they studied was 3,346 with 1,773 X-rays demonstrating

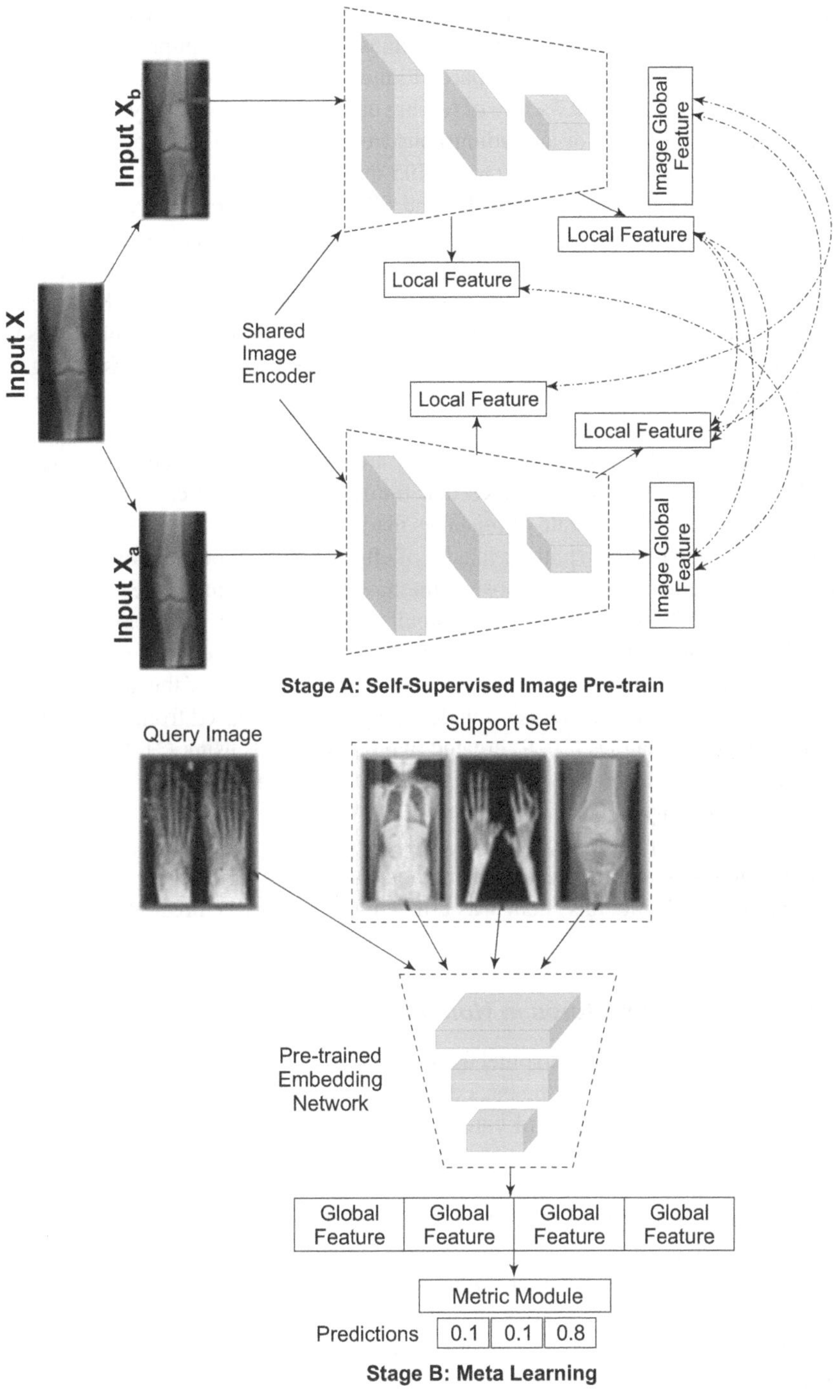

Fig. 5 A visual representation of self-supervised learning.

fractures and 1,573 X-rays demonstrating no fractures. The model was tested using the scores of five orthopedic physicians. There was an improvement in the performance of the model as compared to the orthopedic surgeons. According to them, a 96% accuracy to 92% free of relying on 97% to 57% accuracy of 94 to 88% compared to pre trained organ radiographs were utilized by Cheng et al. (2019) to create a CNN model, amounting to 25,505 images. The model was also accurate in diagnosis of hip fractures with 91 and 98% accuracy, respectively. The false negative rate of this model is very low; it is 1.8 and hence it is a better screening tool. Adams and co-authors created a model to examine the break of the thigh bone (Adams et al., 2019) with accuracy of 91% and AUC value of 0.98. To detect femoral fractures, Balaji and his associates (2020) developed a CNN model using 175 x-ray images to train a system on the data with the objective of classifying the breakage of the femoral shaft as helical, transverse, or comminuted. The model has a 90.7 accuracy, specificity of 92.4 and 86.6.

Fractures in the lower part of the body are uncommon, particularly in trauma patients. Recent research indicates that the rate of mistakes caused by various factors is 44%, while the rate of mistakes made by radiologists is 66%. That is the reason why scientists are putting in a lot of effort to teach models in order to assist radiologists in accurately diagnosing fractures. Kitamura and colleagues (2019) suggested a CNN model that utilizes a small set of ankle x-ray pictures (298 normal and 298 fractures). This model was taught to identify fractures in the front part of the foot, middle part of the foot, back part of the foot, side of the shinbone, and thigh bone. The model's precision in detecting fractures varied from 76% to 81%. Pranatha and colleagues (2019) created two CNN models using CT X-ray images to categorize ankle breaks. The suggested model demonstrates an accuracy of 0.791, a specificity of 0.725, and a sensitivity of 0.828, indicating its potential as a valuable tool for future computer-aided diagnostics. Rahmaniar and colleagues (2019) suggested a computer-based method for identifying calcaneus fractures in CT scans. The Saunders system was utilized to classify fractures. In this system, the calcaneus fragments.

2.5 Vertebrae Fractures in Human Body

The percentage of undetected spinal fracture ranges between 19.4 and 44% according to studies. The CT scans of the back and chest were used by Burns and colleagues (2017) to detect, identify and categorize the fractures in the spine vertebrae, and determine the level of bone density in the lower spine. The recognizing and pinpointing fractures had a score of 0.957, and a positivity rate of 0.29 per patient. Tomita and co-authors (2018) came up with CNN architecture that is used to identify X-ray features of CT scans of spinal fractures as a result of osteoporosis. The images of 1,432 CT have been trained according to this technique 10546 of which are side views and the accuracy is 89.2. In 59 CT scans of patients with insufficiency fractures of the vertebra, a model was advanced by Mueehlematter and colleagues (2019) to determine the susceptibility to the fracture cases. A total of 120 cases (59 healthy vertebrae and 61 unhealthy vertebrae) were used in this research. Nevertheless, the precision with which it could have identified the healthiness or unhealthiness of spinal bones was poor with AUC = 0.51.

3. Fracture Detection Using Deep Learning

Many studies have indicated that deep learning is effective in detecting fractures. In (Kim & MacKinnon, 2018), the investigators used transfer learning to identify abnormalities on the x-rays of hands. A CNN that was originally trained on unrelated x-ray images was used. The CNN models 1, 2, and 3 were trained on non-x-ray images to compete in the ImageNet competition. The upper layers of the original V3 model were changed to binary classification using a manually labeled dataset of 1,389 x-rays. This method attained a test set of 139 x-rays AUC of 0.95, accuracy and precision scores of 0.88 and 0.90, respectively. These results were better than the traditional computer models that are based on edge detection, segmentation and feature extraction that usually have sensitivity and specificity values of 75–85. Nonetheless, the study was burdened with weaknesses including the lack of correspondence between training and validation accuracy, and this was probably as a result of high computational requirements. Various approaches can be used to overcome these shortcomings.

Chung et al., 2018 used front-back (AP) shoulder x-rays to test how well DL can detect and classify upper arm bone fractures. The results from the deep CNN model were compared with the opinions of experts (bone doctors, general doctors, and medical imaging specialists). Their collection of data included 1,891 AP X-rays of the shoulder. They used the modified ResNet-152 model on their similar humerus fracture model. The CNN model excels in identifying common shoulder and arm fractures. In addition, significant findings were made in identifying the kind of break on AP shoulder x-rays. The CNN model improved the skills of general surgeons, medical specialists, and cancer specialists. This is about the capability of using computerized testing to recognize and classify fractures and other complex illnesses using simple X-ray images.

Tomita and his team (2018) conducted a study that investigates the past events and tests the capabilities of DL in identifying osteoporotic vertebral fractures in the CT images and suggested a machine learning-based system. It relies on a complex neural network architecture to identify OVFs (open virtualization formats) in CTs. Their OVF detection system was based on a two-part system: a extraction component based on a convolutional neural network and an RNN component that can integrate the features obtained and provide a final evaluation. They employed ResNet deep residuals to extract and analyze idiosyncratic scans of CT. They had the training, confirmation, and test set of 1,157 CT scans, 135 CT scans, and 129 CT scans, respectively. This automatic search system has the capability of saving time and effort that radiologists would have to use to scan manually to detect OVF.

CT scan pictures were utilized to identify breaks in the neck spine. Because CT scans offer greater pixel data than X-rays, pre processing methods such as windowing and Hounsfield Unit conversion were used to enhance the visibility of tissue abnormalities. Nevertheless, when using X-rays to identify breaks in the upper and lower extremities, a considerable amount of pixel data is not captured, leading to reduced precision in comparison to identifying fractures in the cervical spine. The upper limbs, especially the femur, have higher bone densities compared to other limbs. This enables them to bear the full weight of the body. Figure 6 shows a pie graph demonstrating the use of different techniques and advanced learning models.

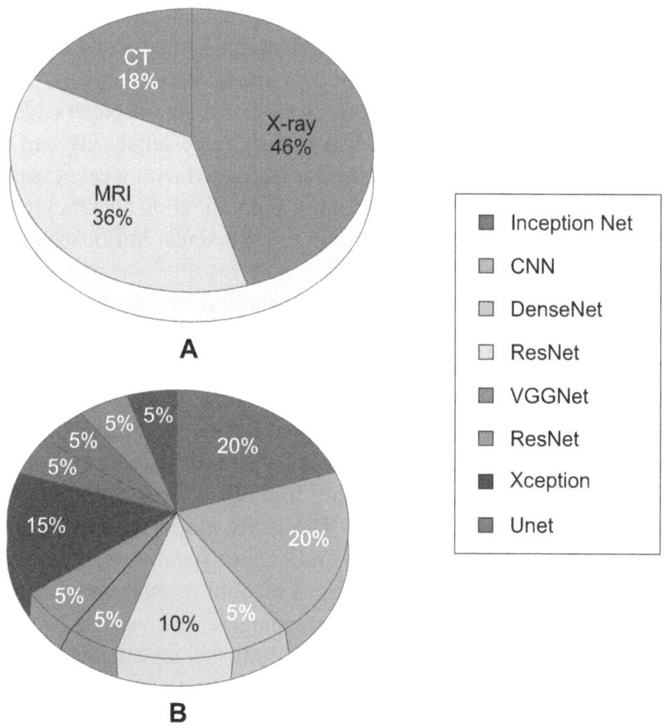

Fig. 6 (A) Refers to the use of different methods in deep learning. (B) Use of deep learning algorithms to detect fractures.

4. Obstacles to Distance Learning in Radiology and Challenges

Several individuals believe that DL will be involved in the future of radiology, especially in X-ray and MRI. Some individuals believe that sophisticated teaching techniques can manage everyday responsibilities, allowing radiologists to focus on more complex mental challenges. Some professionals predict that radiologists will work together with deep learning programs to achieve better performance than they would on their own. Ultimately, some individuals believe that sophisticated learning programs will ultimately replace radiologists entirely. Utilizing DL in radio comes with many challenges. Some of these are outlined below.

4.1 Difficulties in Obtaining Data

The main problem is technical difficulty. Although DL has proven to be effective in various image-related activities, it has not shown that it can outperform radiologists in the field of radiology. There is a large quantity of medical information in the x-ray field that has the potential to be used for training AI. Nevertheless, this information needs to go through a "curation" procedure, in which it is sorted by patient group studies, divided to concentrate on AI analysis-relevant areas, and screened to guarantee precision in capture and portrayal, among other responsibilities.

Annotating the dataset takes a lot of time and effort, and verifying the accuracy of the original diagnosis must be very strong. Rare discoveries are a weak point because if a condition or discovery is very uncommon, it is hard to gather enough samples to properly train the algorithm to identify it with certainty. At times, the sound could be confused with other sounds, causing unwanted disturbance. Furthermore, if the training dataset is inherently prejudiced (such as by race, age, or gender), the algorithm will exclude data gathered from a specific population. various clients.

4.2 Legal and Moral Dilemmas

Another challenge is who is responsible for the mistakes the machine makes. This is very difficult to answer. Similar problems arose from the introduction of other technologies such as elevators and automobiles. Based on the idea that they will affect the nature of human activity, those problems will be investigated, and the answers will be given to them in the years to come. People like to implement Isaac Asimov's "Three Principles of Robotics in Radiography for Artificial Intelligence", where a "robot" is an "intelligent medical imaging bottle". Asimov's three laws are as follows:

- A robot must not hurt a person or let a person be harmed by not doing anything.
- A robot is required to follow the commands given to it by humans, unless these commands go against the First Law.
- A robot needs to ensure its own survival if doing so doesn't go against the First or Second Laws.

Per the initial rule, machine learning tools can accurately detect illnesses, thus improving healthcare. However, computer slow performance, glitches, or failure can result in medical errors, putting a patient's life at further risk. The second rule is that DL must be effectively taught to produce suitable and therapeutically applicable results, and radiologists should oversee the learning process of any artificial intelligence system. When thinking about the certainty and eventual failure of any DL systems, the third law may become problematic. Due to the rapid advancement of scanning technology, simply training the DL system with specific image sequences may not be enough when a new modality or an upgraded version of an existing modality (such as X-ray, MRI, CT, nuclear medicine, etc.) is introduced for clinical use.

4.3 Getting a Lot of Medical Data Needs

To create and train DL models, a lot of medical data must be available. This is a significant drawback for DL model creation. Software engineers utilize a variety of techniques to get training data sets. While some have access to academic or institutional repositories, others work directly with patients. Consent is required for the use of any patient data by third parties, and it may also be obtained if the data is used again in a different way. Additionally, different regions have different copyright ownership policies for radio broadcasts. Patients still have the right to their private information in several nations. However, with the patient's permission, they may be kept at a hospital or radiological facility. Data anonymization must be ensured. It must be confirmed that the patient cannot be identified again using DICOM chips, tracking systems, or other methods because this does not count as de-identification.

5. Restrictions and Limitations of Deep Learning Application in Clinical Environments

In the healthcare industry, DL is still a long way from being able to function autonomously. Thorough thinking is necessary for the DL model to be implemented successfully. While not suitable for regular medical use, recent publications show the potential and usefulness of the suggested diagnostic models, even though they are experimental. Additionally, since the information and software utilized to teach the models are not accessible to the public, it is difficult to replicate the published work. Moreover, the recommended method must be connected to image databases and information systems, along with clinical information systems, to achieve success. Regrettably, there is not sufficient evidence to support this correlation. Additionally, showing the safety of these devices to government officials is an important initial step toward clinical application and widespread use. Additionally, it's undeniable that DL is quickly changing and getting better.

Overall, the new DL age, notably CNN, has proven to be more excellent, imaginative, and accurate than the previous one. These dating techniques have shown to be highly useful, and we believe they will soon outperform human specialists. Additionally, it might provide patients with a more exact diagnosis.

5.1 Future Aspects

The question of whether DL technology belongs in decision support systems has been debated for decades. We expect further areas of greater utility soon as DL technology's use in orthopaedic radiography and traumatology increases. It is well accepted that DL enhances diagnostic performance when incorporated into radiography and imaging techniques (Recht & Bryan, 2017; Gyftopulps et al., 2019) Additionally, it is recommended that these devices undergo a comprehensive assessment and examination before being incorporated into medical decision-making procedures. Given that radiologists typically concentrate on cognitively demanding tasks, Jha et al. (2016) suggested that DL may be utilized to address recurrent pattern recognition issues. Radiologists generally need to be educated.

A thorough understanding of DL and DL-based models/tools is required; nevertheless, these technologies are not intended to replace radiologists' responsibilities or to confine their function to reviewing DL results. Instead, radiologists can use these technologies to supplement their findings and clarify doubts. More study is needed to determine how to train and motivate radiologists to use DL tools and evaluate their results, hence encouraging a productive interaction between DL and radiologists. It is also critical that DL technologies broaden their range of clinical applications. As presented in this article, several promising research shows how DL can improve clinical tasks like fracture classification, treatment decision support, and fracture diagnosis on radiographs and CT scans.

5.2 DL in Radiology Training

A radiologist's competence is developed over several years of training, requiring a doctor to assess various tests using both written and clinical knowledge. The depth and precision of radiographic analysis and characterization are critically important for interpretive skills. DL can process photographs to extract both visual features and quantitative data, such as photo biometrics and radio frequency signatures, that humans cannot perceive. We will include deep learning into our imaging and analysis capabilities. If computers are used frequently during training, beginners may struggle to analyze independently, thus impeding skill development. Additionally, DL helps practitioners make more informed decisions and interpretations. However, overreliance on DL aid raises concerns about future radiologists and may have undesirable implications. Therefore, establishing DL in radiology requires a beginner to know how to effectively integrate DL into diagnostic procedures, so a DL course and specific analysis should be included in radiology training programs.

Radiologists must analyze a wide range of tests using both written and clinical knowledge, which requires years of study to master. Interpretive abilities are strongly reliant on the breadth and precision of radiographic analysis and characterization. DL can extract visual features as well as quantitative information beyond human vision, such as photo biometrics and radio frequency signatures. However, frequent computer use during training may hinder novices' ability to do independent analysis, thus impeding skill growth. Furthermore, DL enables practitioners to make better decisions and interpretations. However, relying excessively on DL support raises concerns for aspiring radiologists and may have negative consequences.

5.3 Can Deep Learning Serve as a Radiologist for Free?

Radiologists are afraid that DL will replace their role in the future. This is untrue, though. The answer to this question is quite straightforward: never. Nevertheless, the tasks of radiologists will undergo significant transformations in the era of artificial intelligence. Deep learning algorithms can speed up and improve many scheduled tasks in radio processing. Nonetheless, the work of a radiologist is difficult as it involves handling intricate medical issues (Debojyoti et al., 2022). Automated labeling (Ko et al., 2022) can assist radiologists in making more precise diagnoses. Embracing the unavoidable change in the radiological field as deep learning becomes integrated into radiology procedures is the true challenge, instead of resisting the implementation and use of automation in day-to-day operations. The concept that "we will follow instructions from a machine because we are fascinated by technology and trust it to make important choices" is one of the most believable concerns. By educating themselves and their future colleagues about the advantages of DL working with academics to ensure its correct, secure, practical, and relevant implementation, and making sure that its use is exclusively for the benefit of patients, radiologists may reduce this. DL could improve radiography and enable doctors to constantly boost their importance and value.

Diagnosing children using X-rays, as well as complex cases of osteoporosis and bone cancers, is always a mental challenge for radiologists. Complex circumstances make analysis tough, but computers can help the programmer make the optimal decision and identify cases that are difficult or overlooked. When it comes to osteoporosis, for example, the tools can predict whether the illness will deteriorate in the future and whether preventative actions should be taken. Children's bones continue to grow until they are between 15–18 years old, which is another reason for X-rays. A radiologist must be consulted to determine whether this is normal in this circumstance. The radiologist does not need to be replaced as a result, but the two elements can cooperate to support the decision-making process.

6. Conclusion

In this article, we looked at various algorithms for finding and categorizing defects. It is evident that CNN models, especially InceptionNet and XceptionNet, excel in fault detection. The categorization of radiologists can be a tiring and lengthy process, but it can be automated by a machine using error detection methods. Numerous professionals think that the main obstacle to creating an effective classification system is the absence of sufficient training information. There is still no established model that can be used with the current data. An effort was made to show how deep learning can be used in medical imaging to assist radiologists in accurately identifying diseases. In radio, it's usually hard to fully release a DL because employees are afraid of getting fired. Our aim is to assist the coder's work, not to replace it.

References

Adams, M., Chen, W., Holcdorf, D., McCusker, M.W., Howe, P.D., Gaillard, F. Computer vs. human: Deep learning versus perceptual training for the detection of neck of femur fractures. *J. Med. Imaging Radiat. Oncol.* **2019**, *63*, 27–32.

Al Ghaithi, A., Al Maskari, S. Artificial intelligence application in bone fracture detection. *J. Musculoskelet. Surg. Res.* **2021**, *5*, 4.

Anand, I., Negi, H., Kumar, D., Mittal, M., Kim, T., Roy, S. ResU-Net Deep Learning Model for Breast Tumor Segmentation. In *Magnetic Resonance Images*; Computers, Materials & Continua, Tech Science Press: Henderson, NV, USA, 2021; Volume 67, pp. 3107–3127.

Balaji, G.N., Subashini, T.S., Madhavi, P., Bhavani, C.H., Manikandarajan, A. Computer-Aided Detection and Diagnosis of Diaphyseal Femur Fracture. In *Smart Intelligent Computing and Applications*; Satapathy, S.C., Bhateja, V., Mohanty, J.R., Udgata, S.K., Eds.; Springer: Singapore, 2020; pp. 549–559.

Burns, J.E., Yao, J., Summers, R.M. Vertebral body compression fractures and bone density: Automated detection and classification on CT images. *Radiology* **2017**, *284*, 788–797.

Cheng, C.T., Ho, T.Y., Lee, T.Y., Chang, C.C., Chou, C.C., Chen, C.C., Chung, I.; Liao, C.H. Application of a deep learning algorithm for detection and visualization of hip fractures on plain pelvic radiographs. *Eur. Radiol.* **2019**, *29*, 5469–5477.

Choi, J.W., Cho, Y.J., Lee, S., Lee, J., Lee, S., Choi, Y.H., Cheon, J.E., Ha, J.Y. Using a dual-input convolutional neural network for automated detection of pediatric supracondylar fracture on conventional radiography. *Investig. Radiol.* **2020**, *55*, 101–110.

Chung, S.W., Han, S.S., Lee, J.W., Oh, K.S., Kim, N.R., Yoon, J.P., Kim, J.Y., Moon, S.H., Kwon, J., Lee, H.-J., et al. Automated detection and classification of the proximal humerus fracture by using deep learning algorithm. *Acta Orthop.* **2018**, *89*, 468–473.

Debojyoti, P., Reddy, P.B., Roy, S. Attention UW-Net: A fully connected model for automatic segmentation and annotation of chest X-ray. *Comput. Biol. Med.* **2022**, *150*, 106083.

Frigenti, L., Beyer, T., Fitzgerald, M. and Chrisney, M. D. (2022). The New Technology Frontier for Developing Economies: Digital Transformation to Achieve the Sustainable Development Goals. Available at SSRN 4138717.

Gan, K., Xu, D., Lin, Y., Shen, Y., Zhang, T., Hu, K., Zhou, K., Bi, M., Pan, L., Wu, W., et al. Artificial intelligence detection of distal radius fractures: A comparison between the convolutional neural network and professional assessments. *Acta Orthop.* **2019**, *90*, 394–400.

Gulshan, V., Peng, L., Coram, M., Stumpe, M.C., Wu, D., Narayanaswamy, A., Venugopalan, S., Widner, K., Madams, T., Cuadros, J., et al. Development and Validation of a Deep Learning Algorithm for Detection of Diabetic Retinopathy in Retinal Fundus Photographs. *JAMA* **2016**, *316*, 2402–2410.

Gupta, T., Arora, P., Rani, R., Jaiswal, G., Bansal, P. and Dev, A. (2022, December). Classification of flower dataset using machine learning models. In *2022 4th International conference on artificial intelligence and speech technology (AIST)* (pp. 1-6). IEEE.

Gyftopoulos, S., Lin, D., Knoll, F., Doshi, A.M., Rodrigues, T.C., Recht, M.P. Artificial Intelligence in Musculoskeletal Imaging: Current Status and Future Directions. *AJR Am. J. Roentgenol.* **2019**, *213*, 506–513.

Hallas, P., Ellingsen, T. Errors in fracture diagnoses in the emergency department—Characteristics of patients and diurnal variation. *BMC Emerg. Med.* **2006**, *6*, 4.

Heimer, J., Thali, M.J., Ebert, L. Classification based on the presence of skull fractures on curved maximum intensity skull projections by means of deep learning. *J. Forensic Radiol. Imaging* **2018**, *14*, 16–20.

International Osteoporosis Foundation. *Broken Bones, Broken Lives: A Roadmap to Solve the Fragility Fracture Crisis in Europe*; International Osteoporosis Foundation: Nyon, Switzerland, 2019; Available online: **https://ncdalliance.org/news-events/news/** (accessed on 20 January, 2022).

Jaiswal, G., Sharma, A. and Yadav, S.K. (2022). DFD-SS: document forgery detection using spectral–spatial features for hyperspectral images. *Journal of Visual Communication and Image Representation, 89*, 103690.

Jha, S., Topol, E.J. Adapting to artificial intelligence: Radiologists and pathologists as information specialists. *JAMA* **2016**, *316*, 2353–2354.

Johari, M.; Esmaeili, F., Andalib, A., Garjani, S., Saberkari, H. Detection of vertical root fractures in intact and endodontically treated premolar teeth by designing a probabilistic neural network: An ex vivo study. *Dentomaxillofac. Radiol.* **2017**, *46*, 20160107.

Kabiraj, A., Meena, T., Reddy, B., Roy, S. Detection and Classification of Lung Disease Using Deep Learning Architecture from X-ray Images. In Proceedings of the 17th International Symposium on Visual Computing, San Diego, CA, USA, 3–5 October 2022; Springer: Cham, Switzerland, 2022.

Kim, D.H., MacKinnon, T. Artificial intelligence in fracture detection: Transfer learning from deep convolutional neural networks.*Clin. Radiol.* **2018**, *73*, 439–445.

Kim, H.E., Cosa-Linan, A., Santhanam, N., Jannesari, M., Maros, M.E., Ganslandt, T. Transfer learning for medical image classification: A literature review. *BMC Med. Imaging* **2022**, *22*, 69.

Kitamura, G., Chung, C.Y., Moore, B.E., 2nd. Ankle fracture detection utilizing a convolutional neural network ensemble implemented with a small sample, de novo training, and multiview incorporation. *J. Digit. Imaging* **2019**, *32*, 672–677.

Ko, S., Pareek, A., Ro, D.H., Lu, Y., Camp, C.L., Martin, R.K., Krych, A.J. Artificial intelligence in orthopedics: Three strategies for deep learning with orthopedic specific imaging. *Knee Surg. Sport. Traumatol. Arthrosc.* **2022**, *30*, 758–761.

Krizhevsky, A., Sutskever, I.; Hinton, G.E. ImageNet Classification with Deep Convolutional Neural Networks. In Proceedings of the NIPS'12: Proceedings of the 25th International Conference on Neural Information Processing Systems, Red Hook, NY, USA, 3–6 December 2012; pp. 1097–1105.

Krupinski, E.A., Berbaum, K.S., Caldwell, R.T., Schartz, K.M., Kim, J. Long Radiology Workdays Reduce Detection and Accommodation Accuracy. *J. Am. Coll. Radiol.* **2010**, *7*, 698–704.

Lin, Q., Li, T., Cao, C., Cao, Y., Man, Z., Wang, H. Deep learning based automated diagnosis of bone metastases with SPECT thoracic bone images. *Sci. Rep.* **2021**, *11*, 4223.

Lindsey, R., Daluiski, A., Chopra, S., Lachapelle, A., Mozer, M., Sicular, S., Hanel, D., Gardner, M., Gupta, A., Hotchkiss, R., et al. Deep neural network improves fracture detection by clinicians. *Proc. Natl. Acad. Sci. USA* **2018**, *115*, 11591–11596.

Majkowska, A., Mittal, S., Steiner, D.F., Reicher, J.J., McKinney, S.M., Duggan, G.E., Eswaran, K., Chen, P.-H.C., Liu, Y., Kalidindi, S.R., et al. Chest radiograph interpretation with deep learning models: Assessment with radiologist-adjudicated reference standards and population-adjusted evaluation. *Radiology* **2020**, *294*, 421–431.

Marwa, F., Zahzah, E.-H., Bouallegue, K., Machhout, M. Deep learning based neural network application for automatic ultrasonic computed tomographic bone image segmentation. *Multimed. Tools Appl.* **2022**, *81*, 13537–13562.

Muehlematter, U.J., Mannil, M.; Becker, A.S., Vokinger, K.N., Finkenstaedt, T., Osterhoff, G., Fischer, M.A., Guggenberger, R. Vertebral body insufficiency fractures: Detection of vertebrae at risk on standard CT images using texture analysis and machine learning. *Eur. Radiol.* **2019**, *29*, 2207–2217.

Olczak, J., Fahlberg, N., Maki, A.; Razavian, A.S., Jilert, A., Stark, A., Sköldenberg, O., Gordon, M. Artificial intelligence for analyzing orthopedic trauma radiographs. *Acta Orthop.* **2017**, *88*, 581–586.

Papandrianos, N.I., Papageorgiou, E.I., Anagnostis, A., Papageorgiou, K., Feleki, A., Bochtis, D. Development of Convolutional Neural Network-based Models for Bone Metastasis Classification in Nuclear Medicine. In Proceedings of the 2020 11th Inter- national Conference on Information, Intelligence, Systems and Applications (IISA), Piraeus, Greece, 15–17 July 2020; pp. 1–8.

Pranata, Y.D., Wang, K.C., Wang, J.C., Idram, I., Lai, J.Y., Liu, J.W., Hsieh, I.-H. Deep learning and SURF for automated classification and detection of calcaneus fractures in CT images. *Comput. Methods Programs Biomed.* **2019**, *171*, 27–37.

Rahmaniar, W., Wang, W.J. Real-time automated segmentation and classification of calcaneal fractures in CT images. *Appl. Sci.* **2019**, *9*, 3011.

Rayan, J.C., Reddy, N., Kan, J.H., Zhang, W., Annapragada, A. Binomial classification of pediatric elbow fractures using a deep learning multiview approach emulating radiologist decision making. Radiol. *Artif. Intell.* **2019**, *1*, e180015.

Recht, M., Bryan, R.N. Artificial intelligence: Threat or boon to radiologists? *J. Am. Coll. Radiol.* **2017**, *14*, 1476–1480.

Roy, S., Bandyopadhyay, S.K. A new method of brain tissues segmentation from MRI with accuracy estimation. Procedia Comput. Sci. 2016, 85, 362–369.

Roy, S., Bhattacharyya, D., Bandyopadhyay, S.K., Kim, T.-H. An improved brain MR image binarization method as a preprocessing for abnormality detection and features extraction. *Front. Comput. Sci.* **2017**, *11*, 717–727.

Roy, S., Mitra, A., Roy, S., Setua, S.K. Blood vessel segmentation of retinal image using Clifford matched filter and Clifford convolution. *Multimed. Tools Appl.* **2019**, *78*, 34839–34865.

Roy, S., Whitehead, T.D., Quirk, J.D., Salter, A., Ademuyiwa, F.O., Li, S., An, H., Shoghi, K.I. Optimal co-clinical radiomics: Sensitivity of radiomic features to tumour volume, image noise and resolution in co-clinical T1-weighted and T2-weighted magnetic resonance imaging. *eBioMedicine* **2020**, *59*, 102963.

Roy, S., Shoghi, K.I. Computer-Aided Tumor Segmentation from T2-Weighted MR Images of Patient-Derived Tumor Xenografts. In *Image Analysis and Recognition*; ICIAR 2019. Lecture Notes in Computer Science; Karray, F., Campilho, A., Yu, A., Eds.; Springer: Cham, Switzerland, 2019; Volume 11663.

Roy, S., Whitehead, T.D., Li, S., Ademuyiwa, F.O., Wahl, R.L., Dehdashti, F., Shoghi, K.I. Co-clinical FDG-PET radiomic signature in predicting response to neoadjuvant chemotherapy in triple-negative breast cancer. *Eur. J. Nucl. Med. Mol. Imaging* **2022**, *49*, 550–562.

Russakovsky, O., Deng, J., Su, H., Krause, J., Satheesh, S., Ma, S., Huang, Z., Karpathy, A., Khosla, A., Bernstein, M., et al. ImageNet Large Scale Visual Recognition Challenge. *Int. J. Comput. Vis.* **2015**, *115*, 211–252.

Sanaat, A., Shiri, I., Ferdowsi, S., Arabi, H., Zaidi, H. Robust-Deep: A Method for Increasing Brain Imaging Datasets to Improve Deep Learning Models' Performance and Robustness. *J. Digit. Imaging* **2022**, *35*, 469–481.

Sarvamangala, D.R., Kulkarni, R.V. Convolutional neural networks in medical image understanding: A survey. *Evol. Intell.* **2022**, *15*, 1–22.

Shah, P.M., Ullah, H., Ullah, R., Shah, D., Wang, Y., Islam, S.U., Gani, A., Joel, J.P., Rodrigues, C. DC-GAN-based synthetic X-ray images augmentation for increasing the performance of EfficientNet for COVID-19 detection. *Expert Syst.* **2022**, *39*, e12823.

Strauss, C., Cavanagh, K., Oliver, A. and Pettman, D. (2014). Mindfulness-based interventions for people diagnosed with a current episode of an anxiety or depressive disorder: a meta-analysis of randomised controlled trials. PLOS one, 9(4), e96110.

Tomita, N., Cheung, Y.Y., Hassanpour, S. Deep neural networks for automatic detection of osteoporotic vertebral fractures on CT scans. *Comput. Biol. Med.* **2018**, *98*, 8–15.

Tyson, S., Hatem, S.F. Easily Missed Fractures of the Upper Extremity. *Radiol. Clin. N. Am.* **2015**, *53*, 717–736.

Urakawa, T., Tanaka, Y., Goto, S., Matsuzawa, H., Watanabe, K., Endo, N. Detecting intertrochanteric hip fractures with orthopedist-level accuracy using a deep convolutional neural network. *Skelet. Radiol.* **2019**, *48*, 239–244.

Wang, X., Xu, Z., Tong, Y., Xia, L., Jie, B., Ding, P., Bai, H., Zhang, Y., He, Y. Detection and classification of mandibular fracture on CT scan using deep convolutional neural network. *Clin. Oral Investig.* **2022**, *26*, 4593–4601.

Yu, J.S., Yu, S.M., Erdal, B.S., Demirer, M., Gupta, V., Bigelow, M., Salvador, A., Rink, T., Lenobel, S., Prevedello, L., et al. Detection and localisation of hip fractures on anteroposterior radiographs with artificial intelligence: Proof of concept. *Clin. Radiol.* **2020**, *75*, 237.e1–237.e9.

Zhang, H., Goodfellow, I., Metaxas, D., Odena, A. Self-Attention Generative Adversarial Networks. In Proceedings of the 36th International Conference on Machine Learning (ICML 2019), Long Beach, CA, USA, 9–15 June 2019; pp. 7354–7363.

4 Transforming Healthcare with AI
An Introduction to Machine Learning and Deep Learning Techniques

Rajkumar Teotia[1], Utkarsh Kumar Verma[2], Ananta Narayana[3], Richa Srivastava[4], Arvind Mewada[5]* and Mohd. Aquib Ansari[6]

The medical sphere is evolving with the help of AI, which is transforming the healthcare industry into a more efficient, accurate, and personalised form. On that note, it is proposed that this chapter provides a background on how AI has been implemented in healthcare, specifically the approaches of ML and DL. The discussion will discuss the most basic ideas in the area of AI, namely, the creation of algorithms in the field of machine learning and modification of models in the field of deep learning, which has found its placement in many fields, including healthcare, such as disease forecasting, medical imaging, and management of patient care, and also drug discovery. It gives an overview of some of the most prominent studies in the fields of ML and DL applications, their advantages, disadvantages, and the problem of AI implementation in healthcare systems. It reviews the challenges of data privacy, fairness, and transparency within the framework of ethical concerns and regulatory processes related to AI in healthcare. Numerous potential AI-driven changes in healthcare practice are on the horizon. The given piece of work provides an overview of where AI can be applied in healthcare and offers insight into how ML and DL technologies will be integrated into clinical practices in the future.

1. Introduction

The fastest and advanced variant of solving complex health-related problems is Artificial Intelligence (AI). It assists healthcare systems in working with massive amounts of data, forecasting previously unknown trends, and enhancing diagnoses. In this way, it enhances the precision of diagnosis and, above all, patient care with the help of high-tech techniques such as Machine Learning (ML) and Deep Learning (DL). The potential uses of AI can be limited to the prediction and

[1] DMSC, HRIT University, Ghaziabad India.
[2] School of Business, Galgotias University, Greater Noida, India.
[3,4] SBM, Noida International University, Greater Noida, India.
[5] SCET, Bennett University, Greater Noida, India.
[6] SCSE, Galgotiyas University, Greater Noida, India
email: rajkumarteotia@gmail.com[1]; utkarsh.verma@galgotiasuniversity.edu.in[2]; ananta.narayana20@gmail.com[3]; dr.richa2000@gmail.com[4]; aquib.ansari@galgotiasuniversity.edu.in[6]
* Corresponding author: mewadabpl@gmail.com

DOI: 10.1201/9781003655121-4

diagnosis of diseases, designs of the treatment for the patient, images, and even direct observations of the patients. AI will likely revolutionise disease management at all levels of the healthcare sector, as it will reduce human error and increase efficiency. Many opportunities also come with a number of challenges that come with the realisation of these concepts, such as data security and privacy, ethical issues, and regulations for the implementation structure. The chapter focuses on the role of AI in healthcare, which has evolved over the years due to advancements in ML and DL , and explores sustainable solutions for the future of healthcare.

1.1 Overview of AI in Healthcare

The introduction of AI in the healthcare sector is a complete revitalisation of medical service delivery, diagnosis, and treatment procedures. It is a term that has a wide range of technologies, including but not limited to ML, DL, and natural language processing (NLP), which allow computers to be programmed to mimic human intelligence, thus executing tasks that are commonly believed to need human intelligence. Diagnostic assistance, custom-made treatment plans, medical imaging, drug development, and development of patient monitoring systems are some of the applications of AI in healthcare (Topol, 2019; Esteva et al., 2017). Over the past few years, there has been a considerable increase in AI advancements, driven by the growth of healthcare data, improved computing power, and algorithm innovations that have revealed the potential for enhancing patient care (Jiang et al., 2017). In certain instances, these AI-driven medical systems are able to analyse large quantities of medical data, detect trends in large datasets and come up with more precise forecasts and suggestions than human clinicians (Miotto et al., 2018). The transformations influence the level of personalisation, effectiveness, and accessibility of the provided health models.

1.2 Importance of AI Technologies in Transforming Healthcare Systems

The technologies of AI are transforming the healthcare industry, delivering a qualitative service, reducing the costs of work, and improving patient outcomes. To begin with, AI-based systems address issues such as misdiagnosis, suboptimal workflow, and the shortage of medical professionals. Utilising AI in the medical sector can assist the clinical decision-making process by delivering factual insights that help make more precise diagnoses and informed treatment choices (Shah & Movahed, 2020). Actually, the DL-based models have demonstrated superiority over researchers in identifying the early detection of diseases, including cancer, using medical imaging (Esteva et al., 2017). The modern world is no exception, as predictive healthcare is applicable, and AI will be able to process data related to patients and predict the likelihood of developing diabetes, heart failure, and sepsis. It allows for intervention at the simplest levels of possible steps and enhances preventive care to a significant extent (Wang & Preininger, 2018). The adoption of AI, however, automates administrative procedures, reducing the number of errors and making healthcare delivery as efficient as possible. According to Verghese and Shah (2018), AI-based chatbots and virtual assistants help medical workers to effectively manage patient requests and appointments, thus creating more time to focus on patient care-related issues. AI improves clinical and administrative processes, and consequently, the administration of healthcare services.

2. Artificial Intelligence Principles

AI is a branch of computer science where scientists envision systems capable of performing tasks that a human brain can in terms of decision-making, problem-solving, language understanding, and recognising patterns. Algorithms, data, and computing power constitute the core of AI, which permit machines to simulate cognitive capabilities. ML is a subset of AI that allows systems to learn and improve their performance with data over time without explicit programming. The second subset from ML is DL, which applies this model by using neural networks on large data sources to reveal underlying complex patterns. The rapid advancement of computing and the increasing availability of big data have made AI increasingly applicable to diverse sectors, including healthcare. AI technologies shall bring a change in the method of diagnostics, customised treatments, and managing the entire care for patients. Therefore, this section will provide a practical elaboration on the basic differences among other subfields of AI that have had an influence across various sectors, especially the healthcare sector, and how this shifts methods of practising healthcare.

2.1 What is Artificial Intelligence?

AI can be defined as the ability of machines to perform tasks that are normally within the reach of a human, including learning from experience, determining natural language, identifying specific patterns, making complex decisions, and solving problems. In a nutshell, AI represents the development of systems designed to automate or execute tasks that humans perform with their intellectual capabilities efficiently, on a large scale, and in an automated manner (Ansari & Singh, 2021; Ansari & Singh 2022). For the sake of simplification, AI can broadly be categorised into two categories. One is known as narrow AI, also termed as weak AI, which has the ability to perform only a single task. On the other hand, strong AI is capable of performing intellectual tasks (Jiang et al. (2017) argue that AI applications in the healthcare sector are gaining increasing popularity, particularly in clinical decision-making, medical image analysis, drug discovery, and patient management systems. Due to the creation of AI systems, their potential use and implications are applicable to every industry that requires big data processing and the identification of latent trends.

2.2 History and Evolution of AI

The history of AI can be traced back thousands of years, following human curiosity and desire to comprehend the world. Nevertheless, the contemporary AI assumed a more specific form in the middle of the previous century, with the introduction of computers and the creation of algorithms. AI was a term coined by John McCarthy at the Dartmouth Conference in 1956, although a group of scientists had been discussing the prospect of machines approaching intelligent behaviour in a simulation (McCarthy et al., 1956). Initial methods of AI were symbolic and involved constructing machines that simulated human experience in narrow and focused fields during the 1970s and 1980s, an era known as the expert systems era. Nevertheless, it was much more difficult to scale up and implement such solutions to practical issues in later decades. Nevertheless, until the late 1990s and the early 2000s, ML and DL became a reality in application, bringing new changes to research in the field of AI. Large datasets, combined with high-level algorithmic methods, have significantly enhanced the power of AI due to increased computational power. Significant advancements in AI have been observed in the 21st century, as exemplified by the emergence of self-driving vehicles, AI virtual assistants, and innovations in healthcare diagnostics (LeCun, Bengio, and Hinton, 2015). The healthcare industry has transformed AI technologies into practical and real-world implementations, further enhancing advances in patient care, operational efficiency, and study productivity (Topol, 2019).

2.3 Key AI Subfields: Machine Learning and Deep Learning

ML is a subfield of AI because systems are enabled to learn from data while also improving their performance over time, making predictions or decisions. In ML, there should be algorithms explicitly intended to detect patterns and then infer conclusions about large datasets. Hence, the system learns from its performance through experience. Some of the applications of ML techniques in healthcare include disease prediction, clinical decision support, and risk stratification. Some of the popular ML algorithms used are regression, decision trees, support vector machines, and k-nearest neighbours (Rajkomar, Dean, & Kohane, 2019). DL is one of the subdomains in ML that targets deep networks responsible for processing large datasets through multiple layers of computation. The quantity of attention that DL research has received lately is due to its ability to examine large datasets, such as images, speech, or even text, that cannot be accommodated within traditional models of ML analysis. Feature engineering is not applied here because DL systems allow learning hierarchical representations of the data itself. This makes DL very effective for applications like image recognition, where it can spot patterns in medical images, such as CT scans, MRIs, and X-rays, with an incredibly high degree of accuracy. Models have broad applications in healthcare, including disease diagnosis, analysis of patient records, and discovery of new drugs (Esteva et al., 2017; LeCun et al., 2015). Indeed, ML and DL, in general, form the skeleton of AI technologies. As such, it enables a system to learn autonomously from data and make decisions automatically, thereby augmenting human ability in almost all markets, particularly in healthcare.

2.4 *Impact of AI on Varying Industries, with Specific Emphasis on Healthcare*

AI has revolutionised most industries, including financial services, retail, transportation, and entertainment. In the healthcare sector, AI solutions transform it from better clinical decision-making to improved resource utilisation, along with the personalisation of care. At its core, AI is making a significant difference in medical imaging. Now, AI models, especially DL, are used in medical image analysis, including X-rays, MRIs, and CT scans, which are diagnosed at much faster speeds and with far greater accuracy than traditional diagnosis. This is the case when AI models were trained to accurately determine conditions such as cancer, heart disease, or neurological disorders, even surpassing the accuracy of human experts (Esteva et al., 2017). This is especially useful in regions where skilled doctors are not available in large numbers, and therefore, AI can be employed as a support system to augment diagnoses. Predictive analytics will also feature AI in the near future. Here, depending on the patient data that has been analysed, the machine learning algorithms will look forward to predicting or anticipating the breakout of diseases in areas, identifying high-risk patients, and suggesting personalised treatments. From big data, AI would identify a trend that a human physician does not and, therefore, better results for patients and also the effectiveness of treatment delivery (Wang & Preininger, 2018). In addition to this, AI enhances research in discovering drugs through the analysis of genetic data, determining the potential effects of new drugs, and optimising clinical trials to expedite the introduction of new drugs to the market (Zhou et al., 2020). Not only for clinical purposes, but AI-enhanced healthcare management through automation scheduling, billing, and patient administration. AI-driven chatbots and virtual assistants enable patients to schedule appointments, ask medical questions, and track their health and well-being, thereby alleviating the burden on healthcare providers (Verghese & Shah, 2018). Such an action frees health workers to take on more complex jobs, thereby making their efforts in organisations that provide care much more efficiently. Generally, AI has a profound impact on healthcare, bringing innovation to both the clinical and operational aspects of the industry. Consequently, its influence on the impact effects that alter healthcare delivery changes will increase with advances made in AI technologies.

3. Literature Review

The rising interest in the practical applications of AI within healthcare has been notable over the past decade. Almost all such studies highlight that it has marvellous prospects to transform the way of the sector. Indeed, in recent years, AI technologies such as ML and DL have been promising innovations for increasing the precision of diagnostics, forecasting patient outcomes, and optimising treatment plans (Topol, 2019; Esteva et al., 2017). In addition to the above, ML models have been utilised in thousands of clinical applications for disease prediction and personalised medicine, including decision trees, support vector machines, and random forests (Shah & Movahed, 2020; Miotto et al., 2018). Techniques of DL, particularly CNNs (convolutional neural networks) and RNNs (recurrent neural networks), have proven particularly well-suited for applications related to extracting insights from unstructured sources of medical imaging data, as well as NLP applications (Rajpurkar et al., 2017; Shen et al., 2017). With these successes, however, many challenges remain, including data privacy issues, the issue of algorithmic bias, and the integration of AI systems into the existing healthcare infrastructure (Obermeyer et al., 2016; Wang & Preininger, 2018). Despite these challenges, AI has shown promise in transforming healthcare delivery and thereby improving patient outcomes.

3.1 Historical Perspective of AI in Healthcare

This technology traces its roots back to some decades of use in healthcare, with expert systems emerging early. These systems were developed primarily to help physicians determine why and what their patients might be suffering from. The 1970s witnessed the development of the MYCIN and INTERNIST-1 systems, which aimed to mimic doctors' diagnostic thinking abilities based on patient information (Topol, 2019). These early systems have developed into the foundation of some of the most advanced AI technologies developed in recent years. However, it was only in the late 1990s and early 2000s that, with increased computing power and rising access to data, AI finally began finding much-needed applications within medical fields, including image diagnostics, predictive analytics, and clinical decision-making (Jiang et al., 2017). It is only when breakthroughs occur in ML and DL that the new ability to learn without intervention, from large amounts of data, emerges. Healthcare transformed ML and DL from simple decision support systems into sophisticated algorithms for disease diagnosis with accuracy close to the human level (Rajkomar et al., 2019). Today, AI is being applied in almost every aspect of healthcare, including diagnosis, treatment planning, patient management, and operational efficiency (Wang & Zhang, 2018).

3.2 Machine Learning and Deep Learning for Healthcare: The History and Context

The history of ML in healthcare started when the classical statistical models, like linear regression and decision trees, were used to solve both predictive modelling and risk assessment (Rajkomar et al., 2019). However, these classical approaches had a fundamental limitation in their ability to handle complex, high-dimensional data, which is common in health applications, ranging from medical images to genomics. DL, a subcategory of ML that requires multi layered neural networks, significantly transformed the modelling and analysis capabilities of such data, which has since led to tremendous strides in the various realms of medical image analysis, disease prediction, and recommendation of appropriate treatment (LeCun et al., 2015). The DL has revolutionised medical image analysis over the past decade, with AI systems now outperforming humans. For example, it has been shown to be comparable to dermatologists in skin cancer classification from images (Esteva et al., 2017) and to radiologists in the detection of pneumonia through chest X-ray analysis (Rajpurkar et al., 2017). This translated into significant performance advantages for diagnostics, and therefore for patients, due to the use of DL. Those DL models were successful in the healthcare sector, involving learning from vast annotated datasets. A good reason is that high performance is required for recognising any pattern in images. In contrast, various forms of data, including clinical data, medical image data, and geneticomic data, are utilised (Shah & Movahed, 2020).

3.3 Major Research Articles on Machine Learning in Healthcare

It has been widely accepted that the automation of clinical work and the capability of machine learning to assist healthcare settings in decision-making and predicting health risks. This category encompasses some of the most prominent applications, including disease prediction, diagnosis, and patient monitoring and management.

***Disease Prediction and Diagnosis*:** ML algorithms are becoming more and more visible in their predictive analysis of diseases and diagnoses, with the positive outcomes of the diagnoses being achieved at higher levels of accuracy. Specifically, the risk prediction of developing heart failure and others was implemented in terms of the early detection of diabetes using ML models (Choi et al., 2016; Rajkomar et al., 2019). These applications are used to predict disease onset using patient information, medical history, laboratory results, and imaging, making it easier to carry out interventions and treatment plans at an earlier stage. As an example, in oncology, to predict cancer progression and choose the most relevant interventions in connection with genetic composition and type of tumour, ML algorithms are already used (Rajkomar et al., 2019). It is because predictions of disease courses and customised treatment advice transform how medical professionals have been and still are assisted in treating their patients.

***Patient Monitoring and Management*:** It has been particularly helpful in further enhancing the monitoring and management of patients. ML-based systems have supported the real-time tracking of patient vitals from sensors and wearable devices, thereby informing healthcare providers of abnormalities (Wang & Preininger, 2018). For example, predictive models of ML for condition-based patients have been shown to be very effective in a monitoring ICU where they predict actual complications that help in better outcomes, even for patients, since they give early interventions (Shah & Movahed, 2020). After observation, the usage of ML should be implemented in a way that allows for the application of prediction models to identify a patient's tendencies for readmission; this can provide the basis for preventive care plans for patients (Miotto et al., 2018). They are helping care providers make better decisions to reduce readmission rates of hospitalised patients through efficient treatment procedures.

3.4 Key Studies on Deep Learning in Healthcare

DL has the power to learn from large datasets, which is increasingly integrated into the healthcare domain in two significant areas: medical imaging and NLP. Several pioneering studies have shown impressive DL capability in augmenting diagnostic accuracy with better healthcare.

***Medical Imaging and Diagnostics*:** DL has revolutionised medical imaging to the extent that, in some areas, it is even more advanced than traditional methods and is capable of even surpassing a human expert in disease diagnosis. Esteva et al. (2017) demonstrated that training deep neural networks can classify skin cancer images with the same accuracy as dermatologists. Rajpurkar et al. (2017) successfully applied DL to develop the CheXNet algorithm, which can scan chest X-rays to identify pneumonia cases with a performance nearly as accurate as that of radiologists. Other researchers have also made use of DL models to predict diabetic retinopathy. It is an ailment that, if left untreated for such long periods, would render a person completely blind. Huang and Song (2019) elaborated on how a system utilising CNNs can classify images of the retina, enabling accurate predictions regarding the presence of disease and facilitating appropriate treatment and diagnosis for the patient.

***Natural Language Processing in Healthcare*:** Another area where DL is performing exceptionally well is in the fields of health and NLP. It has been applied in natural language processing techniques for extracting useful information from unstructured clinical text, such as physician notes, discharge summaries, and EHRs (electronic health records). The existing technologies, which are based on RNNs and transformers as their primary choice for processing and understanding complex medical language, enable healthcare providers to generate value from the vast amounts of clinical data (Shickel et al., 2018). As has been noted, unstructured clinical data is used to diagnose the conditions in a patient and offer a potential treatment plan, which is achieved through the use of unstructured clinical data and the employment of DL-based NLP models, resulting in increased capacities to make decisions and achieve improved operational efficiencies within healthcare systems (Bardhan & Thouin, 2020).

3.5 Literature Gaps

Despite the enormous potential in AI, ML, and DL in healthcare, as well as promising innovations, a number of gaps and challenges need to be addressed to ensure that these applications can adequately exploit their potential in these technologies.

***Data Privacy and Security*:** The biggest problem with an AI-based healthcare system is the security of all this information, and more specifically, information related to patients. In the case of such large systems that deal with sensitive information, data privacy and security are the primary concerns. According to new research, it is essential to ensure the use of secure encryption and to maintain active compliance with follow-up on privacy protection laws, such as HIPAA, to ensure the confidentiality of patient information (Rajpurkar et al., 2017). The security of patient information is directly compromised by data breaches of cloud storage facilities. Therefore, healthcare service providers must always prioritise security issues.

Practical Application of AI in Infrastructures Related to Health: The most significant issues pertain to the practical application of AI models in healthcare-related infrastructures. In summary, AI systems perform well in controlled research environments; however, their application to clinical settings is hindered by concerns over the loss of modelling ability, as well as a lack of clarity and clinical validation. For instance, the proper implementation of AI into the healthcare process involves meeting the requirements of regulatory aspects and the advantages related to outcomes, including patient care and process efficiency, according to Rajkomar et al. (2019). More research into integrating AI into the existing frameworks of the healthcare environment would be recommended to enable humans and computers to work in harmony, as the authors suggest.

4. Machine Learning in Healthcare

Simply put, ML is an AI subdomain in which systems have the capability to improve their performance by acquiring experience automatically. In healthcare, data analysis is used when the data sizes are large and a pattern exists for making predictions. Three primary categories of ML consist of three types: namely, supervised, unsupervised, and reinforcement learning.

Supervised Learning: ML falls into a broader category of supervised learning. In this, an input data set with pairs of the learning system is applied to the correct output, which is labelled. Patient demographics and medical histories would be paired with disease diagnoses and the success of treatments. An algorithm learns the mapping of its input features to output during training; otherwise, it can predict output for unseen data. Common supervised learning algorithms are decision trees, support vector machines, and neural networks (Wang & Zhang, 2018).

Unsupervised Learning: In the case of unsupervised learning, the model is given unlabelled data. It identifies the pattern or structure of the data given to it. It is particularly useful when there is very little labelled data available. Some of the most popular techniques utilised under unsupervised learning include clustering and dimensionality reduction techniques, such as k-means clustering and principal component analysis. These techniques are often employed in medical applications to identify similar patient profiles where there are no obvious results or discernible grouping patterns in the medical data (Rajpurkar et al., 2017).

Reinforcement Learning: This is one kind of ML, in which an agent learns to make and perform decisions by acting in environments, with feedback coming from rewards or penalties. This approach is applied in dynamic and uncertain environments, such as healthcare, where the results of past actions serve as the foundation for determining treatment plans. Reinforcement learning also becomes interesting with applications such as personalised treatment planning and robotic surgery (Esteva et al., 2017).

5. Deep Learning in Healthcare

The newest influential healthcare technology has demonstrated the potential to have tremendous capabilities for analysing large volumes of complex data. Unlike the classical ML approaches, deep models such as NNs (neural networks), CNNs, and RNNs can learn to extract features hierarchically from raw data rather than needing to be done manually. This endows such models, especially in niche applications, with the ability of medical image analysis or NLP (LeCun et al., 2015; Esteva et al., 2017). For example, CNNs have been shown to mimic dermatologists' performance in detecting skin cancer (Esteva et al., 2017). Pneumonia can be predicted in chest X-rays using CNNs (Rajpurkar et al., 2017). Then, RNNs hold much promise for analysing clinical notes, with the ability to predict patient outcomes (Choi et al., 2016). Despite all these promises, issues such as large annotated datasets and computational resources still hinder the proliferation of DL in healthcare, as considerations for model interpretability and transparency are made (Shen et al., 2017). However, DL continues to develop innovations in personalised medicine, automated diagnosis, and patient care.

5.1 Important Deep Learning Models

DL is one form of NN models that was designed specifically for solving a class of problems. Some of the important DL models, along with their applications, are as under:

***Neural Networks*:** A neural network is a simple form of a DL model that is composed of several layers of interconnected nodes, or "neurons ". Networks are layer-based: there must be an input layer, and there can be one or more hidden layers, and finally, there's an output layer. NNs can model patterns in data because they calculate weights and biases given labelled datasets (Goodfellow et al., 2016). In medical practice, simple NNs have been applied to subtasks such as disease diagnosis, risk assessment, and predicting a patient's prognosis. Although DNNs are applied more frequently to complex problems, basic NNs are used for tasks involving less complex data or problems that are relatively easier.

***Convolutional Neural Networks* (*CNNs*):** Convolutional Neural Networks are a subclass of deep learning models designed for processing structured grid data, such as images. CNN automatically learns spatial hierarchies of features by applying convolutional filters to images. This task is particularly suitable for this list, involving the detection of specific patterns, such as tumours or lesions, on X-ray, CT, or MRI images. CNNs have been widely utilised in the healthcare sector for the diagnosis of tumours, radiological image interpretation, and diabetic retinopathy diagnoses (Esteva et al., 2017). The automatic extraction of features by a system without human interference will make CNNs quite useful in medical image diagnostics, where minor texture or geometrical differences often reveal much about the disease.

Recurrent Neural Networks (RNNs): In fact, though, RNNs are designed to handle sequential data. Whereas traditional NNs consider the fact that inputs are independent of each other, RNNs have a memory that considers the input processed earlier as part of the current input. Thus, the inclusion of RNNs becomes significantly important for time-series data, which essentially comprises the temporal factor, such as speech, text, or patient vital signs (Goodfellow et al., 2016). It mainly includes application domains in health, such as, but not limited to, the following: predictive analytics of any type, for instance, patient deterioration risk forecasts, disease progression forecasts, or sequential health-related information analysis extracted from wearable devices. One of the variants of RNN is LSTM (long short-term memory), which has been used heavily in healthcare for predicting the risks of heart failure and analysing clinical time-series data.

Generative Adversarial Networks (GANs): GANs are a kind of NN architecture which comprises two competing networks. One is the generator and the other is the discriminator. The generator should produce synthesised data that is indistinguishable from real data; however, the role of the discriminator is to test the synthesised data to check whether it is real or fake. It causes the generator to continuously produce data that it cannot distinguish from the real one. Most commonly, GANs are applied for image generation or augmentation. However, as of now, they have extensive use in the healthcare sector. Applicative-Healthcare GANs were utilised for the synthetic generation of medical images, where the DL models for training had very limited amounts of annotated data. For instance, the application of GANs in producing artificial MRI or CT scans would enhance access to existing data and models, which are used in these use cases when arriving at a diagnosis (Frid-Adar et al., 2018).

5.2 Use Cases of Deep Learning in Healthcare

DL has a wide range of applications in healthcare, as it can be applied to complex, high-dimensional data, which enhances diagnosis, patient care, and clinical operations. The key areas where DL makes a huge difference are presented below.

Medical Image Processing (X-ray, CT Scan, MRI): DL models have proven to be very useful in analysing and interpreting medical images with almost absolute accuracy. For example, CNNs have become very popular in identifying pneumonia symptoms from chest X-rays (Rajpurkar et al., 2017). Similarly, CNNs have gained significant popularity for identifying retinal disease types, such as diabetic retinopathy, through fundus images (Huang & Song, 2019). These DL models detect subtle patterns in medical images that a human radiologist would likely miss. Faster and more accurate diagnoses can follow this. DL models can be used for organ and lesion segmentation, treatment planning, and surgical navigation.

Natural Language Processing in Healthcare (Clinical Notes Analysis): The NLP techniques, especially DL-based models, are increasingly being used to analyse unstructured healthcare text such as clinical notes, discharge summaries, and EHRs. Free-text clinical notes can also be utilised with deep models, such as RNNs and transformers, to extract valuable information about diseases, medications, and planned treatments (Bardhan & Thouin, 2020). It enables the processing of massive amounts of unstructured data to extract knowledge regarding service providers in the healthcare sector, aiding in enhanced clinical decision-making and even automating tasks such as coding and documentation. The other approach it presents is the predictability of models using features derived from clinical text, for example, predicting patients' outcomes or early signs of diseases (Shickel et al., 2018).

***Predictive Analytics in Patient Care*:** Other DL techniques, especially those based on time series, have been applied in the predictive analytics of patient care. Using past and present health measurements, including vital signs and lab results, as well as EHRs, they are able to foresee the worsening of the patient, readmission risks, and disease advancement. To illustrate, cardiovascular events, sepsis, and numerous other acute medical cases have already been studied with the help of DL models, which suggest early intervention that can positively affect patient outcomes (Rajpurkar et al., 2017). DL models monitor and observe patient information; in cases where there is a likelihood or an emerging problem, it will be indicated, thereby providing proactive care with minimal chances of complications.

***Robotic Surgery and Automation*:** DL has also been used in robotic surgery. The applications include real-time image guidance for surgical robots, enabling improved accuracy and autonomous navigation during the procedure. DL algorithms have provided real instrumentation image guidance as well as tissue recognition during surgical interventions. Live clinical scanning and DL techniques enable robots to perform highly complex operations with minimal human intervention (Esteva et al., 2017). Automation of simple operations, such as patient health statistics entry and medical facility administration activities like booking and workflow, is also made possible by DL, thereby increasing the productivity of health services.

5.3 Challenges in Healthcare and Obstacles in Deep Learning Implementation

Although DL possesses numerous beneficial attributes, its application in healthcare is hindered by several barriers and constraints.

***Data Quality and Availability*:** DL models require enormous amounts of high-quality labelled data to train, and medical data is often partial, unorganised, or not retrievable due to restrictions on patients' personal information. To add that most healthcare organisations tend to operate in silos, integrating other datasets aimed at training better models becomes an almost impossible task (Rajpurkar et al., 2017).

***Interpretability and Explainability*:** Most deep learning models, especially CNNs and GANs, are "black-box" models due to the complexity of their decision-making processes. In healthcare, the opacity of this process can raise significant concerns because the reasoning behind a diagnosis or treatment recommendation is crucial to clinical trust and regulatory approval (Shickel et al., 2018).

Integration with Clinical Workflows: The integration of deep learning applications in healthcare systems is challenging to realise. Most healthcare systems are still using legacy technologies, and it's even hard to imagine those being easily integrated into advanced DL models. It is also noted that "health care professionals will be very slow to adopt new AI-based tools without proof of their effectiveness and reliability", as Rajkomar et al. (2019).

Ethical and Legal Considerations: The application of deep learning in healthcare raises several ethical and legal concerns, including patient consent, data privacy, and accountability. With the increased level of autonomy in deep learning models, questions arise as to who should be held liable in the event of a misdiagnosis or treatment error made by an AI system (Bardhan & Thouin, 2020).

6. Incorporation of Machine Learning and Deep Learning in Healthcare Systems

It would be quite possible to change clinical practices and patient care, and take the benefits of both technologies in their integral form by incorporating ML with DLK into healthcare systems. ML can be used for structured data, such as patient demographics and laboratory reports, because it can classify and accurately predict models concerning diseases. DL can process and extract features from unstructured data, including medical images, clinical notes, and genomic data. These have sophisticated and precise diagnostic instruments (Rajpurkar et al., 2017; Esteva et al., 2017). Some merging methods that the health system can adopt include those that integrate diagnostic, predictive, and therapeutic features within a single structure. For example, ML can be applied in disease identification, and DL algorithms can be used for image interpretation or incorporated into an analysis of EHRs to determine the proper treatment for each patient. Examples include IBM Watson Health and Google Health, whose implementations have been successful, thus showing improved patient outcomes and operational performance (Shah & Movahed, 2020; Ching et al., 2018). However, standardising the data remains one of the challenges, as does interpreting a model and ensuring the integrated system fits into clinical practice in real life.

6.1 Case Study Examples of Successful ML/DL Integration

The following are the most significant case studies of when ML/DL have successfully been integrated to make high-impact health.

Watson Health: The first case of application has been Watson Health. A medical venture that has embodied all the integration of AI, ML, and DL. The Watson Health platform integrates both ML and DL to process big data coming from multiple sources, such as literature, clinical trials, patients' records, and medical images. Thirdly, Watson Health uses ML, which allows the system to extract actionable insights from structured data. DL models are analysed as DNNs in the case of analysing medical images and complex unstructured data. The Watson for Oncology use case is the best illustration, allowing oncologists to make more accurate diagnoses and locate personalised treatment. CNNs are also involved in the processing and analysis of medical images, such as CT scans, to identify cancerous lesions within the system. With NLP, Watson derives patient data, including medical records and clinical notes, and compares the findings to extensive databases of medical literature to provide a tailored treatment based on the latest evidence-based analysis findings. This system of end-to-end AI has also enabled oncologists to make more informed and accurate decisions (Jiang et al., 2017).

***Google Health*:** Another significant player is Google Health, which has integrated ML and DL with the aim of propelling healthcare. Google Health has also created certain AI-enabled applications based on ML and DL, which are used in medical case diagnosis, patient treatment, and research. A few notable examples include the research partnership between Google Health and radiologists on breast cancer, among others. Google AI is based on both methods of ML and DL: it utilises ML algorithms to detect patterns in data, and it leverages the models of DL, namely CNNs, in medical image processing, particularly in mammogram classification. It is trained on millions of labelled images to detect precancerous signs, which leads to more accurate and punctual predictions. Secondly, Google Health is expected to provide patients with more access to treatment and research, as AI is already being used to predict the presence of diseases like diabetic retinopathy using retinal scans. ML and DL integration have enabled Google Health to develop an automated system that facilitates the early detection of diseases, leading to improved patient outcomes and reduced healthcare expenses (Esteva et al., 2017).

The case studies demonstrate the potential of ML and DL in healthcare, including more accurate diagnostic predictions, personalised treatment prescriptions, and improved patient management. These case studies demonstrate the potential of ML and DL in healthcare, including more accurate diagnostic predictions, individualised treatment recommendations, and improved patient management.

7. Ethical Issues and Regulatory Concerns

The topic of ethical issues and regulations has gained considerable importance in the field of healthcare, particularly in the application of AI. Privacy, equity, and decision-making in the healthcare field can be affected by these technologies. The privacy of data is another issue. It is the safeguard of a patient's sensitive health information by introducing regulatory provisions, including HIPAA and GDPR, among others, to secure the privacy and safety of sharing healthcare data (Rajpurkar et al., 2017; Verghese & Shah, 2018). Herein lies a significant challenge: managing massive amounts of data, which could include personal health information, and ensuring data governance is taken seriously to prevent misuse and breaches. The other problem is AI model bias, which, even if the training data are free of bias, can lead to discrimination in medical decision-making (Obermeyer et al., 2016; Esteva et al., 2017). Fairness and transparency are key to preserving confidence in AI decision-making systems. Regulatory bodies should also be able to veto the approval of AI technologies by ensuring they are safe, efficient, and innovative enough (Kassianos & Goutte, 2019; Wang & Preininger, 2018). All these ethical and regulatory concerns should be addressed with care so that AI can be applied optimally in medicine and risks are minimised.

8. Future Trends and Innovations

AI is likely to play a significant role in the diagnosis and management of diseases in the future by leveraging deep learning and advanced technologies, including genomics and precision medicine. The combination of AI, genomics, and precision medicine is one of the most potent tendencies, as it implies that genetic information will be used to inform analysis and assist people in obtaining personalised treatment plans. This would actually enable diseases to be diagnosed and treated in a highly personalised way (Shickel et al., 2018; Wang & Zhang, 2018). AI will be able to predict individual patient risks based on genetic, lifestyle, or other environmental factors, thereby revolutionising preventative care strategies. Another area of innovation involves population management through AI. With an ageing world population, AI-integrated systems may have the potential to manage chronic diseases, forecast when health could begin to deteriorate, or supervise the elderly community (Liu et al., 2019; Topol, 2019). In other aspects, these AI abilities will complement various aspects of robotic surgery, imaging for improved operational efficiency, and natural language processing for a higher potential capacity in diagnosis. The application in healthcare will also change in response to the challenges that face the world, such as pandemics. During the COVID-19 pandemic, AI demonstrated its potential in real-time diagnostics, resource allocation, and predictive modelling that could forecast the spread of the virus (Rajkomar et al., 2020). Furthermore, AI technologies will continue to play a critical role in building stronger healthcare systems and achieving better outcomes while addressing health issues worldwide.

9. Conclusion

In summary, AI, powered by ML and DL, is transforming healthcare through improved diagnostic accuracy and enhanced patient management, thereby activating new treatment options. Introducing AI into healthcare systems will not only make medical practice more efficient but will also open new avenues for personal care and preventive medicine. The future of AI, driven by improved decision-making, faster diagnosis, and personalised therapy, continues to hold promise for healthcare. However, data privacy concerns and problems with biased algorithms, as well as ambiguous regulatory frameworks that hinder the accountability and ethics of AI, must be addressed. Future AI in genomics, precision medicine, and elderly care research may identify issues that will then help solve some of the world's most challenging health problems. Future innovations will take these technologies into the future, moulding healthcare in new ways that bestow deep benefits on patients and providers alike. Further exchange among AI researchers, healthcare practitioners, and policymakers holds the key to realising the full potential of AI in healthcare.

9.1 Summary of Key Takeaways from the Chapter

Discuss here in one chapter on the transformative role played by AI in health care: A history tracing back the origins of its development in the different historical developments and major breaks brought about from the beginning in health care to the very different applications, which are mainly in ML and in various DL techniques in its differential application fields in health care across diagnostics, patient care, imaging of medical fields, and more prominently in medicine.

Some of the major areas in which AI has rightly been proven to make a difference include:

1. **AI-Based Diagnostic:** Here, we discussed how AI, along with its D models, have also proven to help in disease diagnoses similar to or even more effectively than physicians. Applications in medical imaging, dermatology, and radiology have indeed been among the most successful for the diagnosis of cancer and heart diseases.
2. **Patient Monitoring and Outcome Forecasting:** The idea was AI for real-time patient monitoring with wearables that have predictive capabilities to foretell the outcomes of patients. Chronic patients are more manageable in care, and the AI system reduces hospital admissions. Serious events related to the patient are also predicted, such as a cardiomegaly arrest or a disaster due to diabetes.
3. **Machine Learning in Health Care Delivery Systems:** We had discussed how ML can be integrated with the healthcare delivery systems to enhance administrative work activities, patient record management, and clinical decision-making capabilities. And we have also discussed how AI will create personalised treatment plans and precision medicine.
4. **Future Potential and Challenges:** Certain challenges have been identified for the selected. These include data privacy issues, concerns about algorithmic bias, the inability to interpret an AI model, and the need to ascertain safe and ethical use; regulatory frameworks also require soundness.

9.2 Future Potential of AI: Existing State and Future Possibility

Of course, AI is revolutionising health because it transforms the accuracy of diagnostics, the care provided to patients, and the operational efficiencies of health systems. Various technologies in AI are already in developmental stages, where they are applied to early disease detection, individualised treatment, and jobs involving paper forms in administration. Meanwhile, significant strides are being made with the integration of ML/DL models in medical imaging, patient monitoring, and drug development. The possibilities of AI in healthcare are virtually unimaginable. Future healthcare providers will depend on the steps that AI models take towards a more personalised, data-driven decision, culminating in better patient outcomes and a more efficient healthcare system. AI is likely to play a crucial role in identifying novel therapeutic approaches in genomics and precision medicine, based on the profile of genetic and molecular individual data.

Furthermore, AI will manage the geriatric population, along with chronic diseases, and the quality of life of aged patients using tools for monitoring and forecasting. AI machines will predict the onset of diseases and produce enhanced surgical robots, along with entirely tailored treatment algorithms. Long-term research in AI healthcare will fill gaps within present-day capabilities. Thus, accessibility, equity, and efficiency of healthcare will be accessible.

9.3 Conclusion of Thoughts on the Impact of AI in Improving Patient Care, Efficiency, and Healthcare Outcomes

There are indeed strong indications that AI will play a significant role in the future of healthcare. Improves patient care, promotes efficiency in the healthcare sector, and enhances treatment outcomes. As an illustration, the enhancement of health workers' capacity will facilitate faster diagnosis and precision in diagnosis, as well as customised treatment and improved management of long-term ailments. These considerations focus on the well-being of the patient and the optimal utilisation of resources within a medical facility. This alone will deliver a more proactive, preventive-care model with a smaller healthcare system and better quality-of-life cost. The AI tools may also be used to eliminate healthcare disparities by making good diagnostic tools equally accessible and reducing geographical and socioeconomic barriers to a minimum. Nonetheless, to achieve full AI implementation in the healthcare sector, it is necessary to pay special attention to the issues of ethics, privacy, and regulation. The future of AI implementation in healthcare will require collaboration among stakeholders, including healthcare providers, policymakers, and technologists, to create systems that are accurate, fair, and safe, ultimately benefiting the entire society. This way, AI will lead to a total revolution in healthcare, offering solutions to existing issues and new horizons in personalised and precision medicine, disease prevention, and patient care. With the right structures and mechanisms in place, AI will likely usher in a new era in healthcare that is more efficient, accessible, and patient-centric than ever before.

References

Ansari, M.A. and Singh, D.K. (2022). ESAR, an expert shoplifting activity recognition system. *Cybernetics and Information Technologies*, *22*(1), 190–200.

Ansari, M.A. and Singh, D.K. (2021). Human detection techniques for real-time surveillance: A comprehensive survey. *Multimedia Tools and Applications, 80*(6), 8759–8808.

Bardhan, I.R. and Thouin, M.F. (2020). Healthcare applications of artificial intelligence: A literature review. *Health Information Science and Systems, 8*(1), 1–11. HTTPS://DOI.ORG/10.1007/s13755-020-00303-w.

Ching, T., Himmelstein, D.S., Beaulieu-Jones, B.K., Kalinin, A.A., Do, B.T. and Ferrero, E. (2018). Opportunities and obstacles for deep learning in biology and medicine. *Journal of The Royal Society Interface, 15*(141), 20170387. https://doi.org/10.1098/rsif.2017.0387.

Choi, E., Schuetz, A. and Stewart, W.F. (2016). Using recurrent neural networks for early detection of heart failure. *Journal of Machine Learning Research, 17*, 1–24.

Esteva, A. and Kuprel, B. (2017). Dermatologist-level classification of skin cancer with deep neural networks. *Nature, 542*(7639), 115–118. https://doi.org/10.1038/nature21056.

Esteva, A., Kuprel, B., Novoa, R.A., Ko, J., Swetter, S.M. and Blau, H.M. (2017). Dermatologist-level classification of skin cancer with deep neural networks. *Nature, 542*(7639), 115–118. HTTPS://DOI.ORG/10.1038/NATURE21056.

Goodfellow, I., Bengio, Y., Courville, A. and Bengio, Y. (2016). Deep learning (Vol. 1, No. 2, pp. 1-800). Cambridge: MIT press. https://doi.org/10.4258/hir.2016.22.4.351

Huang, G.B. and Song, Y. (2019). Applications of deep learning in medical image analysis. *Medical Image Analysis, 59*, 101565. HTTPS://DOI.ORG/10.1016/J.MEDIA.2019.101565.

Jiang, F., Jiang, Y. Zhi, H., Dong, Y., Li, H., Ma, S. and Wang, Y. (2017). Artificial intelligence in healthcare: Past, present, and future. *Seminars in Cancer Biology, 1*(1), 10–18.

Kassianos, A.P. and Goutte, G. (2019). Artificial intelligence in health: Current challenges and future directions. *Health Information Science and Systems, 7*(1), 34–41. https://doi.org/10.1007/s13755-019-0267-0.

LeCun, Y., Bengio, Y. and Hinton, G. (2015). Deep learning. *Nature, 521*(7553), 436–444. HTTPS://DOI.ORG/10.1038/NATURE14539.

Liu, Y., Chen, P.H. and Krause, J. (2019). Deep Learning for Healthcare: A Review of Opportunities and Challenges. *Nature Medicine, 25*(1), 68–76. HTTPS://DOI.ORG/10.1038/s41591-018-0313-z.

McCarthy, J., Rochester, N. and Shannon, C. (1955). Dartmouth workshop. Summer Research Project on.

Miotto, R., Wang, F., Wang, S., Jiang, X. and Chen, X. (2018). Deep Learning for Healthcare: A Review of Opportunities and Challenges. *Briefings in Bioinformatics, 19*(6), 1236–1246. HTTPS://DOI.ORG/10.1093/BIB/BBX044.

Miotto, R., Wang, F. and Wang, S. (2018). Deep Learning for Healthcare: A Review, Opportunities, and Challenges. *Briefings in Bioinformatics, 19*(6), 1236–1246. HTTPS://DOI.ORG/10.1093/BIB/BBX044.

Obermeyer, Z., Powers, B.W., Vogeli, C. and Mullainathan, S. (2016). Dissecting racial bias in an algorithm used to manage the health of populations. *Science, 366*(6464), 447–453. HTTPS://DOI.ORG/10.1126/SCIENCE.AAX2342.

Rajkomar, A. and Dean, J. (2020). Machine learning for healthcare applications: Challenges and opportunities. *IEEE Transactions on Biomedical Engineering, 67*(6), 1799–1807. HTTPS://DOI.ORG/10.1109/TBME.2019.2919930.

Rajkomar, A., Dean, J. and Kohane, I. (2019). Machine learning in medicine. *New England Journal of Medicine, 380*(14), 1347–1358. HTTPS://DOI.ORG/10.1056/NEJMRA1814259.

Rajpurkar, P., Irvin, J., Zhu, K., Yang, B., Mehta, H., Duan, T. and Pang, J. (2017). CheXNet: Radiologist-level pneumonia detection on chest X-rays with deep learning. *arXiv preprint arXiv:1711.05225.*

Shah, P.M. and Movahed, M.R. (2020). AI in healthcare: A review of current applications and future trends. *Journal of Medical Systems, 44*(5), 123. HTTPS://DOI.ORG/10.1007/s10916-020-01553-0.

Shickel, B., Tighe, P.J., Bihorac, A. and Rashid, H. (2018). Deep EHR: A survey of recent advances in deep learning techniques for electronic health record (EHR) analysis. *IEEE Journal of Biomedical and Health Informatics, 22*(5), 1589–1604. https://doi.org/10.1109/JBHI.2018.2851200.

Topol, E.J. (2019). *Deep Medicine: How Artificial Intelligence Can Make Healthcare Human Again*. Basic Books.

Verghese, A. and Shah, S. (2018). Artificial intelligence in healthcare: Separating fact from fiction. *Annals of Internal Medicine, 169*(10), 702–710. https://doi.org/10.7326/M18-2186.

Wang, F. and Preininger, A. (2018). Machine learning for healthcare applications: Challenges and opportunities. *Biomedical Engineering Letters, 8*(2), 92–103. https://doi.org/10.1007/s13534-018-0085-9.

Wang, L. and Zhang, X. (2018). A survey of deep learning in healthcare applications. *Journal of Healthcare Engineering, 2018*. https://doi.org/10.1155/2018/6571738.

Zhang, Y. and Wang, L. (2019). Applications of deep learning in healthcare: A survey. *Journal of Healthcare Engineering, 2020*. https://doi.org/10.1155/2020/8480351.

5 Semi-Supervised Image Segmentation Techniques for Medical Image Analysis

Deepika Vatsa[1*], Anshika Arora[2], Prachi Singh[3], Aakash Sharma[4], Hardik Bhardwaj[5] and Pratham Jaiswal[6]

Semi-supervised image segmentation has recently shown to be a practical substitute for medical imaging tasks which usually involve limited and expensive annotated data. Learning from both the labelled and unlabelled datasets, such methods boost the performance of the models without as much demand on large, annotated datasets. However, critical challenges in medical image segmentation include data imbalance, domain adaptability, and error propagation through pseudo-labels. Generalization, efficiency, and flexibility of the model in future developments are expected to be improved on various medical imaging datasets. Techniques applied include cross-learning, few-shot and zero-shot learning, and hybrid supervision.

1. Introduction

Image segmentation is an elementary activity in computer vision which divides an image into multiple regions or segments. The partitioning of an image into many different areas that are distinguishable is known as segmentation. These areas are also known as segments that contain pixels (Joshi et al., 2021) with similar properties such as colour, texture, or intensity that differ from other areas in the image. The aim of the process is to have image representation with a greater meaning plus ease of analysis for better interpretation. Haralick and Shapiro discussed most of the techniques found for image segmentation, starting with traditional ones to newer state-of-the-art computer vision ones (Haralick and Shapiro, 1985). Image segmentation found its application in several research areas. The use of tumor location, identification of organs and cells aid in diagnosing and operating more effectively and efficiently. In the traffic environment, segmentation is utilised for lane detection, pedestrians' detection, and object detection to ensure road safety while driving. In the satellite, segmentation helps track land-use and

[1] School of Computer Science Engineering and Technology, Bennett University, Greater Noida, UP, India.

[2] Department of Computer Science and Engineering, Delhi Technological University, New Delhi, India.

[3-6] School of Computer Science Engineering and Technology, Bennett University, Greater Noida, UP, India.

* Corresponding author: deepika.vatsa@bennett.edu.in

DOI: 10.1201/9781003655121-5

changes, monitors natural catastrophes, and observes growth in urban regions. In agriculture, segmentation monitors crop health, detects diseases, and thus allows precision farming.

Image segmentation can be categorised into three categories: Semantic Segmentation, Instance Segmentation, and Panoptic Segmentation. Figure 1 shows visual representation of different segmentation categories on an image. Semantic segmentation divides an image into semantically meaningful regions, where every pixel can be classified with a class label, for instance, 'car', 'tree', or 'road' in a street scene (Garcia-Garcia et al., 2018). On the contrary, instance segmentation is considered a variant of both object detection and semantic segmentation since, if there are two or more instances of a class, it performs instance identification; and it also assigns a different identity (ID) to each pixel. Panoptic Segmentation, however, assigns a specific instance ID that presents each pixel of the image with instance segmentation and a class label, i.e., semantic segmentation.

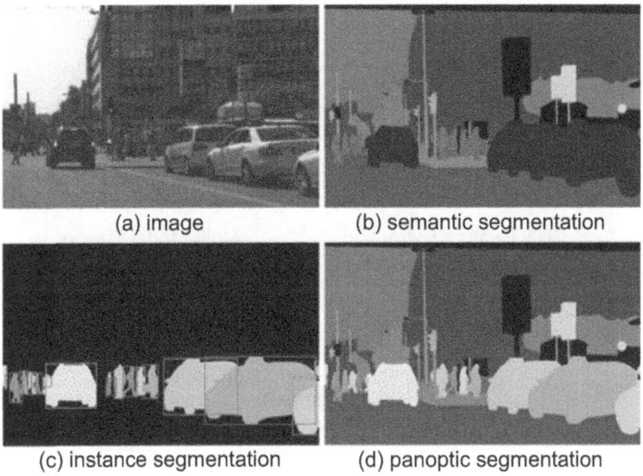

Fig. 1 Visualization of segmentation paradigms (a) original image, (b) semantic segmentation, (c) instance segmentation, and (d) panoptic segmentation. ***Credits***: Kirillov et al. (2019).

Although image segmentation has been effective in many applications, several issues remain unsolved. There are problems in precision when images involved are complex and contain overlapping or ill-defined objects. If the data are noisy, or the object boundaries are not well defined, segmentation will turn out poor (Dhaundiyal et al., 2020).

Given these challenges, Semi-Supervised Learning (SSL) has become a viable approach. SSL has proven to be useful in areas such as medical imaging and remote sensing, where gathering labelled data is expensive or highly time-consuming. SSL improves performance of the model and boosts its accuracy without requiring large, annotated datasets by using abundant unlabelled data. In medical imaging,

SSL helps to segment tumours or organs from Magnetic Resonance Imaging (MRI) and Computed Tomography (CT) scans (Diwakar et al., 2021). In general, such scan data is scarce, and requires expertise for labelling which is not easy. Liu et al. (2018) present their SSL framework on several medical image datasets including brain MRI scans and lung CT scans (Liu et al., 2018). They said the SSL model would be stronger than the trained traditional supervised models with the same amount of unlabelled data. When applied to an autonomous car scenario, SSL allows object detection by partitioning pedestrians, cars, and road signs given relatively fewer counts of images labelled. It is crucial in satellite imaging and agriculture by separating crop health or even the monitoring of land use.

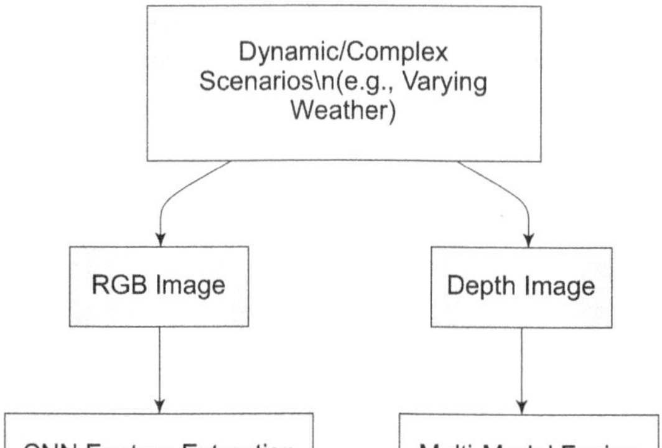

Fig. 2 Multimodal Segmentation Pipeline.

Future trends will suggest that semi-supervised image segmentation methods can be more advanced. Some deep learning models including Convolutional Neural Networks (CNNs), transformers, and Generative Adversarial Networks

(GANs) may further be integrated to improve segmentation accuracy. These will primarily occur in more dynamic and complex scenarios. Further enhancement of the segmentation model may be based on the multi modal fusion of data, for instance (Joshi et al., 2019), RGB (red, green, blue) and depth images, especially in challenging situations like varying weather conditions. One such pipeline for multi modal segmentation is presented in Figure 2.

In summary, image segmentation remains a highly relevant area of application, though augmentation of these applications requires the strengthening of weak points of traditional approaches. More accessible and efficient models have developed for SSL. This is one of the most influential techniques in further reducing the dependence on significant amounts of labelled data. Deep learning and SSL methods will spur further innovation in the field as the area matures and fosters more accurate and efficient algorithms for segmentation.

2. Semi-Supervised Learning Methods

SSL algorithms of image segmentation are designed to make use of the very small amount of labelled data and a much greater amount of unlabelled data so that the performance of models increases. Such methods are useful if it is hard or even expensive or time-consuming to obtain fully labelled datasets. Here are a few of the popular SSL techniques:

2.1 Consistency Regularization

Consistency regularization, especially in tasks such as image segmentation, is a method that trains models to make predictions with uniformity even when minor changes or transformations on inputs are altered. These changes might be the application of distorted types, spinning, turning upside down, or input additions of noise. The model must be invariant to such transformations, so that even slight changes in the input data should not significantly change the output predictions. This forces generalisation of the model to the new data by requiring its predictions to be coherent. The method doesn't learn specifics of individual training samples but instead learns patterns and features of underlying data that would be necessary for a segmentation task.

Example: Even though the transformation may alter the car's visual look, a car that is segmented in the original image should likewise be consistently segmented as such in the flipped or rotated version of the image. The model would be penalised for inconsistency if it predicted a different label for the same object in the enhanced photos, such as identifying the car as a pedestrian in the rotated version.

2.2 Self-Training

A model gets trained initially using a small collection of labelled data in a process known as self-training. The model is then used to produce predictions, or pseudo-labels, for the unlabeled data following this first training. The model can treat the unlabelled data as though it were labelled thanks to these pseudo-labels, even though their accuracy isn't guaranteed. Next, both the freshly pseudo-labelled data and the original labelled data are used to retrain the model.

Example: Consider a model that was first trained to distinguish between cats and dogs using a tiny, labelled dataset of 1,000 photos as an example of self-training. Ten thousand (10,000) unlabelled photos are then subjected to label prediction using the model. Selecting high-confidence predictions (e.g., over 90%), like "cat" images with a confident label, adds them to the initial labelled collection. Using the enlarged dataset, the model is iteratively retrained to increase its accuracy and generalisation without the need for more manual labels.

2.3 Adversarial Learning

The use of GANs in adversarial learning improves the quality of output segmentation. The discriminator distinguishes between segmentation maps of the unlabelled data and segmentation maps of the labelled data. The generator, i.e., the segmentation model, generates the segmentation maps. Simultaneous training of both networks encourages the generator to produce segmentation outputs that are realistic and precise.

Example: Imagine that a model has been trained to identify and categorize cancers in medical images. To confound the segmentation model, a "generator" adds tiny perturbations, like faint noise or distortions, to produce slightly altered images. The "discriminator" assesses whether the noise has changed, or the segmented output is accurate. By learning to accurately forecast tumour boundaries despite these adversarial perturbations, the segmentation model (generator) becomes more resilient to changes and guarantees accurate segmentation in noisy, real-world medical datasets.

2.4 Graph-based Methods

By taking advantage of the connections between labelled and unlabelled data, graph-based techniques are important in semi-supervised segmentation. Each pixel, voxel, or image is represented as a node in these algorithms, which consider the dataset as a graph. The edges between nodes indicate how similar or close they are to one another. The main concept is to use the graph structure to ensure that similar nodes have similar labels by spreading label information from a small number of labelled nodes to the whole graph. To improve the segmentation results, label propagation techniques are used to move labels from tagged nodes to unlabelled ones.

Example: Graph-based methods are particularly effective in medical imaging, remote sensing and biological microscopy. Each voxel in a brain MRI segmentation can be represented as a node in a graph, with edges joining voxels that are close to one another or have comparable intensity values. The entire brain is divided into regions of interest by propagating labels from a small number of manually labelled voxels (such as tumor locations) throughout the graph.

2.5 Contrastive Learning

The goal of the self-supervised learning method known as contrastive learning is to learn representations by differentiating between similar and dissimilar data points. The main objective is to push different data farther apart and bring comparable data closer together in the feature space. It is frequently used to develop meaningful representations without a lot of labelled data in a variety of disciplines, such as computer vision and natural language processing.

Example: A positive sample in image recognition could be an enhanced image of the same "cat", such as one that has been cropped or rotated. A negative example could be a picture of a "dog". In the feature space, the model learns to push the negative far away while mapping the anchor and positive near together.

2.6 Co-training

Co-training uses several perspectives or representations of the same data to enhance model performance. Co-training is the process of training two or more models at the same time, each with a distinct perspective on the data. These models exchange predictions on unlabelled data to iteratively teach one another. When the available data is naturally split into different views, like in online classification tasks where one view might be the content on a webpage and another could be the hyperlinks linking to it, co-training is especially helpful.

Example: Co-training can be applied to medical imaging to enhance the precision of disease diagnosis by combining various modalities, such as CT and MRI images. Similar to this, co-training can combine many features, such as texture and form, to improve segmentation results in object detection.

Table 1 An overview of Semi-Supervised learning techniques for segmentation tasks.

Technique	*Core Idea*	*Key Features*	*Applications*	*Challenges*
Consistency Regularization	Ensures stable predictions under input variations (noise, flips, rotations).	Invariance to data augmentations; improves generalisation.	Medical imaging, environmental mapping.	Sensitive to augmentation quality.
Self-Training	Uses model predictions on unlabelled data as pseudo-labels for further training.	Iterative improvement; expands labelled data pool.	Satellite imagery, autonomous driving.	Risk of propagating incorrect labels.

Contd...

Table 1 *Contd...*

Technique	*Core Idea*	*Key Features*	*Applications*	*Challenges*
Adversarial Learning	Employs a discriminator to differentiate between real and generated segmentations.	Generates robust features; adversarial network refines output.	Autonomous driving, medical segmentation.	Training can be unstable and sensitive to hyperparameters.
Graph-Based Methods	Constructs graphs where nodes represent data points, and edges capture similarity.	Exploits structure in data; propagates labels using graph connectivity.	Social networks, medical imaging.	Computationally intensive for large datasets.
Contrastive Learning	Learns by maximising agreement between similar data points in feature space.	Focuses on learning discriminative representations.	Instance segmentation, image retrieval.	Requires careful selection of positive and negative pairs.
Co-Training	Trains multiple models on different views of the data, allowing them to teach each other.	Diverse perspectives improve learning; leverages multiple feature sets.	Natural language processing, image fusion.	Requires datasets with distinct, complementary views.

3. Medical Datasets

3.1 ISIC (International Skin Imaging Collaboration)

The ISIC dataset is a vital resource for dermatology researchers when it comes to identifying and classifying skin lesions like melanoma. It is one of the largest publicly accessible collections for skin cancer research, with thousands of high-quality dermoscopic photos taken under controlled conditions. It is a useful tool for creating and evaluating segmentation algorithms in the context of skin cancer diagnosis because the photos come with thorough annotations that enable the examination of distinct skin lesions and the detection of cancers. To improve the training and validation of deep learning models (Sharma et al., 2021) for automated skin lesion segmentation and classification, the ISIC library provides both photos and segmentation masks that emphasize tumor locations.

ISIC Archive - https://www.isic-archive.com/

3.2 BRATS (Brain Tumour Segmentation)

The BRATS dataset is utilised for the segmentation of brain tumours in MRI scans. Multi modal brain MRI scans, such as T1-weighted, T2-weighted, and post-contrast T1-weighted images, are included in this collection. Each of the scans offers vital details about various types of brain tissue. It is elaborated based on specific regions of interest such as the core of the tumour, enhancing tumour, and oedema. The BRATS challenge has become a benchmark to measure segmentation techniques in medical images that prompt further work on brain tumour segmentation. The BRATS dataset is meant to support the development, tuning, and validation of models that will be used to automatically classify and identify brain tumours in clinical scenarios by providing raw and pre processed data.

BRATS dataset – https://www.med.upenn.edu/cbica/brats2020/data.html.

3.3 LIDC-IDRI (Lung Image Database Consortium and Image Database Resource Initiative)

The LIDC-IDRI data set is primarily used when working on any lung cancer issues, especially pulmonary nodule-related studies. The database is a collection of images of thoracic CT scan annotated by radiologists. All these annotations describe different types of lung diseases and even lung nodules, both need to develop models which could recognise and classify lung cancer. The dataset is quite useful for determining the strength of image segmentation algorithms regarding problem detection in lungs.

LIDC-IDRI Dataset - https://wiki.cancerimagingarchive.net/display/Public/LIDC-IDRI.

3.4 CAMELYON (Cancer Metastases in Lymph Nodes)

They include digital WSIs from the lymph node biopsies of patients who were clinically diagnosed with breast cancer to detect lymph node metastases in breast cancer. This included samples of normal tissue and annotated regions displaying metastatic lesions. This is an important benchmark for detection in cancer histopathology since the development of deep learning algorithms that target the detection and classification of metastatic cancer in lymph nodes.

CAMELYON dataset - https://www.camelyon16.grand-challenge.org/.

3.5 ChestX-ray14

Also known as the ChestXray14, it is one of the biggest collections of chest X-ray images to the disease's category for pneumonia and other kinds of lung diseases. It contains more than 100,000 anterior view chest X-rays annotated with 14 types of illnesses. The data includes several conditions like pulmonary tuberculosis, pneumonia, lung nodule, etc. Most researchers use to train a variety of deep learning algorithms that deal specifically with the segmentation and classifications that go into chest disease segmentation.

ChestX-ray14 dataset - https://nihcc.app.box.com/v/ChestXray-NIHCC.

3.6 OAI (Osteoarthritis Initiative)

The OAI dataset is helpful to carry out an analysis on the progression of osteoarthritis using medical imaging techniques such as MRI and X-rays of the knee. It gives joint health information in general, on pictures of knee joints, taken over time. It is useful for research on joint degeneration and for developing algorithms that will automatically estimate knee joint deterioration for the diagnosis of the disease and predicting its course.

OAI dataset - https://oai.epi.ucsf.edu/datarelease/.

3.7 ACDC (Automated Cardiac Diagnosis Challenge)

Automatic Cardiac Diagnosis Challenge, or ACDC proposes the division of the heart and many other parts of it, like left and right ventricles and myocardium as part of segmentation where focus is on the cardiac MRI images. Algorithms that can autonomously segment heart structures and aid in the diagnosis of cardiac disorders are frequently developed using this dataset. It includes a range of cardiac diseases, such as dilated cardiomyopathy, myocardial infarction, and normal.

ACDC dataset - https://www.creatis.insa-lyon.fr/Challenge/acdc/databases.html.

Several research works have been done using SSL techniques on the above-mentioned medical datasets (Laine & Aila 2017; Xie et al., 2020; Lee, 2013; Berthelot et al., 2019; Goodfellow et al., 2014; Salimans et al., 2016; Zhu & Ghahramani, 2002; Li & Zhang, 2017; Chen et al., 2020; He & Sun, 2020; Blum & Mitchell, 1998; Dasgupta & Hsu, 2008)

4. Related Work

SSL has gained a lot of traction in the medical picture segmentation field due to its effectiveness with both labelled and unlabelled data. A semi-supervised deep learning method for medical image segmentation using a stacked U-Net architecture called UNet++ was proposed by Zhou et al. (2019). The model showed remarkable accuracy in detecting organs and cancers in CT and MRI scans, with an accuracy of 90%. Liu et al. (2018) extended the applicability of SSL to medical image segmentation with the possibility of training deep learning models on labelled and unlabelled data (Liu et al., 2018). Their technique outperformed state-of-the-art approaches when tested in several medical datasets, offering improved accuracy in segmentation for an additional portion of unlabelled images within the training stage. In organ segmentation tests, the model performed much better than traditional fully-supervised methods, with an accuracy of 87%. The use of

SSL in combination with adversarial learning for medical image segmentation was also examined by Yang et al. (2018). When evaluated on CT scans, their method improved tumor segmentation using both labelled and unlabelled data. By using adversarial training, which enhanced the model's ability to learn from a smaller set of labelled data, it was able to generate realistic picture samples. As a result, the model was able to identify cancers in CT images with 93% accuracy. Chen Y. et al. (2020) introduced a self-training method for SSLK in medical image segmentation, particularly for lung tumour segmentation (Chen et al., 2020). As the model was being trained, it generated labels for unlabelled data using a technique known as pseudo-labelling. Our method demonstrated the effectiveness of SSL techniques in reducing the demand for large, labelled datasets without compromising performance, with an 89% segmentation accuracy for lung tumours. Isensee et al. (2019) introduced a SSL system based on deep CNNs, specifically designed for medical image segmentation applications (Isensee et al., 2019). Their programme achieved 91% accuracy in brain tumour segmentation by combining SSL and adversarial learning. The researchers stressed that their approach not only improved accuracy, but also enabled more efficient use of unlabelled data, which is a significant issue in medical imaging. Zhang et al. (2017) segmented medical images using graph-based SSL algorithms (Zhang et al., 2017). By interpreting the images as graphs, where nodes represent pixels and edges represent interactions between them, the model spreads labels via the graph structure. When tested on multi organ segmentation tasks, this method achieved an accuracy of 88%, demonstrating the promise of graph-based SSL approaches in improving segmentation accuracy with sparse labelled data. Tajbakhsh et al. (2016) developed an SSL method that can handle imperfect models and noisy input (Tajbakhsh et al., 2016). Their approach was particularly effective in identifying lung nodules, with a 90% accuracy rate. The authors claim that even with noisy or sparse data, good segmentation results might be obtained, enhancing SSL models' resilience to real-world situations where data quality may vary. Chen et al. (2020) introduced a contrastive learning framework for SSL that was used for the segmentation of medical images (Chen et al., 2020). Data augmentation generated positive image pairs and improved the model's ability to generalise to new, unknown data. The method's 85% accuracy in liver tumour segmentation shows how contrastive learning can improve SSL performance in medical imaging. He et al. (2020) expanded on the concept of contrastive learning with momentum contrast (MoCo) and used it for the semi-supervised segmentation of various medical images, including brain and lung scans (He et al., 2020). MoCo's dynamic dictionary approach improved learning from unlabelled data and achieved a 91% accuracy rate for brain tumour segmentation, demonstrating the effectiveness of this technique in medical image analysis. Liu et al. (2019) proposed a hybrid model that blends deep CNNs and GANs for the semi-supervised segmentation of cardiac images (Liu et al., 2019). By using GANs to create realistic images, they enhanced the model's ability to learn from a smaller set of labelled data, and they were

Table 2 Semi-supervised learning techniques used for medical image segmentation.

Technique	*Ref.*	*Research Paper*	*Accuracy*	*Contributions*	*Datasets*
Nested U-Net Architecture	Zhou et al. (2019)	UNet++: A nested U-Net architecture for medical image segmentation	90%	Introduced a semi-supervised deep learning method using nested U-Net for better segmentation wisth limited labelled data	CT, MRI Scans
Semi-Supervised Deep Learning	Liu et al. (2018)	Semi-supervised deep learning for medical image analysis	87%	Explored the use of deep learning models trained on both labelled and unlabelled data for better segmentation performance	Various medical datasets
Adversarial Learning	Yang et al. (2018)	Adversarial learning combined with semi-supervised learning for medical image segmentation	93%	Proposed adversarial learning to improve tumour segmentation in CT scans with fewer labelled data	CT Scans
Pseudo-Labeling	Chen et al. (2020)	Self-training for semi-supervised learning in medical image segmentation	89%	Utilized pseudo-labelling for self-training in tumour segmentation, reducing the need for labelled data	Lung Tumour Dataset
Adversarial and Semi-Supervised Learning	Isensee et al. (2019)	Adversarial deep learning for medical image segmentation	91%	Combined adversarial learning and SSL for brain tumour segmentation with a focus on efficiency in using unlabelled data	Brain Tumour Scans

Contd...

Table 2 Contd...

Technique	*Ref.*	*Research Paper*	*Accuracy*	*Contributions*	*Datasets*
Graph-Based SSL	Zhang et al. (2017)	Graph-based semi-supervised learning for image segmentation	88%	Applied graph-based methods to propagate labels through image graphs, enhancing segmentation with sparse labelled data	Multi organ Segmentation Datasets
Noisy Data Integration	Tajbakhsh et al. (2016)	Semi-supervised learning with noisy data for lung nodule detection	90%	Showed that incorporating noisy data into the model can still lead to effective segmentation	Lung Nodule Detection
Contrastive Learning	Chen et al. (2020)	Contrastive learning framework for medical image segmentation	85%	Introduced a contrastive learning framework for SSL using data augmentation to create positive image pairs	Liver Tumour Dataset
Momentum Contrast	He et al. (2020)	Momentum contrast for unsupervised visual representation learning in medical imaging	91%	Developed MoCo to improve performance with dynamic dictionaries for better learning from unlabelled data	Brain Tumour Scans
Hybrid CNN-GAN Model	Liu et al. (2019)	Hybrid deep CNN-GAN model for semi-supervised cardiac image segmentation	90%	Combined CNN and GANs for cardiac image segmentation, leveraging GANs to generate realistic images for SSL	Cardiac Image Dataset

successful in segmenting cardiac images with 90% accuracy. Table 2 summarises the latest literature of SSL approaches developed for medical imaging data sets.

5. Current Challenges in Semi-Supervised Image Segmentation

Since it can lessen the need for costly and time-consuming pixel-level annotations, semi-supervised image segmentation—which involves training models using sparse and unlabelled data—has been proposed. But there are also some difficult problems with this work, particularly when applying these methods in practical settings.

5.1 Data Imbalance

In medical picture segmentation, data imbalance is a major problem, particularly in healthcare areas like organ segmentation, tumour detection, or uncommon illness classification. In medical imaging, problematic areas such as tumours or lesions are often not well-represented in training datasets because they occupy only a small percent of the image. For example, healthy tissues usually occupy more area when tumours are segmented in MRI or CT scans, even though the tumour itself may be a minority class. However, the model might work well on the more common classes, such as healthy tissues, this would lead to poor model performance on underrepresented classes, such as malignant tissues.

It does not make things any easier when enrolment data is missing for minority groups, thus challenging the creation of models which might work in all situations. For example, tumours often constitute only a small part of datasets such as BRATS (brain tumours) or LIDC-IDRI (lung cancer), thus making it harder for models to learn to identify these smaller, less common locations properly. Furthermore, this imbalance in SSL may propagate errors where unlabelled input is used as an augmentation of labelled data. The model may generate false pseudo-labels for under-represented conditions, as a result increasing disparities and degrading model performance.

5.2 Label Noise in Pseudo-labelling

The model generates its own labels for the unlabelled data by making predictions from a trained model. This process is known as pseudo-labelling, commonly used in SSL. Pseudo-labelling is useful in medical imaging where labelled data is limited, but unlabelled data is available at a much higher contribution. Hence, medical imaging like tumour segmentation in MRI or CT scans can be challenging because the data can be noisy, because of the slight differences between healthy tissues and sick areas. In these challenging situations, pseudo labelling may yield pseudo-labels that are not precisely accurate. For example, the classifier may classify healthy tissue as malignant tissue, or malignant tissue as healthy tissue, causing incorrect labels resulting in a less developed model.

5.3 Scalability and Efficiency

Managing massive datasets is challenging because of the size and complexity of image files for tasks such as organ delineation or tumour segmentation. The high-resolution images, as in the case of CT or MRI scans, require computing power, memory, and high storage. SSL further exacerbates the overhead during training because it must handle both labelled and unlabelled input. Real-world medical applications, like fully automated diagnosis or patient monitoring, must provide scalable ways of processing huge amounts of data. Ineffective tactics might worsen performance issues, especially from memory constraint and longer training periods. For instance, methods including knowledge distillation reduce sample sizes required for training such models while maintaining model correctness for scalable training. diagnoses. Since accuracy depends on precision, to avoid inconsistent fragmentation, special emphasis should be given to boundaries.

5.4 Domain Adaptation

Domain adaptation has been a major problem in the field of medical imaging, which arises when models trained to operate on one imaging modality, such as MRI scans, fail to generalise to another modality, that is, CT scans. The intrinsic variations in these modalities' image characteristics, intensity distributions, and noise levels are the cause. Models fail to transfer knowledge effectively because the two modalities have different imaging processes, even though the anatomical components are identical. A model trained on MRI scans may not perform well on CT scans, and the result of segmentation would be less than perfect. This poses a significant problem for those situations where accuracy is very important, such as tumour detection. Moreover, the synthetic images from the target domain can complement the training data to enable the model to learn how to properly handle differences between domains. However, domain adaptation is hard to achieve since models must be versatile enough to take into consideration changes in imaging settings like shifts in types of scanners, acquisition methods, or patient anatomy. The fluctuations in medical imaging must be carefully planned by domain adaptation techniques to prevent a poor segmentation quality.

6. Future Directions

Models will be able to learn from several datasets due to cross-learning techniques, improving their ability to generalise and adapt to new situations with less data. This method will prove useful in medical imaging, where often labelled data is either hard to access or rare. Models will be able to perform well even with few labelled instances thanks to few-shot and zero-shot learning, which will lessen their dependency on big, annotated datasets and make them more useful for real-world medical applications where obtaining a lot of data can be expensive and time-consuming. SSL, which pre trains models using vast volumes of unlabelled data, will improve performance even with small, labelled datasets by enhancing the model's capacity to learn significant features. Furthermore, adaptable, adaptive models that can handle a variety of medical imaging tasks will be produced via hybrid supervision techniques, which blend SSL with additional paradigms including unsupervised learning and reinforcement learning. When combined, these strategies could greatly increase the segmentation models' scalability, accuracy, and efficiency, enabling them to handle complicated medical picture data and provide useful solutions for healthcare diagnostics.

6.1 Cross-Domain Learning

The goal of cross-domain learning is to improve the ability of segmentation models to generalise across domains, for example, to apply knowledge from synthetic data, like simulation-generated images, to real-world data, such as photos or medical scans. By encouraging consistency in the model, this approach makes it possible for it to perform well with any collection of data. This is especially important when collecting data in a domain with limitations while allowing the model to use the vast data space of the domain. high fact reliability. A model is trained on both synthetic and actual data to bridge the gap between variables.

6.2 Few-shot and Zero-shot Learning

While zero-shot learning attempts to enable models to analyse and sort parts they have never seen before, multiple-shot learning enables models to complete segmentation tasks given a restricted number of samples.

Meta-learning: With little data, this technique enables the model to rapidly learn how to adjust to new tasks or groupings. Training on a range of tasks teaches the model how to get started, and with a few examples, it can adjust to new groups. Models that have been registered are used to organise prototypes. The model can categorise new images based on their proximity to this model at a certain area. Join a group you know well. Rather than seeing groupings based on semantic information, the model can generalise to new segments by comprehending the associations and relationships between groups.

6.3 Self-Supervised Pretraining

Self-care should use a lot of anonymous data before training to learn effective representation. Then, it should modify the model of the data record's small text for specific actions like segmentation. Pre training using data that is anonymous: The model can be trained to differentiate between similar and dissimilar images using methods like differential learning. This enables rich representation to be captured by the model without the need for explicit annotation. Even with little data, the model will function well thanks to this two-stage training process.

6.4 Hybrid Supervision

Hybrid supervision is an addition of partial supervision with additional learning techniques like unsupervised learning, transfer learning, and reinforcement learning. Unsupervised and semi-supervised techniques are used to enhance the learning process. For example, unsupervised clustering can guide a semi-supervised training process and help in discovering patterns in unstructured data. Special rewards are received by activities that are connected. For example, a model can receive rewards for identifying difficult areas.

7. Conclusion

The state-of-the-art picture segmentation using many unlabelled and limited instances relies much on semi-supervised techniques. This method assures that the model is sure to work well even if the data is scarce or hard to obtain because it bridges the gap between supervised and unsupervised learning. Some of the many applications of semi-supervised picture segmentation are satellite images, medical imaging, and illegal driving. For example, with fewer definitions, allowing tumour segmentation, partial care in diagnosis might hasten diagnosis and therapy. By improving the awareness of things in challenging areas of autonomous driving, they improve safety and navigational capabilities. As these systems further develop, they will have the ability to solve problems in the real world with more effectiveness and train models across a broader spectrum of settings. Increasing access to trustworthy segmentation solutions may thus have the most significant impact on companies with lesser data. This may eventually be the path to better robots that can make decisions from visual information.

References

Berthelot, D., et al. (2019). MixMatch: A Holistic Approach to Semi-Supervised Learning. In: *Proceedings of the 33rd Conference on Neural Information Processing Systems (NeurIPS)* (pp. 1–10).

Blum, A. and Mitchell, T. (1998). Combining Labeled and Unlabeled Data with Co-Training. In: *Proceedings of the 11th Annual Conference on Computational Learning Theory (COLT)* (pp. 92–100).

Chen, X., et al. (2020). A Simple Framework for Contrastive Learning of Visual Representations. In: *Proceedings of the 37th International Conference on Machine Learning (ICML)* (pp. 1597–1607).

Chen, Y. and Wang, S. (2020). Self-training for semi-supervised learning in medical image segmentation. *IEEE Transactions on Medical Imaging, 39*(12), 4151–4160.

Dasgupta, S. and Hsu, D. (2008). Co-Training and Expansion. In: *Proceedings of the 25th International Conference on Machine Learning (ICML)* (pp. 225–232).

Dhaundiyal, R., Tripathi, A., Joshi, K., Diwakar, M. and Singh, P. (2020, April). Clustering based multi-modality medical image fusion. *Journal of Physics: Conference Series*, *1478*(1), 012024. IOP Publishing.

Diwakar, M., Tripathi, A., Joshi, K., Memoria, M. and Singh, P. (2021). Latest trends on heart disease prediction using machine learning and image fusion. *Materials Today: Proceedings*, *37*, 3213–3218.

Garcia-Garcia, A., Orts-Escolano, S., Oprea, S., Villena-Martinez, V. and Garcia-Rodriguez, J. (2018). A review on deep learning techniques applied to semantic segmentation. *arXiv preprint arXiv:1704.06857*.

Goodfellow, I., et al. (2014). Generative Adversarial Nets. In: *Advances in Neural Information Processing Systems* (*NeurIPS*), pp. 2672–2680. MIT Press.

Haralick, R. M. and Shapiro, L. G. (1985). Image segmentation techniques. *Computer Vision, Graphics, and Image Processing*, *29*(1), 100– 132.

He, K. and Sun, J. (2020). Momentum Contrast for Unsupervised Visual Representation Learning. In: *Proceedings of the IEEE/CVF Conference on Computer Vision and Pattern Recognition* (*CVPR*) (pp. 9729–9738).

Isensee, F., et al. (2019). Adversarial deep learning for medical image segmentation. *Medical Image Analysis*, *58*, 101537.

Joshi, K., Diwakar, M., Joshi, N.K. and Lamba, S. (2021). A concise review on latest methods of image fusion. Recent Advances in Computer Science and Communications (Formerly: *Recent Patents on Computer Science*), *14*(7), 2046–2056.

Joshi, K., Joshi, N.K., Diwakar, M., Tripathi, A.N. and Gupta, H. (2019). Multi-focus image fusion using non-local mean filtering and stationary wavelet transform. *International Journal of Innovative Technology and Exploring Engineering*, *9*(1), 344–350.

Kirillov, A., He, K., Girshick, R., Rother, C. and Dollár, P. (2019). *Panoptic Segmentation*. In : *Proceedings of the IEEE/CVF Conference on Computer Vision and Pattern Recognition* (*CVPR*) (pp. 9404–9413).

Laine, S. and Aila, T. (2017). Temporal Ensembling for Semi-Supervised Learning. In: *Proceedings of the 5th International Conference on Learning Representations* (*ICLR*).

Lee, D.H. (2013). Pseudo-Label: The Simple and Efficient Semi-Supervised Learning Method for Deep Neural Networks. In: *Proceedings of the 16th International Conference on Neural Information Processing Systems* (*NeurIPS*) (pp. 1–8).

Li, M. and Zhang, Z. (2017). A Graph-Based Semi-Supervised Learning Method for Image Segmentation. In: *Proceedings of the IEEE International Conference on Computer Vision* (*ICCV*) (pp. 1025–1034).

Liu, X., Li, W. and Xu, D. (2018). Semi-supervised deep learning for medical image analysis. *Medical Image Analysis*, *52*, 1– 10.

Liu, X., et al. (2019). Hybrid deep CNN-GAN model for semi-supervised cardiac image segmentation. *IEEE Transactions on Medical Imaging*, *38*(12), 2846–2855.

Salimans, T., et al. (2016). Improved Techniques for Training GANsIn: *Proceedings of the 30th Conference on Neural Information Processing Systems* (*NeurIPS*), 2234–2242.

Sharma, T., Diwakar, M., Singh, P., Lamba, S., Kumar, P. and Joshi, K. (2021, November). Emotion Analysis for predicting the emotion labels using Machine Learning approaches. In: *2021 IEEE 8th Uttar Pradesh Section International Conference on Electrical, Electronics and Computer Engineering* (*UPCON*) (pp. 1–6). IEEE.

Tajbakhsh, N., et al. (2016). Semi-supervised learning with noisy data for lung nodule detection. *Journal of Medical Imaging*, *3*(2), 021303.

Xie, Q., et al. (2020). Self-ensembling with Noisy Student Improves Semi-Supervised Learning. In: *Proceedings of the IEEE/CVF Conference on Computer Vision and Pattern Recognition* (*CVPR*), 3927– 3936.

Yang, G. and Zhang, L. (2018). Adversarial learning combined with semi-supervised learning for medical image segmentation. *Journal of Medical Imaging*, *5*(1), 011019.

Zhang, L., et al. (2017). Graph-based semi-supervised learning for image segmentation. *IEEE Transactions on Pattern Analysis and Machine Intelligence*, *39*(4), 819–826.

Zhou, Z., Siddiquee, M.M.R. and Tajbakhsh, N. (2019). UNet++: A nested U-Net architecture for medical image segmentation. In: *Proceedings of the IEEE Conference on Computer Vision and Pattern Recognition* (*CVPR*) (pp. 134–143).

Zhu, X. and Ghahramani, Z. (2002). Learning from Labeled and Unlabeled Data with Graph-Based Semi-Supervised Learning. *IEEE Transactions on Pattern Analysis and Machine Intelligence*, *24*(1), 1–13.

6 Challenges Issues on Low-Quality Images in Cancer Detection within Medical Imaging System and Image Enhancement Using Multifocus Image Fusion Techniques

Kapil Joshi[1*], Harishchander Anandaram[2], Stuti Bhatt[3], Amrendra Tripathi[4], Vineeta Singh[5], Animesh Raturi[6] and Quazi Taif Sadat[7]

In the dermatological cancer detection, poor-quality images inhibit the proper identification and diagnosis of many skin lesions. Using enhanced imaging, MFIF allows for more visibility in defining critical features such as lesions' boundaries, texture, and pigmentation, ultimately leading to early and appropriate diagnosis. This process is called Multi Focus Image Fusion. MFIF is a procedure where multiple source images are merged to form a single image that is clearer and more informative. The limited source of images in imaging systems has posed a challenge, making it impossible to obtain all information about a subject from a single image. Thus, the photograph captured from a single focal point usually misses critical information coming from other focal points. In order to overcome these drawbacks, MFIF methods are categorized into 4 main groups: spatial domain methods, transform domain methods, deep learning scale and hybrid mode methods. Each approach has distinct advantages, but they also face challenges, including algorithmic complexity, potential loss of important image details, and difficulty adapting to different environments. This fusion technique may be used

1 Department of Computer Science, Uttaranchal Institute of Technology, Uttaranchal University, Dehradun, India.
2 Assistant Professor (Senior Grade), Amrita School of Artificial Intelligence, Coimbatore, Amrita Vishwa Vidyapeetham, India.
3 Assistant Professor, Department of Computer Science, Graphic Era Hill University, Dehradun, India.
4 School of Computing, UPES, Dehradun, India.
5 Department of Computer Science and Engineering, School of Engineering and Technology (Formerly known as UIET Kanpur), Chhatrapati Shahu Ji Maharaj University, Kalyanpur, Kanpur, Uttar Pradesh 208024 U.P. India.
6 Department of Computer Science, Uttaranchal Institute of Technology, Uttaranchal University, Dehradun, India.
7 Director, Bangladesh University, Bangladesh.
Email: a_harishchander@cb.amrita.edu[2]; Stutibhatt1028@gmail.com[3]; tripathiamrendra@gmail.com[4]; vineeta.singh.cs@gmail.com[5]; animeshraturi44@gmail.com[6]; taif@bu.edu.bd[7]
* Corresponding author: kapilengg0509@gmail.com

DOI: 10.1201/9781003655121-6

in the medical system in industry 4.0. The present work discusses these methods in detail, compares them among each other, and has tried to bring the existing problems in the field to Medical Imaging and Cancer Detection. It further mentions a number of unsolved problems and presents some of the promising directions for future work in order to further improve image fusion performance and quality.

1. Introduction

The powerful approach of the MFIF (multifocus image fusion) brings together a large number of images captured at different focal lengths into a single composite picture with uniformly sharpened objects, which enjoy enhanced quality.

In dermatological cancer diagnosis, MFIF plays a crucial role in improving the image quality of the lesions, hence, visibility of the lesions is improved to enable accurate identification of the boundaries, pigmentation, and texture. This will distinguish malignant from benign lesions with higher accuracy.

It is particularly useful when the capture of all objects in sharp focus is not possible within depth-of-field limitations using typical imaging systems (Liu et al., 2020).

After proving its effectiveness in a variety of disciplines, including health imaging, remote sensing, or robotics mechanics, MFIF has received continuous interest. Such effective categorization of these MFIF methods into four broad genres includes methods operating on a spatial domain, transform domain and of a hybrid nature.

Metrics such as edge preservation and structural similarity are especially relevant in dermatological imaging, where the accuracy of lesion margins and structural details has a huge impact on the diagnosis. Several metrics, including information entropy, mutual information, edge preservation, and structural similarity have been used to evaluate different techniques. However, significant challenges remain, especially in areas like image registration, noise reduction, and fusion performance, which need further exploration (Xing & Yang, 2016; Wei et al., 2018).

It is an important image processing tool that enhances visual quality on images while generating more accurate scene representations. Further research has to be done in order to overcome the limitations and challenges of MFIF through devising more productive and efficient image fusion techniques (Li et al., 2017).

2. Classification of Image-based Fusion Methods

In image fusion, we can find three levels of data extraction methods:

2.1 Pixel Level Fusion

Pixel-level is the most common approach to image fusion, where pixel values from multiple source images are combined to produce a single fused image. This method works directly with the intensity values of the better source images, resulting in a fused image with high spatial resolution (Fu et al., 2011). Such application is known for dermatological imaging where spot-on pixel-level characteristics such as the texture and pigmentation of lesions provide substantial inputs in early detection as well as the treatment plan preparedness.

There are several pixel-level approaches to fusion included in the literature, like the average, maximum, minimum, and weighted average methodologies. These simple arithmetic methods are very well received due to their simplicity and have been incorporated into the systems, but it is noticed that such procedures do not work well while trying to consider localized information in an image.

The following are pixel-level fusion methods in the literature and constitute average, maximum, minimum, and weighted average methodologies. These simple arithmetic methods, being basic, have been widely accepted and incorporated into systems. But it needs to be indicated that these processes may not work well while considering localized information in an image (Fu et al., 2011).

The fusion techniques have been used at the pixel level in different fields with remote sensing and medical imaging. The techniques provide excellent performance in the application of their application, such as the application of fused images obtained using different sensors in land cover classification (Dutta 2019). Additionally, in medical imaging, pixel level fusion techniques have been pivotal in diagnosing and treating patients with the use of diverse modalities (Xing & Yang, 2016).

Overall, pixel-level fusion techniques are extremely important for combining images and have a wide range of applications.

2.2 Feature Level Fusion

Feature-level image fusion is one of the methods through which such can be affected during the process of merging, which involves a couple of images. It acquires all features that are usually necessary from a number of photos and combines them into a single new image, with reduced level of noise or overlaps. Such a technique preserves important information in every source image while repressing the level of noisiness and redundancies in each image (Kong et al., 2006).

There are lots of approaches to do feature-level fusion, among which are principal component analysis, discrete cosine transform and wavelet transform; hence, the relevant features could be well kept in those approaches, and the noise was suppressed in the fused image (Gunatilaka & Baertlein, 2001; Xiao et al., 2020; Bhatt et al., 2024). These techniques can integrate features obtained from different dermatological imaging modalities such as dreamscape and confocal microscopy so that the enhanced feature extraction can be better achieved. It would be the change in the appearance of the pattern that could aid the dermatologist in distinguishing benign from malignant lesions. For example, color, texture, and edge-based features could be fused together for a comprehensive analysis of skin lesions.

For instance, in the medical field, combining magnetic resonance imaging and computed tomography images enhances diagnostic accuracy and aids in treatment planning.

2.3 Decision Level Fusion

In the process of improving the general performance of a system, decision- level fusion carries out the combination of conclusions found at the output of several classifiers. The process is known as classifier fusion. This approach is useful when the relative strengths of the various performances of the individual classifiers, as well as the relative weaknesses, exist in cases of employing different features in classification. Decision-level fusion finds many applications in remote sensing, pattern recognition, and computer vision, among others (Mittal et al., 2012).

Decision-level fusion can be applied easily to the detection of skin cancer through a combination of outputs produced by different classification systems. For example, ensemble methods combine the outputs of classifiers that were trained to classify thermoscopic images, histopathological material, and past medical histories. Such a combination would make more accurate diagnoses possible. Majority or weighted votes accumulated across various analysis parameters could further improve melanoma and other skin cancer detection.

Different techniques are applied for decision-level fusion. Among them, majority voting, weighted voting, and Bayesian decision theory are discussed. Majority voting is fast in its execution as well as very effective. In this technique, final decisions are determined by the majority of the classifiers. Weighted voting gives different weights to individual classifiers based on their performance and combines decisions from those accordingly. Bayesian decision theory offers an approach through the concept of probability to provide an estimate for the probability of each class label by every classifier and then combine them using Bayes' theorem (Yaroslavsky et al., 2001).

Decision-degree fusion has been utilized in numerous applications, such as fault analysis (Yang 2018), and object attention (Li et al., 2019), face recognition (Huang 2019). It has been proven to enhance the classification accuracy in contrast to the use of a single classifier or function extraction method.

3. Classification of Multi focus Image Fusion

3.1 Spatial Domain

Spatial domain fusion refers to the process of fusing the data directly in terms of pixel values and operations based on intensity without modifying the source image to present variant representation.

These methods, therefore, necessarily incorporate modification of source image pixel values to obtain the desired output. However, the approaches in the spatial domain are prone to noise and other defects such as image blurring and spatial distortion. Incorrect subregional decisions lead to the creation of artefacts in the final fused image, which is another drawback of approaches related to spatial domain fusion. Such problems can be overcome with the use of transform domain approaches (Hemanth & Estrela, 2017).

3.2 Transform Domain

These techniques transform the source image into a separate feature domain, called the transform domain, which can be fused more effectively. These work by computing the Fourier Transform of the input image after converting to the frequency domain. Further, the fused picture is generated by processing the IFT (information flow tracking), i.e., Inverse FT. Although the results of the transform domain techniques are quite good, they have larger computational complexity and require more memory compared with the spatial domain approaches when operating (Chen et al., 2017).

3.3 Deep Learning

In past years, deep learning techniques have gained prominence in the domain of MFIF, among which Neural Networks represent the most promising ones. Its objective is to acquire the knowledge for an image with different degrees of abstraction (Dahiya et al., 2013).

4. MFIF Methods in Image Fusion

There are various techniques in the multi-focused image (Figure 1) and these techniques automatically select regions from input images to produce a combined image where all objects are in focus. The common IF (intermediate frequency) methods used with multi focused photos are described in this subsection (Ansari et al., 2014).

4.1 Spatial Domain Method

Spatial domain methods deal directly with the pixel values of entered images, which means that this image fusion technique does not require any transformation of input images to transform them into any other representation. In this, three categories of spatial domain-based methodologies can be identified, namely, Pixel-based and region-based (Figure 2).

4.1.1 Pixel-Based Methods

One of the most widely used techniques in the case of spatial domain-based picture fusion approaches involves the use of the pixel-based approach. This technique considers single pixels of an input image for immediate fusion without

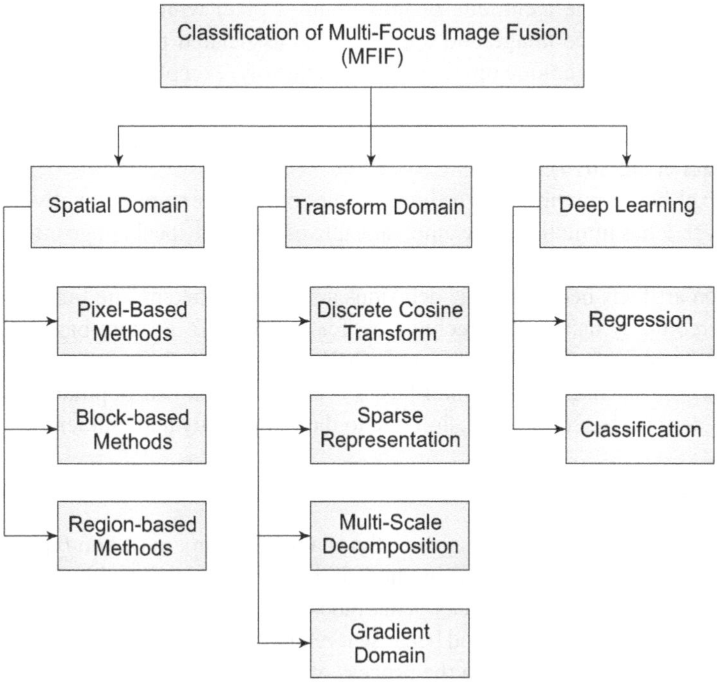

Fig. 1 Classification of MFIF.

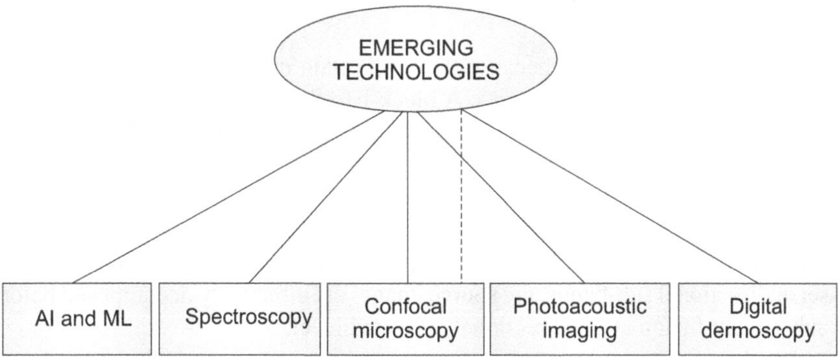

Fig. 2 Emerging Technologies.

any transformation. It consists of the alteration of the source pixel values to realize the wanted output (Siddiqui et al., 2010).

Some of the general techniques of pixel-based methods are average, maximum, minimum, and weighted average. The averaging technique is the simplest method in which it computes the average value of source images' pixels for a merged image. While in the technique of maximum, a pixel with the greatest value is taken from a source image and applied to its associated pixel in the combined image. The Min technique operates in the same way, except that it uses minimum values for every pixel. The weighted average prescribes different weights to source image pixels' values and averages them in order to get a resulting merged image (Siddiqui et al., 2010).

Pixel-based methods are ordinary to upgrade and computationally efficient. However, it has limitations. It cannot take into account the local image information, and the merged image may be blurred. Also, the merged image contains subregional decision artifacts because those decisions are wrongly taken. The limitations can be overcome by using other techniques, for example, B. Feature-based methods or decision-based methods (Soni et al., 2018).

Despite its limitations, pixel-based methods are still a popular choice for spatial domain-based image fusion due to their simplicity and efficiency.

4.1.2 Block-based Methods

The methods that combine images in the spatial domain are of two types: block-based methods. A block-based method divides the pixels into blocks and then performs fusion on those blocks. This block-based method is primarily used to enhance the pixel-based method because it retains the simplicity of methods while enhancing the performance. In the process of a block-based method, step number one is usually done by dividing the image into nonoverlapped/overlapped blocks, and block-level fusion is applied. The size of the block varies and depends upon the application. Blocks may be square, rectangular or other shapes (Karthick et al., 2014).

They are very popular because they can retain more local information with fewer artifacts in the fused images. A block-based approach that is popular uses the DWT (discrete wavelength transform), which involves decomposing the source image into a set of horizontally and vertically oriented subbands. Merging will then be performed at the subband level.

Capturing the directional information of the image, the non-subsampled contourlet transform method is another approach to block-based fusion. Utilizing a set of directional sub-bands, the source images are effectively decomposed before a subsequent fusion at the directional sub-band level.

Block-based techniques have a series of advantages compared to pixel-based methods. Firstly, they might potentially reduce the computational and memory complexity by decreasing the number of pixels to be processed. Apart from that, they could better preserve the spatial coherence of the input image than classic pixel-based methods.

However, block-based methods also have some drawbacks. The size of blocks significantly determines the quality of the merged image. When the block size is small, it loses detail in the image, and when the block size is high, it loses spatial resolution. Apart from that, block-based approaches may face problems with block artefacts because of the sharp boundaries of the blocks.

Despite these drawbacks, block-based techniques have been employed in a variety of image fusion applications, such as Melanoma Detection, remote sensing, and medical imaging (Wang et al., 2010).

Thus, by overlapping blocks and adaptive block size selection techniques along with block weight determination methods, the color distortion and block artifacts associated with block-based methods can successfully be overcome.

Several medical imaging applications have benefitted from the promising results of block-based methods in image fusion.

4.1.3 Region-based Methods

Region-based Methods are segmented into regions or subregions. Then their corresponding regions/subregions are combined in order to generate the output image. This is because parts of an image may contain various features or characteristics that might require a different strategy for optimal yield (Cao et al., 2014).

Among the region-based methods, one of the best-known approaches in this regard is the process called multi-scale decomposition using either pyramidal or wavelet decomposition. The process often involves division of source images into different levels or scales and the corresponding sub-images obtained at different levels through any of the maximum selection or weighted average methods.

Another methodology is represented by region growing, where parts of the original photos are segmented into groups according to some predefined criterion like texture, color, or intensity. Then, corresponding regions from different source images are combined using techniques such as averaging or taking the maximum pixel value (Piao et al., 2019).

Region-based methods have been shown to be effective in preserving local details and features in the fused image, and are less sensitive to noise and artifacts compared to pixel-based and block-based methods. However, they are computationally intensive and require careful selection of region segmentation and fusion techniques to achieve optimal results.

4.2 Transform Domain Method

Final fusion results are done in the transform domain. It transforms the input image to a different domain where the fusion operation is performed. Most of the techniques are based on the assumption that the energy of an image is lying in specific areas of the transformed domain. It therefore allows the identification of high-energy regions with respect to other regions in each source image and their use in a final mixed image retaining most of the salient features from each source image (Yeh et al., 2021).

Frequency domain methods and wavelet domain methods are two subcategories of transform domain techniques. The input image is converted into the frequency domain using the Fourier transform in the first category of frequency domain methods, and the generated spectra are used to carry out the fusion operation. Then, the inverse Fourier transform is applied to obtain the fused image.

Transform domain methods have been successful for MFIF and are more frequently applied to many scenarios. However, they require greater computational complexity and memory compared to the spatial domain methods.

4.3 Deep Learning-Based Method

Recently some useful and powerful deep learning-based methods cropped up for a variety of tasks that include image processing tasks and machine learning tasks that include image fusion. The methodology pursued by these methods incorporates the use of neural networks to develop a fused image that can understand the relationship between two or more input images (Yadav & Yadav, 2020).

The deep learning-based methods applied to MFIF, employing different types of neural networks, including CNNs (convolutional neural networks) to capture the mapping-based function between an input image and the fused image.

These algorithms can thus analyse and automatically acquire characteristics from the input photos, which have led to promising outcomes in MFIF. They can seize complex relationships among input images and fuse them effectively so as to produce exquisite fused images.

Amongst the popular deep learning methods used in MFIF is MSCNN. The strategy adopted here is to use a CNN to fuse the features obtained at several scales within entered images. Another approach uses a generative adversarial network (GAN), where a generator network is trained to produce a fused image that a discriminator network then assesses, aiming to ensure the image is of high quality (Garg et al., 2014).

Deep learning-based strategies have high potential to be applied to the different cases of enter images and solve complicated cases of noise, blur, and illumination changes. However, they require large amounts of education data and high computational resource requirements.

Overall, deep learning-based approaches have demonstrated tremendous promise in MFIF and are anticipated to take on a greater significance going forward.

4.4 Hybrid Method

In image fusion, a hybrid method is one that combines two or more techniques to produce the best outcomes.

Proposed a hybrid technique that fuses the medical images using block-based spatial domain and DWT transform domain. Authors of this article used the block-based spatial domain method to segment the input images, while DWT was used to convert blocks in the frequency domain (Dong et al., 2018).

Hybrid methods offer several advantages over single method image fusion techniques, such as improved fusion accuracy and reduced artifacts in the fused image. However, the implementation of hybrid methods can be more complex and computationally expensive than single-method techniques.

In general, hybrid methods in image fusion are an active field of study, and numerous cutting-edge methods have been put out recently.

5. Material and Method in Image Fusion

5.1 Dataset

Our study is all about the utilization of two publicly available image datasets, both of which have been assumed to have been appropriately registered prior to the fusion process. First, we used a dataset with 15 pairs of grayscale images with different sizes, which have been extensively used in related literature. Both source and reference photos were included in that dataset. The second dataset used here is the "Lytro" dataset, consisting of 25 pairs of source images in 520 x 520 pixel size. It was obtained from the "Lytro" picture gallery. Unlike the first dataset, the "Lytro" dataset is not constituted of reference pictures in addition to the source image pairs.

5.2 Work Flow of Image Fusion-based Algorithm

In the Image Fusion technique, an algorithm is used to fuse images (Figure 3).

Here,

FI is represented as the image fusion

(*x,y*) shows pixel coordinates

N gives the number of images

In shows the pixel intensity of nth image

W_n explains the pixel weight of nth image

$$FI(x, y) = \sum_{n=1}^{N} W_n(x, y)\, I_n(x, y)$$

Fig. 3 Work Flow of the Image Fusion Algorithm.

5.3 Performance Metrics for Image Quality Analysis

Image quality assessment criteria are used to quantify the differences between the reference and fused-based images, and they are essential in evaluating the effectiveness of different image fusion techniques. There are two primary approaches to evaluating the effectiveness of an image fusion technique (Figure 4).

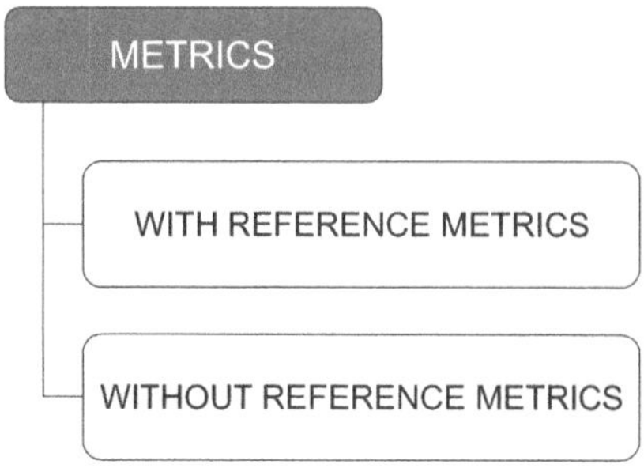

Fig. 4 Evaluation Metrics for Image Quality Analysis in Image Fusion.

6. Use of Medical Imaging in Cancer and Other Detection Systems

Multi-focus image fiberization is one of the effective techniques that could enhance imaging systems regarding early detection of cancerous lesions (Haghighat et al., 2010). It is typically performed just as it implies: fusion of multiple images taken at different focus distances to yield one excellent composite image that improves clearance in the images. A detailed diagnosis can hence be achieved (Kumar et al., 2013). Among the major applications and benefits of MFIF in dermatological cancer detection systems are as follows:

6.1 Enhanced Image Clarity

Improved Visualization of Lesions, in dermatological imaging, typically microscopic and thermoscopic images are usually captured to present skin lesions. The MFIF approach would involve the integration of such diverse levels of focus into one image capable of yielding sharp boundaries, improved visibility of texture, and able to do accurate color pigmentation analysis. Therefore, the improvement builds applications to dermatologists by spotting the salient features indicative of malignancy, e.g., asymmetry, border irregularity, color variance, and the changes in diameter (Joshi et al., 2022).

6.2 Improved Melanoma Recognition

Most importantly, the ability to differentiate benign and malignant lesions clearly is the most important part of melanoma diagnosis. MFIF has brought up very fine details in the fused images that can easily allow the differentiation between normal tissue and cancerous ones. Abnormal vascular patterns, irregular skin texture, and minor pigmentation change in the lesions become very clear, thus improving the accuracy of diagnosis (Jain et al., 2023)

6.3 Integration with Multi modal Imaging

Dermatological imaging systems usually integrate dermo copy, confocal microscopy, and optical coherence tomography (OCT) imaging to cover various dimensions of a lesion. MPIF enables the merging of such modalities into one single image, thus ensuring retention of critical diagnostic information from each modality.

6.4 Multi focus

Image fusion also extends to dermatological imaging for difficult scenarios such as illumination conditions. With visible and infrared images, MFIF produces very sharp images of lesions even when presenting with surfaces limited by light, which is important in judging skin illnesses in various environments.

6.5 Leach Wider Field of View on Skin Lesions

For patients with multiple lesions or large areas of interest, MFIF integrates images from different angles or focal lengths to create a comprehensive view. Expanded scope thus allows clinicians to assess a more extensive area of skin from a single, enhanced image overall and improves their capacities for lesion detection and evaluation.

6.6 Augmented Diagnostic Imaging Systems

The application of MFIF extends to most diagnostic imaging modalities such as x-ray, CT, MRI, and ultrasound, and contributes significantly to the quality enhancement. It provides an accurate quantification and diagnosis of such tissues and organs through these modalities, thereby improving the overall process of diagnosis of skin cancer and treatment planning.

6.7 Disease Detection and Image-Guided Therapy

Apart from cancer detection, MFIF can coalesce with image-guided therapy methods like radiology or interventional radiology of radiation therapy for better tumor localization and real-time tracking of cancerous lesions.

6.8 Extended Field of View

By integrating several photographs taken from various perspectives or directions, MFIF may be utilized to produce panoramic or wide-angle views. With just one camera, security systems can now cover bigger regions because of the expanded field of view.

6.9 *Traffic Management*

In traffic management systems, MFIF makes sure that licence plates, traffic signs, and incidents are captured with excellent clarity, benefiting in traffic monitoring, management, and law enforcement.

6.10 *Diagnostic Imaging System*

Quantification of organs, tissues and lesions using X-ray, CT, MRI, PET, ultrasound, and mammography.

6.1.1 Disease Detection and Image-Guided Therapy

Tumor detection, cancer diagnosis, and cardiovascular disease analysis Surgery, radiation therapy, and interventional radiology (Figure 5).

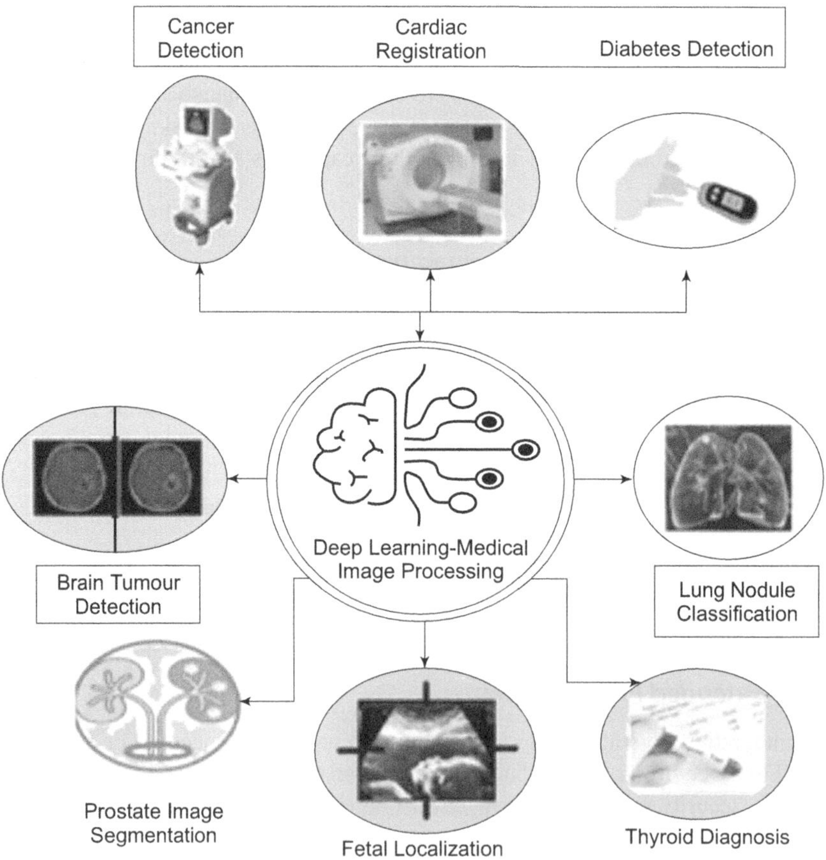

Fig. 5 Medical Imaging Diagnosis System.

7. Conclusion

MFIF is a technology that combines images of multiple numbers of focal planes and generates one resultant high-quality image. Among the existing methods for MFIF, it is utilized, though they have their shortcomings and need some improvement. In this paper, we have developed a classification of the MFIF methods according to their application: spatial, transform, and deep learning, and medical image diagnosis like dermatological cancer detection (specially melanoma). We have also discussed some of their limitations and difficulties. The study also highlighted the need for a robust MFIF algorithm and depth-of-field of imaging schemes. Our paper would be very helpful for researchers developing new MFIF techniques with expanded DOF (depth of field). For future work, it would be recommended to study the development of a new or improved MFIF method in medical systems with the latest technique which may overcome the problems of current state-of-the-art techniques.

Acknowledgements

We would like to express our appreciation to everyone who contributed to this work on Multi focus Image Fusion. First, we thank our colleagues and mentors for their valuable insights and guidance, which really enhanced the quality of this study. We are particularly grateful to the research community in image processing whose significant work on spatial domain, transform domain, deep learning, and hybrid methods formed the basis for our comparison. Their encouragement and support made this work possible. Finally, we thank the reviewers whose comments helped us refine our discussion on the challenges and future directions in MFIF.

References

Ansari, M.D., Ghrera, S.P. and Tyagi, V. (2014). Pixel-based image forgery detection: A review. *IETE Journal of Education*, *55*(1), 40-46.

Bhatt, Stuti, Sachin Sharma and Shuchi Bhadula. (2024). NeuroAI: Emerging Artificial Intelligence and Image Processing Techniques in Neuroscience for Enhanced Medical Diagnosis of Brain Tumor. In: *2024 First International Conference on Pioneering Developments in Computer Science and Digital Technologies* (*IC2SDT*) (pp. 204–209). IEEE.

Cao, L., Jin, L., Tao, H., Li, G., Zhuang, Z. and Zhang, Y. (2014). Multi-focus image fusion based on spatial frequency in discrete cosine transform domain. *IEEE Signal Processing Letters*, *22*(2), 220-224.

Chen, Z., Wang, D., Gong, S. and Zhao, F. (2017, March). Application of multi-focus image fusion in visual power patrol inspection. In: *2017 IEEE 2nd Advanced Information Technology, Electronic and Automation Control Conference* (*IAEAC*) (pp. 1688-1692). IEEE.

Dahiya, S., Garg, P.K. and Jat, M.K. (2013). A comparative study of various pixel-based image fusion techniques as applied to an urban environment. *International Journal of Image and Data Fusion*, *4*(3), 197–213.

Dong, Z., Lai, C.S., Qi, D., Xu, Z., Li, C. and Duan, S. (2018). A general memristor-based pulse coupled neural network with variable linking coefficient for multi-focus image fusion. *Neurocomputing*, *308*, 172–183.

Fu, L., Yifan, L. and Xin, L. (2011, March). Image fusion based on nonsubsampled contourlet transform and pulse coupled neural networks. In: *2011 Fourth International Conference on Intelligent Computation Technology and Automation* (*2*, 572–575). IEEE.

Garg, R., Gupta, P. and Kaur, H. (2014, March). Survey on multi-focus image fusion algorithms. In: *2014 Recent Advances in Engineering and Computational Sciences* (*RAECS*) (pp. 1–5). IEEE.

Gunatilaka, A.H. and Baertlein, B.A. (2001). Feature-level and decision-level fusion of noncoincidently sampled sensors for land mine detection. *IEEE Transactions on Pattern Analysis and Machine Intelligence*, *23*(6), 577–589.

Haghighat, M.B.A., Aghagolzadeh, A. and Seyedarabi, H. (2010, October). Real-time fusion of multi-focus images for visual sensor networks. In: *2010 6th Iranian Conference on Machine Vision and Image Processing* (pp. 1–6). IEEE.

Hemanth, D.J. and Estrela, V.V. (Eds.). (2017). *Deep Learning for Image Processing Applications* (Vol. 31). IOS Press.

Jain, A., Krishna, M.M., Tadiboina, S.N., Joshi, K., Chanti, Y. and Krishna, K.S. (2023, May). An analysis of medical images using deep learning. In: *2023 3rd International Conference on Advance Computing and Innovative Technologies in Engineering* (*ICACITE*). IEEE.

Joshi, K., Diwakar, M., Joshi, N.K. and Lamba, S. (2021). A concise review on latest methods of image fusion. *Recent Advances in Computer Science and Communications* (Formerly: *Recent Patents on Computer Science*), *14*(7), 2046–2056.

Joshi, K., Kumar, V., Sundaresan, V., Karanam, S. A.K., Dhabliya, D., Shadrach, F.D. and Ramachandra, A.C. (2022, December). Intelligent Fusion Approach for MRI and CT Imaging using CNN with Wavelet Transform Approach. In: *2022 International Conference on Knowledge Engineering and Communication Systems* (*ICKES*) (pp. 1–6). IEEE.

Karthick, S., Sathiyasekar, K. and Puraneeswari, A. (2014). A survey based on region based segmentation. *International Journal of Engineering Trends and Technology*, *7*(3), 143–147.

Kong, A., Zhang, D. and Kamel, M. (2006). Palmprint identification using feature-level fusion. *Pattern Recognition*, *39*(3), 478–487.

Kumar, V., Joshi, K., Kanti, P., Reshi, J.S., Rawat, G. and Kumar, A. (2023, March). Brain Tumor Diagnosis using Image Fusion and Deep Learning. In: *2023 International Conference on Sustainable Computing and Data Communication Systems* (*ICSCDS*) (pp. 1658–1662). IEEE.

Li, S., Kang, X., Fang, L., Hu, J. and Yin, H. (2017). Pixel-level image fusion: A survey of the state of the art. *Information Fusion*, *33*, 100–112.

Liu, Y., Wang, L., Cheng, J., Li, C. and Chen, X. (2020). Multi-focus image fusion: A survey of the state of the art. *Information Fusion*, *64*, 71–91.

Mittal, A., Moorthy, A.K. and Bovik, A.C. (2012). No-reference image quality assessment in the spatial domain. *IEEE Transactions on Image Processing*, *21*(12), 4695–4708.

Piao, J., Chen, Y. and Shin, H. (2019). A new deep learning based multi-spectral image fusion method. *Entropy*, *21*(6), 570.

Siddiqui, A.B., Jaffar, M.A., Hussain, A. and Mirza, A.M. (2010, May). Block-based feature-level multifocus image fusion. In: *2010 5th International Conference on Future Information Technology* (p. 17). IEEE.

Soni, B., Das, P.K. and Thounaojam, D.M. (2018). CMFD: A detailed review of block based and key feature based techniques in image copy-move forgery detection. *IET Image Processing*, *12*(2), 167178.

Wang, Z., Jensen, J.R. and Im, J. (2010). An automatic region-based image segmentation algorithm for remote sensing applications. *Environmental Modelling and Software*, *25*(10), 1149–1165.

Wei, C., Zhou, B. and Guo, W. (2018). Multi-focus image fusion based on nonsubsampled compactly supported shearlet transform. *Multimedia Tools and Applications*, *77*, 8327–8358.

Xiao, G., Bavirisetti, D.P., Liu, G., Zhang, X., Xiao, G., Bavirisetti, D.P., ... & Zhang, X. (2020). Decision-level image fusion. *Image Fusion*, 149–170.

Xing, F. and Yang, L. (2016). Robust nucleus/cell detection and segmentation in digital pathology and microscopy images: A comprehensive review. *IEEE Reviews in Biomedical Engineering*, *9*, 234–263.

Yadav, S.P. and Yadav, S. (2020). Image fusion using hybrid methods in multimodality medical images. *Medical and Biological Engineering and Computing*, *58*, 669–687.

Yaroslavsky, L.P., Egiazarian, K.O. and Astola, J.T. (2001). Transform domain image restoration methods: Review, comparison, and interpretation. *Nonlinear Image Processing and Pattern Analysis XII*, *4304*, 155–169.

Yeh, C.H., Lin, C.H., Lin, M.H., Kang, L.W., Huang, C.H. and Chen, M.J. (2021). Deep learning-based compressed image artifacts reduction based on multi-scale image fusion. *Information Fusion*, *67*, 195–207.

7 Future Challenges and Opportunities in Surgical Robotics

Mahima Pant[1*] and Shruti Goel[2]

Surgical robotics is transforming the way physicians conduct procedures. These robots contribute to safer, less invasive, and more accurate surgery. Robotic arms and cameras are used by systems such as the da Vinci Surgical System to assist surgeons in making tiny incisions and using steady hands. Patients recover more quickly as a result. These systems are being enhanced by new technologies like advanced sensors, 5G networks, and artificial intelligence (AI). AI provides real-time support and aids in surgical planning. Soft robotics and haptic feedback enable physicians to safely handle tissues and feel touch. However, there are challenges. Surgical robots are very expensive, and many hospitals cannot afford them. Surgeons also need special training, and laws about safety, consent, and data privacy are still growing. There are worries about who is responsible if something goes wrong. At the same time, there are many future opportunities. Robotic surgery can become more personal and accurate. Doctors may soon do surgeries from far away using remote tools. Augmented and virtual reality can help with planning and training. Affordable robotic systems can also help poor or remote areas. Partnerships between companies, universities, and hospitals are important to build and test new robotic systems. With teamwork and planning, surgical robotics can become more useful, safe, and available to people around the world.

1. Introduction

Surgical robotics is changing how doctors carry out operations. With these tools, the surgeons attain more precision and more control and they are safe during the surgeries. Robotic surgery with a da Vinci Surgical System has been already used during the last 20 years to perform more general operations like urology, women care, and the heart (Herron, 2020). Such systems are composed of small instruments, cameras, and robotic arms that respond to the actions of the surgeons' hands. This makes the incisions smaller and leads to faster recovery of patients

[1] Uttaranchal College of Health Sciences, Uttaranchal University, Dehradun.
[2] Staff Software Engineer, Turo Inc, San Francisco, CA, USA 94104.
Email: reachshrutigoel@gmail.com[2]
* Corresponding author: Mahimapant@uumail.in

DOI: 10.1201/9781003655121-7

(Ballantyne, 2002). Robot surgery is getting more popular, yet it is rife with barriers. Cost is one of the greatest problems: These are highly unaffordable machines, and most hospitals cannot possibly afford them (Barbash & Glied, 2010). Besides, surgeons also need particular training in order to operate these systems, which may take much time. The concern about robots replacing surgeons should not disturb human beings because in the near future, surgeons would be required to train the machines (Lanfranco et al., 2004). Others are concerned with the possibility of a robot crash during a procedure that could be hazardous or cause delays (Alemzadeh et al., 2016).

At the same time, there are wonderful possibilities for enhancement. Among new technologies, such as AI, sophisticated sensors, and high-speed networks such as 5G, robots may be able to do even better (Yang et al., 2017; Hashimoto et al., 2018). Robotic systems will in the future allow doctors to operate while sitting somewhere else, especially in remote areas or during emergencies (Anvari, M. 2002). To make all this a reality, medical researchers and tech companies will have to work together, problem-solving and making the advance of robotic surgery more equitable.

In short, robotic surgery still has a pleasant future. But with precise planning, proper training and team work, we can utilize these systems to make surgery safer, more advanced and available to patients across the world.

2. Current State of Surgical Robotics

2.1 Leading Technologies and Systems

The use of surgical robots is so prevalent in most hospitals today. One of the most famous systems is called the da Vinci Surgical System, and it involves the application of robotic hands that a surgeon can control with the help of a console. This system allows making movements very precise and offers a clear 3D picture. Fewer and shorter incisions are thus necessary to conduct surgical procedures and patients also recover lightly and quickly (Herron, 2020; Ballantyne, 2002). One has several robot systems now besides da Vinci. The more recent alternatives are the MAKO System used in surgeries over joints, and the Versius System by CMR Surgical (Hares et al., 2021). These machines are more flexible to the hospitals as they are often smaller and easier to install in the standard operating rooms.

New technology is also making these systems smarter. AI and machine learning (ML) are being used to help plan surgeries better and support doctors in making quick decisions during operations (Yang et al., 2017; Hashimoto et al., 2018). Some systems now include augmented reality and haptic feedback, which may help surgeons feel more connected to the procedure by simulating a sense of touch (Pratt et al., 2018). In addition, some hospitals are trying telerobotic surgery, where doctors perform operations from far away using robotic systems and fast 5G networks (Anvari, 2002).

2.2 Applications in Different Surgical Specialities

Today surgical robots are used in many surgical operations. They are commonly used in a urological procedure known as prostate removal (prostatectomy) where steady hands and deft movements are paramount in a small operating area (Herron, 2020; Ballantyne, 2002). Robots help in gynaecology in carrying out myomectomy (removal of fibroids) and hysterectomy procedures. With the above procedures, patients usually recover faster and less blood is made to leave the body (Herron, 2020; Lanfranco et al., 2004) In heart surgery, robots also conduct coronary bypasses with small incisions and surgical repair of heart valves (Ballantyne, 2002; Lanfranco et al., 2004). They can assist in general surgery during such procedures as removal of the gallbladder, colon surgery, and repair of hernia (Herron, 2020; Lanfranco et al., 2004). Robotic machinery such as ROSA and MAKOplasty helps doctors to deploy accurate spine and joint surgery in orthopaedics and neurosurgery. Such systems are used in pre surgery planning as well as during surgery (Alemzadeh et al., 2016; Hares et al., 2021).

Even though robotic systems offer many advantages, they still rely on the skill of the surgeon and the support of the surgical team. If the system has a technical issue or is not used correctly, errors can happen (Alemzadeh et al., 2016). This shows how important it is to have strong training, good teamwork, and regular safety checks in all fields where robotic surgery is used.

3. Emerging Technologies in Surgical Robotics

3.1 Artificial Intelligence and Machine Learning Integration

AI is a novel opportunity in surgical robotics. It supports the machines to become better decision- makers based on learning through experience. AI can assist doctors to conduct robotic surgery in many different ways including before, during, and after the surgery (Yang et al., 2017). In a procedure, such as computer vision, AI may determine the organs or blood vessels. Also, it can help to track surgical instruments and propose the following operations based on the plan (Hashimoto et al., 2018). The part of AI, called ML, examines massive amounts of surgical data. This assists in anticipating patient outcomes, betterment in the performance of surgeries, and the reduction of the possibility of complications (Hashimoto et al., 2018). Training tools are also based on AI. These devices monitor the movement of a surgeon and provide helpful feedback to enhance proficiency (Yang et al., 2017). Eventually, AI can also partially handle small tasks such as stitches or cutting tissue though directly under the surgeon.

Even with these exciting changes, AI must be used carefully. Strong rules and ethical checks are needed to make sure these systems work safely and make fair decisions (Yang et al., 2017).

3.2 Haptic Feedback and Tactile Sensors

The absence of touch is one of the drawbacks of the robotic systems in use today. When using robotic arms, surgeons are unable to feel the softness or hardness of a tissue. This is addressed by a new technology called haptic feedback, which uses specialized sensors to provide a sense of pressure or resistance (Pratt et al., 2018). By simulating touch, these devices assist the surgeon in preventing harm to sensitive tissues.

In order to measure things like force, pressure, or texture, tactile sensors are being developed. This increases precision and makes robotic systems safer (Kim et al., 2020). Additionally, haptic feedback aids in training by enabling novice surgeons to practice using their sense of touch more effectively. Numerous businesses are attempting to incorporate haptic systems into surgical robots of the future (Pratt et al., 2018; Kim et al., 2020).

3.3 Miniaturized and Soft Robotics

Minuscule surgical robots which may be inserted into the body through small cuts or at the point of natural entry are called miniature robotics. They are very often used in endoluminal or minimally invasive procedures, when the access is highly limited (Park et al., 2021). The robots can move and bend and turn inside bodily organs such as the heart and colon. Through soft robotics, the hard materials are substituted by bendable ones. They help when one needs to work with them because they are able to smoothly move with them without causing an injury to soft tissues (Rus, & Tolley, 2015]. Soft robotic arms allow a more safe control, and handling tissues exemplifies one area of such manipulation. Capsule robots are also an area of active research, and in this case the capsules, which are small in size, can travel through the digestive tract and provide image or drug delivery services (Park et al., 2021). Such improvements lead to the possibility of not needing big incisions to treat conditions in hard to reach parts of the body.

While still in early stages, miniaturized and soft robotics offer a future where surgeries are even less invasive, with faster recovery and fewer complications.

4. Challenges in Adoption and Integration

4.1 High Cost and Economic Feasibility

The high cost of surgical robotics is one of the main obstacles to its use. With additional yearly maintenance costs, robotic systems such as the da Vinci Surgical System can cost over $2 million (Barbash, & Glied, 2010). Additionally, costly single-use instruments are required for every surgery. Because of this, robotic surgeries are more expensive than conventional ones.

Such systems are frequently out of reach for smaller clinics and hospitals, particularly in developing nations (Barbash, & Glied, 2010). This restricts access to cutting-edge care. Additionally, some studies have questioned whether the higher cost of robotic surgeries results in better outcomes (Barbash, & Glied, 2010). More research is required to demonstrate long-term financial benefits, and cost-effectiveness is still up for debate.

4.2 Training and Learning Curve for Surgeons

Robotic systems require special training. Even experienced surgeons need to learn new skills to use the robotic console, handle instrument arms, and interpret 3D images (Lanfranco et al., 2004). The learning curve can be steep, especially for complex procedures.

Studies show that early cases often take longer and have more complications than later ones (Lanfranco et al., 2004). Without proper training, the chances of errors or inefficiency increase. Simulation-based training and mentorship are helpful but not yet standard everywhere (Yang et al., 2017).

There is also a shortage of certified training centres in many regions, making it harder for new surgeons to learn robotic techniques.

4.3 Standardization and Regulatory Barriers

As of now, there is no international standard for the development, testing, and application of surgical robots. Various nations adhere to distinct regulations, and certain areas continue to lack well-defined guidelines (Yang et al., 2017). Because of this, it is challenging to swiftly and safely introduce robotic systems to the market.

The approval of AI-assisted robots presents additional difficulties for regulators. ML systems that may alter their behaviour in response to data are challenging to evaluate for safety (Yang et al., 2017). Laws pertaining to informed consent, data privacy, and malpractice liability are still being developed (Tack et al., 2012).

Robotic surgeries run the risk of uneven safety and legal ambiguity in the absence of strict regulations.

4.4 System Reliability Error Management

Although surgical robots are advanced, they are not perfect. Technical failures can happen, like power loss, camera malfunction, or robotic arm errors (Alemzadeh et al., 2016). These failures can delay surgeries or force the team to switch to open surgery, increasing risks for the patient (Figure 2).

A study of adverse events in robotic surgery found several cases of mechanical errors and software faults (Alemzadeh et al., 2016). Proper maintenance, checklists, and emergency protocols are needed to reduce these risks. But not all hospitals are prepared for technical failures, especially in smaller centres.

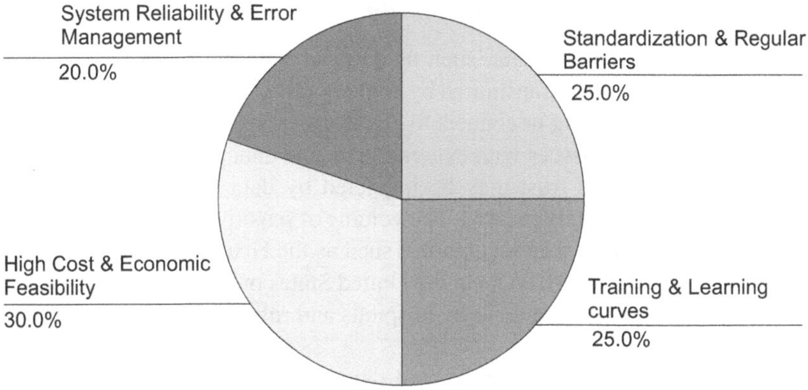

Fig. 1 Shows challenges in adoption and integration of Surgical Robotics (Generated by author).

5. Ethical and Legal Considerations

5.1 Patient Safety and Liability

Patient safety is the most important part of any surgery, including robotic procedures. Even though surgical robots help improve accuracy, errors can still occur due to machine malfunctions, software issues, or surgeon mistakes (Alemzadeh et al., 2016). When something goes wrong, it becomes hard to decide who is responsible—the surgeon, the hospital, or the robot manufacturer.

This creates confusion in legal cases. For example, if an AI feature gives a wrong suggestion, is it the robot's fault or the humans? These questions are still being discussed in courts and among medical experts (Yang et al., 2017; Tack et al., 2012). Clear rules are needed to define liability in robotic surgeries, especially when AI is involved (Amodeo et al., 2018).

5.2 Informed Consent in Robotic Surgeries

Patients are required to provide informed consent prior to any surgery, indicating that they are aware of the procedure's risks and available options. This is more complicated in robotic surgeries. Patients need to be aware that the surgeon will be using a robot and that, if thc surgeon is unfamiliar with the system, there may be technical difficulties or learning curve problems (Lanfranco et al., 2004).

Physicians must explicitly state whether the surgery is conventional or robot-assisted, as well as who will operate the robot and their level of experience (Amodeo et al., 2018). Research indicates that some patients consent to robotic procedures without fully comprehending these issues. Because of this, hospitals should use standard consent forms and improved communication tools (Yang et al., 2017).

5.3 Data Privacy and Cybersecurity

Large volumes of patient data, such as surgical videos, pictures, and medical records, are gathered and transmitted by contemporary surgical robots. Some even enable remote monitoring or connect to cloud systems (Yang et al., 2017; Anvari, 2002). This brings up issues with cybersecurity and data privacy.

Patient safety and trust may be impacted by data breaches or hacking if systems are not adequately secured. The volume of sensitive data rises with the use of more AI tools. Strict data regulations, such as the Health Insurance Portability and Accountability Act (HIPAA) in the United States or comparable local laws in other nations, must be adhered to by hospitals and robot manufacturers (Dinh-Le et al., 2019).

Regular security checks, encrypted data storage, and secure networks are important to prevent such problems. Surgeons and hospitals must also train staff to follow privacy rules while using robotic systems.

6. Opportunities and Future Trends

6.1 Personalized and Precision Surgery

Surgical robotics opens the door to personalized surgery, where treatment is tailored to the unique anatomy of each patient. Using 3D imaging, AI, and robotic tools, doctors can plan and perform surgeries with very high precision (Yang et al., 2017; Hashimoto et al., 2018). For example, robots can help remove a tumor without touching nearby healthy tissues.

AI can also analyse data from previous surgeries to predict the best approach for each patient (Hashimoto et al., 2018). This can reduce complications, shorten surgery time, and improve recovery. As more patient-specific tools like customized implants become available, robotic systems will play a bigger role in delivering precision medicine (Satava, 2020).

6.2 Remote and Telesurgery Potential

Telesurgery means performing surgery when the surgeon is in a different location than the patient, using robots and fast internet. This is already possible in special cases using high-speed connections like 5G (Anvari, M. 2002). Remote surgery can help patients in rural, disaster-hit, or military zones where expert surgeons are not available.

One of the first successful telesurgeries was done in 2001, called the “Lindbergh Operation”, where a surgeon in New York removed a gallbladder from a patient in France (Anvari, M. 2002). Today, robotic systems are more advanced, and 5G technology can reduce time delays and improve control (Marescaux et al., 2001).

6.3 Integration with Augmented Reality and Virtual Reality

Augmented Reality (AR) and Virtual Reality (VR) are becoming powerful tools in surgical robotics. With AR, surgeons can see extra layers of information—like blood vessels or tumour boundaries—over the patient's body during surgery (Pratt et al., 2018). This helps improve accuracy and confidence.

VR simulators are also used to train surgeons without needing a live patient. Surgeons can practice procedures in a virtual setting, making training safer and faster (Yang et al., 2017). Future robotic systems may include AR headsets or 3D overlays that guide surgeons' step by step.

This fusion of robotics and extended reality will greatly improve surgical planning, navigation, and education.

6.4 Robotics in Low-Resource Settings

Surgical robotics is often seen as a luxury, but it can also bring benefits to low-resource settings if made affordable and simple to use. Portable, low-cost robotic systems are being developed for small hospitals and mobile health units (Satava, 2020).

Robots that use battery power, lightweight materials, and modular designs can help bring advanced surgical care to places with limited infrastructure (Satava, 2020; Rivas & Haluck, 2021). AI can also support decision-making in places where trained specialists are few. Organizations and governments must invest in scaling such innovations to close the global surgical gap.

7. Role of Industry and Academia

7.1 Collaborative Innovation

- The growth of surgical robotics depends heavily on partnerships between companies, universities, and hospitals. Industry brings technical knowledge, like building robotic arms, sensors, and software. Academia contributes clinical knowledge, research skills, and medical training (Yang et al., 2017; Satava, 2020).
- Many successful systems, such as the da Vinci robot, were developed through such collaborations. For example, universities often test new robotic tools in clinical trials before they are released for general use (Satava, 2020) These partnerships help ensure that the technology is safe, effective, and based on real surgical needs.
- Government grants and public-private partnerships also support innovation. Together, they help create better, safer, and more affordable robotic systems (Yang et al., 2020).

7.2 Research and Development Strategies

- To keep advancing, the surgical robotics field needs strong research and development (R&D) programs. These focus on areas like AI integration, robotic control systems, miniaturization, and tissue sensing technologies (Yang et al., 2017; Hashimoto et al., 2018; Rus & Tolley, 2015).
- R&D (research and development) teams work to reduce the cost, size, and complexity of robots so they can be used in more places Barbash & Glied, 2010; Satava, 2020). Some teams also explore open-source robotics, which allow developers to share ideas and build affordable systems faster (Yang et al., 2020).
- Academic journals and international conferences like IEEE BioRob or SAGES serve as platforms to share new findings. Industry uses these insights to bring innovations to market.
- To avoid repeating past mistakes, R&D strategies now include safety testing, user feedback, and regulatory input early in the design phase (Yang et al., 2017; Tack et al., 2012).

7.3 Training and Educational Initiatives

- Using surgical robots requires specialized training. Surgeons, nurses, and technicians all need to understand how the robot works, how to troubleshoot problems, and how to switch to manual surgery if needed Lanfranco et al., 2004; Yang et al., 2017).
- Many universities now include robotic surgery training in their medical and surgical programmes. Some hospitals use simulation laboratories and VR to let new surgeons practice before performing real surgeries (Pratt et al., 2018).
- Companies like Intuitive Surgical and Medtronic also run certification programmes for their robotic systems (Satava, 2020). These programmes include hands-on workshops, video-based learning, and team-based simulations.
- Academic–industry partnerships are essential here. Universities provide the learning environment, while companies provide the tools and systems for practice. This combination helps ensure that future surgeons are ready to use robots safely and effectively (Satava, 2020; Yang et al., 2020).

8. Case Studies and Real-World Implementations

8.1 Successful Robotic Surgeries and Outcomes

Robotic systems have been used in many successful surgeries with good patient outcomes. One well-known case is in prostate cancer surgery. The da Vinci robot has helped thousands of surgeons perform robot-assisted prostatectomy with less blood loss, fewer complications, and faster recovery (Herron, 2020; Ballantyne, 2002). Studies show that patients who had robotic prostate surgery returned to normal activities sooner than those who had open surgery (Herron, 2020).

In gynaecology, robotic-assisted hysterectomy has become common for women with fibroids or cancer. It allows for better precision and less pain after surgery Lanfranco et al., 2004). A 2020 study found that robotic hysterectomy patients had shorter hospital stays and lower infection rates compared to traditional methods (Wright et al., 2013).

In cardiothoracic surgery, robotic tools have been used to repair heart valves and perform coronary bypasses through very small incisions. These procedures showed fewer complications, better cosmetic results, and quicker healing (Ballantyne, 2002; Lanfranco et al., 2004).

Even in complex neurosurgical cases, systems like ROSA have helped doctors place electrodes or remove brain tumours more precisely (Hares et al., 2021). These results suggest that, when used properly, surgical robots can lead to better safety and outcomes.

8.2 Institutional Adoption: Success and Results

Many hospitals and medical centres around the world have adopted robotic systems. Institutions like Cleveland Clinic (USA), Apollo Hospitals (India), and Guy's and St. Thomas' NHS Foundation Trust (UK) are leaders in robotic surgery (Satava, 2020; Rao et al., 2021).

The Cleveland Clinic uses robots across specialties, including urology, gynaecology, and general surgery. The hospital has developed detailed protocols, surgeon training programmes, and safety checklists to support robotic procedures (Rao et al., 2021).

In India, Apollo Hospitals introduced robotic surgery in 2006 and now operates one of the largest robotic programs in Asia. Their experience shows that success depends not just on the machine, but also on team training, cost management, and patient education (Rao et al., 2021).

However, not all institutions succeed right away. Some hospitals reported early challenges like high costs, longer operation times, and lack of trained staff (Barbash & Glied, 2010; Lanfranco et al., 2004). But over time, with proper planning and support from both industry and academia, outcomes improved.

Key lessons from these case studies include:

- Start with a few focused specialties
- Invest in structured training
- Track performance data to improve outcomes
- Educate patients on robotic options.

9. Conclusion

9.1 Balancing Technology with Human Expertise

Surgical robotics has brought a major shift in how surgeries are done. Robots now help make surgeries safer, more accurate, and less invasive. However, no matter

Table 1 Outcomes of Real-World Implementations of Robotic Surgery (Generated by author).

Category	*Examples*	*Outcomes*
Successful Robotic Surgeries	Prostatectomy (da Vinci System)	Less blood loss, fewer complications, faster recovery (Herron, 2020; Ballantyne, 2002)
	Robotic Hysterectomy	Shorter hospital stay, lower infection rates, better precision (Lanfranco et al., 2004; Wright et al., 2013)
	Cardiothoracic Surgery	Small incisions, better cosmetic results, quicker healing (Ballantyne, 2002; Lanfranco et al., 2004)
	Neurosurgery (ROSA System)	Precise tumour removal, accurate electrode placement (Hares et al., 2021)
Institutional Adoption	Cleveland Clinic (USA)	Multi-specialty use, structured training, protocols & safety checklists (Rao et al., 2021)
	Apollo Hospitals (India)	Early adopter, large programme, focus on training and cost-efficiency (Rao et al., 2021)
	Guy's & St Thomas' NHS (UK)	Leading UK site, combines research, clinical use, and training (Satava, 2020)
Challenges Faced by Institutions	• High equipment cost • Longer initial operation times • Lack of trained staff	Highlighted need for planning, training, and performance tracking (Barbash & Glied, 2010; Lanfranco et al., 2004)
Key Lessons Learned	• Begin with focused specialties • Invest in structured team training • Monitor data • Educate patients on robotic options	Improved safety, performance, and patient trust over time

how advanced the technology becomes, human expertise remains essential. Robots do not make decisions on their own—they follow the surgeon's commands and require skilled teams to operate safely (Lanfranco et al., 2004; Yang et al., 2017).

The best results come when technology and human judgement work together. Surgeons must understand not just how to operate the robot, but also when it should or should not be used. Proper training, experience, and decision-making are still the foundation of good surgery. As AI becomes more involved, it will be even more important for doctors to supervise, interpret, and guide robotic systems (Yang et al., 2017; Hashimoto et al., 2018).

9.2 *Shaping the Future of Surgery*

Looking ahead, surgical robotics is likely to grow in many ways. New technologies like AI, 5G, haptic feedback, and AR will make surgeries smarter, faster, and more personalized (Yang et al., 2017; Hashimoto et al., 2018; Pratt et al., 2018). Robots may help bring expert care to remote areas through telesurgery (Anvari, 2002; Marescaux et al., 2001). Smaller and cheaper robotic systems may even allow low-resource hospitals to benefit from these advances (Satava, 2020; Rivas & Haluck, 2021).

At the same time, there are challenges. Cost, training, regulation, and patient trust must all be managed carefully. Hospitals, companies, and universities will need to work together to create safe, ethical, and accessible systems for everyone.

In short, surgical robotics is not just about machines—it's about building a future where technology supports human care. With the right balance, we can shape the next era of surgery to be more precise, inclusive, and patient-centred.

References

Alemzadeh, H., Raman, J., Leveson, N., Kalbarczyk, Z. and Iyer, R.K. (2016). Adverse events in robotic surgery: A retrospective study of 14 years of FDA data. *PLoS ONE, 11*(4), e0151470. https://doi.org/10.1371/journal.pone.0151470.

Amodeo, A.M., Patton, C., Avrunin, G.S., Clarke, L.A. and Osterweil, L.J. (2018). Ethical and legal issues in the use of robotic and AI-assisted surgery. In: *Proceedings of the International Symposium on Ethics of Robotics and Artificial Intelligence*.

Anvari, M. (2002). Remote surgery: Robotic telesurgery. *IEEE Engineering in Medicine and Biology Magazine, 21*(3), 94–102. https://doi.org/10.1109/MEMB.2002.1016219.

Ballantyne, G.H. (2002). Robotic surgery, telerobotic surgery, telepresence, and telementoring. *Surgical Endoscopy, 16*(10), 1389–1402. https://doi.org/10.1007/s00464-001-8283-0.

Barbash, G.I. and Glied, S. A. (2010). New technology and health care costs—the case of robotic-assisted surgery. *New England Journal of Medicine, 363*(8), 701–704. https://doi.org/10.1056/NEJMp1006602.

Dinh-Le, C., Chuang, R., Chokshi, S. and Mann, D. (2019). Wearable health technology and electronic health record integration: Scoping review and future directions. *JMIR mHealth and uHealth, 7*(9), e12861. https://doi.org/10.2196/12861.

Hares, L., Roberts, P. and Al-Rubaie, A. (2021). Robotic surgical systems in orthopaedics and general surgery: Current developments and future perspectives. *International Journal of Medical Robotics and Computer Assisted Surgery, 17*(3), e2232. https://doi.org/10.1002/rcs.2232.

Hashimoto, D.A., Rosman, G., Rus, D. and Meireles, O.R. (2018). Artificial intelligence in surgery: Promises and perils. *Annals of Surgery, 268*(1), 70–76. https://doi.org/10.1097/SLA.0000000000002693.

Herron, D.M. (2020). The evolution of robotic surgery. *Surgical Clinics of North America, 100*(2), 295–307. https://doi.org/10.1016/j.suc.2019.11.004.

Kim, Y., Cheng, S., Kim, S., Lee, H., Song, S., Jo, D.H., … & Hahn, S.K. (2020). Recent advances in tactile sensors for intelligent systems. *Advanced Intelligent Systems, 2*(6), 1900188. https://doi.org/10.1002/aisy.201900188.

Lanfranco, A.R., Castellanos, A.E., Desai, J.P. and Meyers, W.C. (2004). Robotic surgery: A current perspective. *Annals of Surgery, 239*(1), 14–21. https://doi.org/10.1097/01.sla.0000103020.19595.7d.

Marescaux, J., Leroy, J., Gagner, M., Rubino, F., Mutter, D. and Vix, M. (2001). Transatlantic robot-assisted telesurgery. *Nature, 413*(6854), 379–380. https://doi.org/10.1038/35096636.

Park, S., Park, S., Song, S.Y. and Kim, B. (2021). Capsule endoscopy and miniaturized robotic devices: Current status and future perspectives. *Biomedical Engineering Letters, 11*, 1–15. https://doi.org/10.1007/s13534-020-00169-5.

Pratt, P., Ives, M., Lawton, G., Simmons, J., Rudarakanchana, N., Yang, G.Z. and Darzi, A. (2018). Through the holographic looking glass: Augmented reality for extremity reconstruction surgery using 3D vascular models with perforating vessels. *European Radiology Experimental, 2*(1), 2. https://doi.org/10.1186/s41747-017-0033-2.

Rao, N.R., Thakar, S. and Kaur, N. (2021). Robotic surgery in India: The way forward. *Journal of Minimal Access Surgery, 17*(4), 453–458. https://doi.org/10.4103/jmas.JMAS_193_20.

Rivas, H. and Haluck, R.S. (2021). Robotic surgery: Review of limitations, clinical impact, and future directions. *American Journal of Surgery, 221*(1), 11–18. https://doi.org/10.1016/j.amjsurg.2020.04.048.

Rus, D. and Tolley, M.T. (2015). Design, fabrication, and control of soft robots. *Nature, 521*(7553), 467–475. https://doi.org/10.1038/nature14543.

Satava, R.M. (2020). Future trends in robotic surgery. *Surgical Endoscopy, 34*(11), 4605–4610. https://doi.org/10.1007/s00464-020-07814-4.

Tack, P., Victor, J., Gemmel, P. and Annemans, L. (2012). The impact of economic and regulatory drivers on the adoption of medical devices: A systematic review. *Health Policy, 106*(3), 231–239. https://doi.org/10.1016/j.healthpol.2012.04.017.

Wright, J.D., Ananth, C.V., Lewin, S.N., Burke, W.M., Lu, Y.S., Neugut, A.I. and Herzog, T.J. (2013). Robotically assisted vs laparoscopic hysterectomy among women with benign gynecologic disease. *JAMA, 309*(7), 689–698. https://doi.org/10.1001/jama.2013.186.

Yang, G.Z., Cambias, J., Cleary, K., Daimler, E., Drake, J., Dupont, P.E., … & Taylor, R.H. (2017). Medical robotics: Regulatory, ethical, and legal considerations for increasing levels of autonomy. *Science Robotics, 2*(4), eaam8638. https://doi.org/10.1126/scirobotics.aam8638.

Yang, G.Z., Nelson, B.J., Murphy, R.R., Choset, H., Christensen, H., Collins, S.H., … & McNutt, M. (2020). Combating COVID-19: The role of robotics in managing public health and infectious diseases. *Science Robotics, 5*(40), eabb5589. https://doi.org/10.1126/scirobotics.abb5589.

8 Artificial intelligence in Cardiac Surgery and Medicine Practice
Hope for the Future

Suresh Babu Kondaveeti[1], Reshabh Saini[2], Kangan Saraswati[3], Jitender Gairolla[4], Ranjay Kumar Chaudhary[5], Sapna[6] and Vivek Kumar Garg[7]*

Modern medicine involves complicated decision-making, which should ideally be founded on structured knowledge, current information, and appropriate analysis within the context of each patient. Clinical decision-making procedures may benefit from the assistance of automated algorithms, sometimes known as artificial intelligence, that can identify and build upon significant trends in data collection. This article reviews clinical cardiology medicine and surgery, both researches that use artificial intelligence. The essay also discusses ethical concerns and future challenges about how automated algorithms will assist physicians in cardiac surgery and medicine more broadly in the future.

1. Introduction

There has been a recent explosion in studies at the nexus of medicine and artificial intelligence (AI). The enormous potential for therapeutic uses of AI is especially likely to benefit cardiovascular care. These tools may enable increased accuracy

[1] Department of Biochemistry, Symbiosis Medical College for Women, Symbiosis International (Deemed University), Pune, India.
[2] University Institute of Pharma Sciences, Chandigarh University, Mohali, Punjab, India.
[3] Chandigarh Group of Colleges, Jhanjeri, Mohali, Punjab, 140307, Chandigarh School of Business, Department of Sciences.
[4] Himalayiya College of Paramedical & Health Sciences, Sparsh Himalaya University, Dehradun, Uttarakhand, India.
[5] Department of Medical Laboratory Sciences, College of applied and Health Sciences, A'Sharqiyah University, P.O. Box-42, Ibra, Sultanate of Oman-400
[6] Saraswati College of Pharmacy, SGC Group, Gharuan-140413, Mohali, Punjab, India.
[7] Department of Medical Lab Sciences (USAHS), Rayat-Bahra University, Mohali, Punjab, India.
Email: ksuresh.babu@smcw.siu.edu.in[1]; dr.reshabhsaini@gmail.com[2]; kangansaraswati97@gmail.com[3]; jeetugairolla1985@yahoo.com[4]; r.choudharymt@gmail.com[5]; sapna92622@gmail.com[6]
* Corresponding author: garg.vivek85@gmail.com

DOI: 10.1201/9781003655121-8

and efficiency, which would improve healthcare for patients as physicians depend more and more on data to make choices. The Covid-19 outbreak also brought attention to the potential of AI developments, particularly the use of remote and high-throughput detection techniques known as healthcare deserts. It will be wise for doctors to comprehend the fundamentals of AI in order to assess the research and technology (Yan et al., 2019).

Medical AI research is advancing at an exponential rate, comparable to the Cambrian explosion in terms of both number and diversity. While some investigations are still in its early phases, others have already started to be used in clinical settings (Nakamura et al., 2022). In the discipline of cardiology, biological data is collected and assessed not only as pictures but also in the form of audio data, such as auscultation, and temporal data, including electrical impulses and electrocardiograms. This characteristic sets cardiology apart from other medical specialties since it makes extensive use of a wide range of biological data (Joshi et al., 2023).

AI is expected to lead to better outcomes for patients, cardiac surgeons, medical professionals, insurance companies, and executive powers globally as it is used more often to solve complicated problems and quantify data. AI holds great promise for helping doctors with risk assessment, medication development, illness treatment, and medical diagnostics (Raman et al., 2023).

2. Artificial Intelligence (AI)

The field of AI is often seen as an engineering discipline that applies innovative ideas to tackle difficult problems. Deep learning (DL) algorithms, a group of automated algorithms that can identify significant patterns in data sets, have been used in a number of domains and have shown revolutionary improvements over current machine learning (ML) algorithms due to the rapidly increasing data requirements in biology and medicine (Xu et al., 2021). As a result, the widespread use of DL algorithms in medicine may produce valuable information and alter the way we develop therapies, classify patients, research diseases, and make decisions. Four biomedical massive information sources are particularly relevant to cardiovascular biomedicine. They include: 1) functional phenotypes, including imaging data, echocardiograms, hemodynamic, demographics, and electrocardiography; 2) biological characteristics obtained from extensive panomics data that have been obtained in clinical settings or big studies; 3) medical information, including patient digital health records that include laboratory test results, doctor's notes, and other data on disease, therapies, and epidemiological research that can be extracted for association research and forecasting on prognosis and drug reactions; and 4) literature skills: it's determined that a new publication in cardiovascular medicine occurs every 2.7 minutes. Although human intellect cannot handle this volume of data, DL systems may be able to mine and organize it (Li et al., 2023).

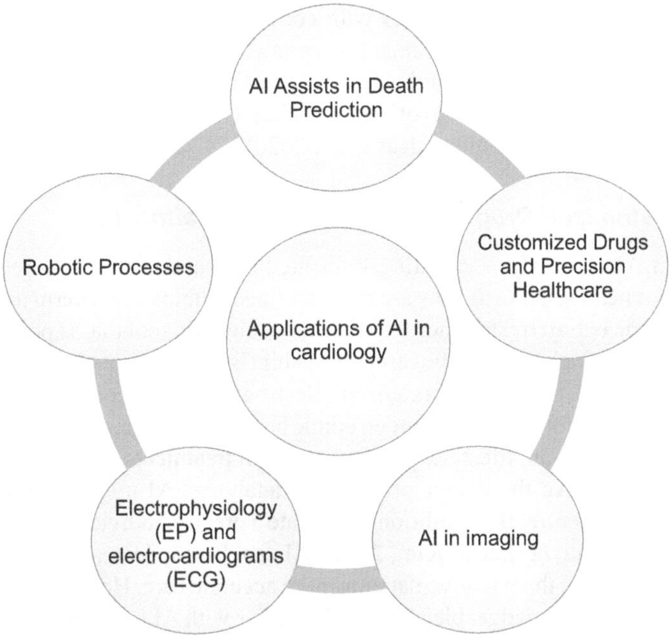

Fig. 1 The various crucial roles of AI in cardiology.

2.1 Artificial Intelligence in Cardiology

In the field of cardiology, promptness, accuracy, and precision are essential to the patient's survival. In addition to saving lives, the doctor's job is to properly comprehend his patient and provide guidance for his general health. A comprehensive AI solution that helps the cardiologist be skilled, quick, and sympathetic to the greater social community can accomplish all of these goals. The following is an overview of the crucial applications of AI in cardiology (Figure 1) (Kulkarni et al., 2021).

2.2 AI Assists in Death Prediction

AI is utilized to accurately forecast the likelihood of a fatality based on data streaming from people's health applications, wearable technology, and patient scan pictures. Techniques used in big data analytics and ML makes these tools feasible (Krishnan et al., 2023).

To calculate the cardiac mortality and myocardial infarction risk, scientists from Cedars-Sinai Medical Center in the USA employed ML in a 15-year prospective ESINER experiment that included 1,912 participants asymptomatically. A myocardial infarction or cardiac mortality occurred in 76 participants throughout the 15-year follow-up time frame for this investigation, which involved the ML integration of diagnostic indicators with coronary artery calcium and automatic epicardial adipose tissue measurement. In contrast to conventional risk assessment, scientists found that ML combining imaging data and clinical risk variables could reliably predict a patient's risk of experiencing a medical condition like cardiac death or heart failure (Commandeur et al., 2020).

2.3 Customized Drugs and Personalized Healthcare

Although AI is slowly permeating both medicine and biology in general, the majority of heart specialists now are more inclined to think of the term as referring to a futuristic extraterrestrial activity than as a scientific tool that is poised to take over medicine, including cardiovascular health (Bonderman et al., 2017).

Based on the patient's unorganized (electronic health record) EHR dataset—which includes information on gender, ethnic background, age, family background, demographic location, lifestyle, previous medical treatments, and vital signs—AI can be used to give the doctor prescriptive analytics. AI might be used by the cardiologist to identify the condition and create a precise, individualized treatment plan for every patient (Lee & Kim, 2021). AI can thereby lessen the workload for doctors and enable them to give patients more accurate care. Health care providers should become knowledgeable about and familiar with AI technology since it can be used to evaluate enormous volumes of data and enhance the identification and management of cardiovascular disease. More AI should ideally be used in precision medicine to offer individualized health care for every patient (Bajwa et al., 2021).

2.4 AI in Imaging

Cardiovascular scanning has emerged as one of the greatest cutting-edge fields of AI study since convolutional neural networks (CNN's) creation and advancement. Although ultrasound echocardiograms (UCGs) are a great non-invasive method for evaluating heart function both quantitatively and qualitatively, the issue is that the sonographer's expertise has a significant impact on how well the UCG is performed. This issue could be resolved using AI. Automatic assessments are performed by an AI system applied to UCG data, while another AI system aids in probe navigation and noise mitigation. Some have previously obtained authorization from the US Food and Drug Administration (FDA) (Lim et al., 2020). Prior to the creation of an AI technology that can detect heart failure with intact ejection fraction, models that can identify heart failure with reduced left ventricular ejection fraction were created. Another excellent illustration of how the AI model may identify anomalies that are invisible to the human eye is this one (Gavaert et al., 2023).

Additionally, image identification in nuclear medicine is evolving quickly. It was shown that ML models using perfusion imaging could determine whether myocardial ischemia was present and forecast how reperfusion therapy would work. The FDA has already given some of them approval for use in clinical settings (Miller et al., 2022).

It is also anticipated that AI would be used in cardiac magnetic resonance imaging (CMR). Atrial fibrillation management is one use of AI for CMR. One of the most interesting developments in CMR is no longer necessary for contrast improvement. The gold standard for noninvasively characterizing cardiac tissue to identify fibrotic or scarred areas is late gadolinium enhancement (LGE) in CMR. However, LGE necessitates the injection of contrast media intravenously, which may be detrimental to individuals with impaired renal function (Villegas-M.M. et al., 2024). Zhang et al. (2021) created virtual native enhancement (VNE)-guided CMR from non-contrast pictures using AI. It produced noticeably higher image quality and had great agreement with LGE in terms of lesion location and quantification. The cardiac computed tomography (CT) system has likewise undergone these developments. Motwani predicted the 5-year all-cause death rate in 10,300 individuals with probable coronary heart disease using deep learning for CT angiography. Doctors and other medical professionals will always be needed, but these advancements will give them more precise tools to identify illnesses, more reliably stratify risk, and improve patient-specific therapy (Zhang et al., 2021).

2.5 Electrophysiology (EP) and Electrocardiograms (ECG)

Due to its non-invasiveness, affordability, and ease of recording and storage, the 12-lead ECG is a frequently utilized modality. When combined with AI, this century-old equipment becomes a cutting-edge tool. All facets of healthcare, including treatment, diagnosis, prognosis, and preventive medicine, can benefit from AI-ECG.

ECG interpretation calls for a particular level of expertise and education. When a cardiologist is not available, rule-based machine diagnosis is frequently utilized. However, there are situations when the precision of traditional rule-based algorithms is insufficient (Martinez-S.M. et al., 2023). Accuracy in diagnosis can be increased by integrating AI into ECG (AI-ECG), and several AI models have been created that perform diagnostically on par with cardiologists. New device development is also being aided by AI-ECG technologies. ECG-compatible smartphones and smartwatches, as well as implantable loop recorders (ILRs), can be utilized as stratification tools to screen the general population for cardiovascular disease and identify high-risk populations. These AI-ECG tools were developed to identify anomalies and align with automated diagnosis to lessen the workload for doctors (Martinez-S.M. et al., 2023).

To demonstrate that AI-ECG can be a diagnostic method for the identification of ventricular abnormalities, Attia et al. developed a CNN model to recognize the individuals without symptoms of left ventricular abnormalities from ECG. In place of neural networks, a related study was carried out using another ML technique (Random Forests). Numerous more intriguing AI models have been documented, such as those that can forecast age, gender, hypokalemia, hypertrophic cardiomyopathy, and other organic heart conditions (Yakamura et al., 2022; Negi et al., 2022).

3. Robotic Processes

AI holds great promise for cardiac procedures such as electrophysiology (EP) for catheter ablation of cardiac arrhythmias and percutaneous coronary intervention (PCI). By automatically maneuvering, AI models may carry out high-precision operations, reducing radiation exposure for medical staff and improving patient safety (Biondi-Z.G. et al., 2025).

The first telerobotic PCI performed on a human was carried out using vascular robotic technology in December 2018 in India. The procedure was carried out remotely, outside of the catheterization lab. Precision cardiac interventional techniques brought achievable by this significant development could be highly beneficial to the patients who have restricted options for cardiovascular treatments. Numerous commercial cardiovascular robotic systems have developed a clinical record for successful robotic PCI treatments in European and African countries. Future devices can carry out vascular interventional procedures with greater precision and safely because of this registry (Kulkarni et al., 2021).

A cutting-edge robotic technology that is popular right now is the da Vinci Surgical technology (Intuitive Surgical, Sunnyvale, California, USA) for heart related surgeries, and have a six degree of freedom. This device's components comprise a side robotic cart having four robotic arms which a doctor controls from a console, an outstanding three dimensional vision system that can expand a picture up to ten times, and a console that the doctor uses during the surgery (Figure 2). The instruments for surgery have connections to three of the robotic arms, whilst the camera is controlled by the fourth arm (Koulazidis et al., 2023).

4. Ethical Considerations and Future Goals

When we are using AI in the medical field, we face many ethical issues like sample collection and patient information should be confidential. For this, strong restrictions and daily monitoring is required. Moreover, as we know AI can misdiagnose or wrongly treat the patients, it can raise many questions of using AI in healthcare (Pham, 2025). The use of AI in Cardiology is also a worrisome situation nowadays. We cannot rely on AI technology for using automated technology in cardiac surgery without human interference.

It's important that we maintain a balanced perspective and use AI as a useful tool instead of as a substitute for medical expertise and judgment. To set up procedures for ongoing human oversight, validation, and meticulous assessment of AI-driven results becomes important (Vanden et al., 2023). Last but not least, while AI techniques excel at assessing well-organized healthcare data, they encounter intrinsic difficulties when it pertains to taking into consideration social aspects

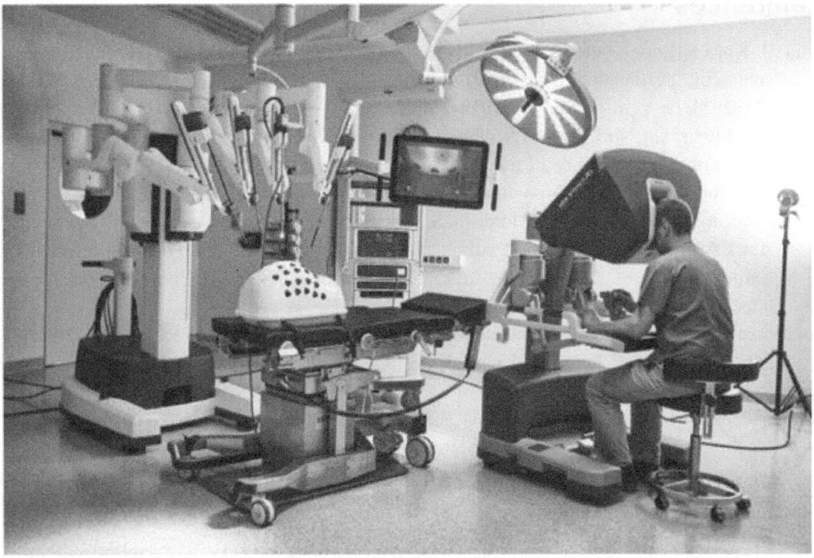

Fig. 2 The da Vinci Surgical System (Sunnyvale, California, USA, Intuitive Surgical) (Koulazidis et al., 2023).

and interpersonal relationships—two outside variables that have a direct effect on health. AI mostly utilizes already accessible healthcare data, often focusing on clinical and biological signs. The role of AI technology in cardiology has a positive future regardless of these difficulties. It is important to establish rules and security procedures so that patient data cannot be breached which ultimately helps in patient privacy (Biondi-Z.G. et al., 2025).

Strict oversight by regulators guarantees that AI technology adheres to the highest standards for reliability, security of information, and integrity. If we can achieve the right balance between technologies and security of the patient data, we may use AI to improve patient care while preserving people's privacy and wellbeing throughout the healthcare system (Farhud & Zokaei, 2021).

5. Conclusion

AI has the ability to revolutionize cardiology as a profession. The benefits of this technology are already being seen in electrophysiology and cardiac imaging. Cardiologists need to employ AI technology to boost workflow efficiency to provide patients precision care. The difficulties of applying AI in medical and research areas should also be understood by clinicians. AI systems should undergo thorough prospective research studies before being applied in cardiology practice. Ethical guidelines should be developed before AI is used, and patients' right to privacy should come first.

References

Attia ZI, Kapa S, Lopez-Jimenez F, McKie PM, Ladewig DJ, Satam G, et al. Screening for cardiac contractile dysfunction using an artificial intelligence-enabled electrocardiogram. Nat Med. (2019) 25:70–4. 10.1038/s41591-018-0240-2.

Bajwa, J., Munir, U., Nori, A. and Williams, B. (2021, Jul.) Artificial intelligence in healthcare: Transforming the practice of medicine. *Future Healthc. J.*, *8*(2): e188–194. [Internet]. [cited 2025 Jun. 24]. Available from: https://pmc.ncbi.nlm.nih.gov/articles/PMC8285156/.

Biondi-Zoccai, G., D'Ascenzo, F., Giordano, S., Mirzoyev, U., Erol, Ç., Cenciarelli, S., et al. (2025, Apr.). Artificial Intelligence in Cardiology: General Perspectives and Focus on Interventional Cardiology. *Anatol. J. Cardiol.*, *29*(4): 152–163. [Internet]. [cited 2025 Jun. 24]. Available from: https://pmc.ncbi.nlm.nih.gov/articles/PMC11965948/.

Bonderman, D. (2017, Dec.). Artificial intelligence in cardiology. Wien Klin Wochenschr., *129*(23–24): 866–868. [Internet]. [cited 2025 Jun. 24]. Available from: https://pmc.ncbi.nlm.nih.gov/articles/PMC5711980/.

Commandeur, F., Slomka, P.J., Goeller, M., Chen, X., Cadet, S., Razipour, A., et al. (2020, Dec.) Machine learning to predict the long-term risk of myocardial infarction and cardiac death based on clinical risk, coronary calcium, and epicardial adipose tissue: A prospective study. *Cardiovasc. Res.*, *116*(14): 2216–2225. [Internet]. [cited 2025 Jun. 24]. Available from: https://pubmed.ncbi.nlm.nih.gov/31853543/.

Farhud, D.D. and Zokaei, S. (2021). Ethical issues of artificial intelligence in medicine and healthcare. *Iran J. Public Health*, *50*(11): i–v. [Internet]. [cited 2025 Jun. 24]. Available from: https://pmc.ncbi.nlm.nih.gov/articles/PMC8826344/.

Gevaert, A.B., Van De Heyning, C.M. and Tromp, J. (2023, Aug.). Artificial Intelligence to Aid Early Detection of Heart Failure with Preserved Ejection Fraction. *JACC Adv.*, *2*(6): 100447. [Internet]. [cited 2025 Jun. 24]. Available from: https://pmc.ncbi.nlm.nih.gov/articles/PMC11198274/.

Joshi, K., Reddy, G.A., Kumar, S., Anandaram, H., Gupta, A. and Gupta, H. (2023). Analysis of Heart Disease Prediction Using Various Machine Learning Techniques: A Review Study. In: *Proceedings IEEE Int. Conf. Device Intell. Comput. Commun. Technol.* (*DICCT*) (pp. 105–109).

Koulaouzidis, G., Charisopoulou, D., Bomba, P., Stachur, J., Gasior, P., Harpula, J., et al. (2023, Sep.). Robotic-Assisted Solutions for Invasive Cardiology, Cardiac Surgery, and Routine On-Ward Tasks: A Narrative Review. *J. Cardiovasc. Dev. Dis.*, *10*(9): 399. [Internet]. [cited 2025 Jun. 24]. Available from: https://www.mdpi.com/2308-3425/10/9/399/htm.

Krishnan, G., Singh, S., Pathania, M., Gosavi, S., Abhishek, S., Parchani, A., et al. (2023). Artificial intelligence in clinical medicine: Catalyzing a sustainable global healthcare paradigm. *Front. Artif. Intell.*, *6*: 1227091. [Internet]. [cited 2025 Jun. 24]. Available from: https://pmc.ncbi.nlm.nih.gov/articles/PMC10497111/.

Kulkarni, P., Mahadevappa, M. and Chilakamarri, S. (2021, Nov.). The Emergence of Artificial Intelligence in Cardiology: Current and Future Applications. *Curr. Cardiol. Rev.*, *18*(3): e191121–198124. [Internet]. [cited 2025 Jun. 24]. Available from: https://pmc.ncbi.nlm.nih.gov/articles/PMC9615212/.

Lee, S. and Kim, H.S. (2021, Sep.). Prospect of artificial intelligence based on electronic medical record. J. Lipid Atheroscler., *10*(3): 282–290. [Internet]. [cited 2025 Jun. 24]. Available from: https://pmc.ncbi.nlm.nih.gov/articles/PMC8473961/.

Li, M., Jiang, Y., Zhang, Y. and Zhu H. (2023). Medical image analysis using deep learning algorithms. *Front. Public Heal.*, *11*: 1273253. [Internet]. [cited 2025 Jun. 24]. Available from: https://pmc.ncbi.nlm.nih.gov/articles/PMC10662291/.

Lim LJ, Tison, G.H. and Delling, F.N. (2020). Artificial Intelligence in Cardiovascular Imaging. Methodist *Debakey. Cardiovasc. J.*, *16*(2): 138–145. [Internet]. [cited 2025 Jun. 24]. Available from: https://pmc.ncbi.nlm.nih.gov/articles/PMC7350824/.

Martínez-Sellés M and Marina-Breysse M. (2023, Apr.). Current and Future Use of Artificial Intelligence in Electrocardiography. *J. Cardiovasc. Dev. Dis.*, *10*(4): 175. [Internet]. [cited 2025 Jun 24]. Available from: https://pmc.ncbi.nlm.nih.gov/articles/PMC10145690/.

Miller, R.J.H., Hauser, M.T., Sharir, T., Einstein, A.J., Fish, M.B., Ruddy, T.D., et al. (2022, Oct.). Machine learning to predict abnormal myocardial perfusion from pre-test features. *J. Nucl. Cardiol.*, *29*(5): 2393–2403. [Internet]. [cited 2025 Jun 24]. Available from: https://pmc.ncbi.nlm.nih.gov/articles/PMC9588501/.

Nakamura, T. and Sasano, T. (2022, Mar.). Artificial intelligence and cardiology: Current status and perspective. *J. Cardiol.*, *79*(3): 326–333. [Internet]. [cited 2025 Jun 24]. Available from: https://www.sciencedirect.com/science/article/pii/S0914508721003361 21.

Negi, S.S., Memoria, M., Kumar, R., Joshi, K., Pandey, S.D. and Gupta, A. (2022). Machine Learning Based Hybrid Technique for Heart Disease Prediction. In: *2022 Int. Conf. Adv. Comput. Commun. Mater.* (*ICACCM*).

Pham T. (2025, May). Ethical and legal considerations in healthcare AI: Innovation and policy for safe and fair use. *R. Soc. Open Sci.*, *12*(5): 241873. [Internet]. [cited 2025 Jun 24]. Available from: https://pmc.ncbi.nlm.nih.gov/articles/PMC12076083/.

Raman, R., Shintre, V., Joshi, K., Prasanthi, G.S.L.B.V., Kaleem, A. and Rajput, K. (2023). Smart Use of Machine Learning in Heart Disease Identification. In: *2023 3rd Int., Conf. Adv. Comput. Innov. Technol. Eng.* (*ICACITE*) (pp. 1169–1174).

Vandenberk, B., Chew, D.S., Prasana, D., Gupta, S. and Exner, D.V. (2023). Successes and challenges of artificial intelligence in cardiology. *Front. Digit. Heal.*, *5*: 1201392. [Internet]. [cited 2025 Jun 24]. Available from: https://pmc.ncbi.nlm.nih.gov/articles/PMC10336354/.

Villegas-Martinez, M., de Villedon de Naide, V., Muthurangu, V. and Bustin, A. (2024, Jul.). The beating heart: artificial intelligence for cardiovascular application in the clinic. *Magn. Reson. Mater. Physics, Biol. Med.*, *37*(3): 369–382. Med [Internet]. [cited 2025 Jun 24]. Available from: https://pmc.ncbi.nlm.nih.gov/articles/PMC11316708/.

Xu, Y., Liu, X., Cao, X., Huang, C., Liu, E., Qian, S., et al. (2021, Nov.). Artificial intelligence: A powerful paradigm for scientific research. *Innovation*, *2*(4): 100179. [Internet]. [cited 2025 Jun 24]. Available from: https://www.sciencedirect.com/science/article/pii/S2666675821001041.

Yan, Y., Zhang, J.W., Zang, G.Y. and Pu, J. (2019). The primary use of artificial intelligence in cardiovascular diseases: What kind of potential role does artificial intelligence play in future medicine? *J. Geriatr. Cardiol.*, *16*(8): 585–591. [Internet]. 2019 [cited 2025 Jun 20]. Available from: https://pmc.ncbi.nlm.nih.gov/articles/PMC6748906/.

Zhang, Q., Burrage, M.K., Lukaschuk, E., Shanmuganathan, M., Popescu, I.A., Nikolaidou, C., et al. (2021, Aug.). Toward Replacing Late Gadolinium Enhancement with Artificial Intelligence Virtual Native Enhancement for Gadolinium-Free Cardiovascular Magnetic Resonance Tissue Characterization in Hypertrophic Cardiomyopathy. *Circulation*, *144*(8): 589–599. [Internet]. [cited 2025 Jun 24]. Available from: https://pubmed.ncbi.nlm.nih.gov/34229451/.

9 The Role of AI and Robotic Aided Plastic Surgery in Skin Cancer Management

D. Jayarajan[1], Sameer Ahmad Sheikh[2], Vivek Chandra Sunori[3], Kangan Saraswati[4], Ranjay Kumar Choudhary[5], Sapna[6] and Vivek Kumar Garg[7*]

Nowadays, an emergent area of study in computer science is artificial intelligence (AI). While AI has been used to predict many diseases, but its use in the dermatology field and robotic surgery procedures is very limited and new. So, this is the need of time for Dermatologists to have solid knowledge about AI as skin disorders, e.g., skin cancer, psoriasis, atopic dermatitis, etc., having a vast dermatoscopic data and images, may be the next great thing in medical AI applications. Apart from plastic surgery, robotic-assisted surgeries have become standard practice in numerous medical specialties throughout the past 20 years. Despite the encouraging outcomes of a number of case series, technological and financial constraints have hindered their implementation in clinical practice. This review article provides a summary on AI recent advancements, its application and ethical issues that are relevant to dermatology and also discuss the possibilities of robotic support in the field of plastic surgery.

[1] Program of Medical Lab Technology, Faculty of Paramedical Sciences, Assam down town University, Sankar Madhab Path, Gandhi Nagar, Panikhaiti, Guwahati, Assam, India, PIN–781026.
[2] Department of Dialysis Therapy Technology, (USAHS), Rayat-Bahra University, Mohali, India 140104.
[3] School of Allied Health Sciences, ARNI University, (Kathgarh), Tehsil Indora, Distt. Kangra, Himachal Pradesh–176401, India.
[4] Chandigarh Group of Colleges, Jhanjeri, Mohali, Punjab,140307, Chandigarh School of Business, Department of Sciences.
[5] Department of Medical Laboratory Sciences, College of Applied and Health Sciences, A'Sharqiyah University, P.O. Box-42, Ibra, Sultanate of Oman-400.
[6] Saraswati College of Pharmacy, SGC Group, Gharuan-140413, Mohali, Punjab, India.
[7] Department of Medical Lab Sciences (USAHS), Rayat-Bahra University, Mohali, Punjab, India-140104.
Email: asairaj123@gmail.com[1]; majeedsameer49@gmail.com[2]; sunorivivek@gmail.com[3]; kangansaraswati97@gmail.com[4]; r.choudharymt@gmail.com[5]; sapna92622@gmail.com[6]
* Corresponding author: garg.vivek85@gmail.com

DOI: 10.1201/9781003655121-9

1. Background

Digital technology, telemedicine, and information technology are increasingly interacting in the area of dermatology. Several efforts have been attempted to use artificial intelligence (AI) for dermatological applications as an outcome of its rising global prominence. In an international survey in 2020, only 23.8% of respondents of 1,271 dermatologists had strong or exceptional knowledge of how to use AI in their field, with 85.1% of respondents being aware of the AI technology use in the area of dermatology (Gamolin et al., 2020). Promoting what dermatologists themselves see as a developing, advantageous, and possibly required component of the field requires informing stakeholders on the current state of AI. So, in this review, we tried our best to provide a basic knowledge about AI and its use in dermatology and how it helps in patient care (Sengupta, 2023).

2. History of Artificial Intelligence

The power of computer systems to acquire information from inputs or retrospective data is known as artificial intelligence (AI), sometimes called machine intelligence (ML). When a machine simulates the cognitive processes associated with learning and problem-solving that are present in the human brain, the term AI is frequently employed. The article, "On Computable Numbers, With an Application to the Entscheidungs Problem", was written by mathematician Alan Turing. A lot of individuals consider this paper as the foundational work of the computer era (Xu et al., 2021). The concept of "effective calculability", which was established as the framework for the computational models known as "algorithm", was defined by Turing and his Princeton colleague Alonzo Church utilizing calculus. The term AI was initially used in 1956 at a renowned conference organized at Dartmouth College. Researchers in the medical field realized that AI could be used in the life sciences around the beginning of the 1970s (De A., et al., 2020). Nevertheless, AI use was further restricted by technological constraints. Improved hardware and software advancements over the past 20 years have increased computer capacity, which allowed us to understand the potential of AI to help improve present medical treatments. Nowadays, many researches are going on in many medical fields, including dermatology. As circumstances evolve and more dermatological AI studies are conducted, it is anticipated that the application of AI technology in dermatology will significantly decrease the distance between clinicians across different hospital levels and increase diagnosis accuracy (Bajwa et al., 2021).

3. Categories and Terminologies of AI

AI can be broadly classified into two categories: weak AI and strong AI. "Artificial general intelligence", or strong AI, gives machine intelligence comparable to that of a person. This intricate device needs to be able to learn how to perform various types of activities on its own. Machines with the ability to think ethically, be conscious, and multitask fall under this wide category. But as of right now, such sophisticated devices are a long way off.

At the moment, we only have weak or narrow AI, where a machine learns to accomplish a particular action. It is necessary to develop distinct programs to carry out distinct jobs when AI is weak (Sufyan et al., 2023).

4. Analytics, Training, Confidence

In analytics, artificial neural networks (ANN) are adaptable algorithms or mathematical models that can find intricate nonlinear relationships in big information. When mistakes made in response to small algorithmic changes are fixed (training), machines learn and the accuracy of the predictive model (confidence) gradually increases (Kantidakis et al., 2022).

4.1 Machine Learning (ML)

ML is a branch of AI that focuses on developing computer algorithms that can acquire knowledge from data and make choices or forecasts on their own. These models constantly improve their accuracy by using learned data. Arthur Samuel coined the term "machine learning" in 1959 to refer to "the ability of computers to learn without programming new skills directly" (Yazici et al., 2023). An ML algorithm that is backed by a mathematical model produces predictions or certain conclusions based on the datasets that are available. Supervised and unsupervised learning are the two primary categories of ML. In a supervised setting, datasets of problems and their solutions are supplied into the system. Through trial and error, machines are able to determine the right answer. Machines evaluate input data in unsupervised learning without a predetermined solution (Kufel et al., 2023).

4.2 Deep Learning (DL)

One ML method that instructs computers and other devices to function logically is called deep learning (DL). It draws inspiration from the human brain's structure. After decades of studies and development, DL—which started out as ANNs—has become significantly more efficient than conventional ML methods (Taye, 2023). By continuously evaluating data in accordance with a predetermined logical structure, DL algorithms seek to reach judgments that are comparable to those made by humans. DL enables machines to perform human-like activities by manipulating text, audio, or image information similarly to humans. Neural networks are a multi layered structure of algorithms used in DL to do this. DL entails delving deeply into a network's many layers, including its hidden layer. Complex information is gleaned when one delves deeper. The iterative learning techniques used in DL expose computers to enormous amounts of data (Manakitsa et al., 2024).

4.3 Artificial Neural Network (ANN)

ANNs which are made up of several perceptrons, or "neurons", that process and send data, are similar to the human brain. Finding out how they work starts with entering data, including text, voice, or pictures. Before arriving at the output, this data is processed by the network's successive layers of perceptrons. The input data is handled by many neurons in each layer. Neural networks find extensive application in speech identification, picture identification, natural language processing, and stock price prediction (Kufel et al., 2023).

5. AI Use in Dermatology Y

The most practical use of AI in dermatology is the analysis of photographs, mainly for psoriasis, ulcers, and possible skin malignancies. Specialists can increase the effectiveness and precision of their diagnosis by using AI based on image recognition, even if typical dermatological assessments are dependent on manual observation, which can be subjective and challenging to quantify.

5.1 Recognition of Cancers

An extensive and expanding collection of studies shows that AI applications can successfully differentiate between benign nevi and melanoma in the early stages. These applications are based on the fundamental idea that lesions in dermatoscopic or non-dermatoscopic pictures can be dissected into separate pixels for analysis. Jafari et al. provide a representative example of an application that analyzes photos pixel by pixel and extracts 60 attributes to forecast the categorization of diseases (Li et al., 2022). The capacity of these applications to accurately diagnose lesions is usually compared to that of qualified dermatologists in order to validate them. Using 48 melanoma-screening tools, Safran et al. reviewed photo recognition applications and found that the average sensitivity was 87.60% and the average specificity was 83.54%. Because of the increased interest in this subject, an international skin imaging competition was established in 2016 and has been held yearly ever since. Despite the increased robustness of these applications, there are still few prospective clinical trials and ongoing discussions about recognized implementation difficulties (Gomolin et al., 2020).

Additionally, a growing number of original investigations have started to categorize non-melanoma skin malignancies (also called keratinocyte carcinomas) as distinct from pre-malignant and benign lesions. An AI model created by Spyridonos et al., for instance, has a sensitivity of 91.7% and a specificity of 89.8% in distinguishing between actinic keratosis and healthy skin. Overall, the majority of research on skin cancer shows both the expanding evidence for therapeutic benefit and technological viability. It has still to be proven whether or not these technologies can be used and depended upon in routine clinical practice (Melarkode et al., 2023).

AI has been applied to more than just photo identification. In addition to processing picture pixels, apps can also extract trends by processing numerical values in different sequences. Tan et al., for instance, presented an application that used initial evaluation visit data, such as patient age and tumor size, to predict the complexity of micrographic Mohs surgery. They were able to develop an early model that might be applied to prioritize Mohs referrals and triage patients. Despite the fact that photo identification algorithms form the basis of the majority of AI and skin cancer research, there are additional options (Pinto-C.L., 2023).

5.2 *Skin Inflammatory Disorders*

To the detection of skin inflammatory disorders such as psoriasis, dermatitis and acne (Figure 1) AI can be used for the categorization and examination of dermatological images. Additionally DL methods have been used to predict the effectiveness of biological treatments. This is achieved by including essential clinical data such as patient demographic data, past medical history and the occurrence of comorbidities, which enables more effective and personalized therapies (Goessinger et al., 2024).

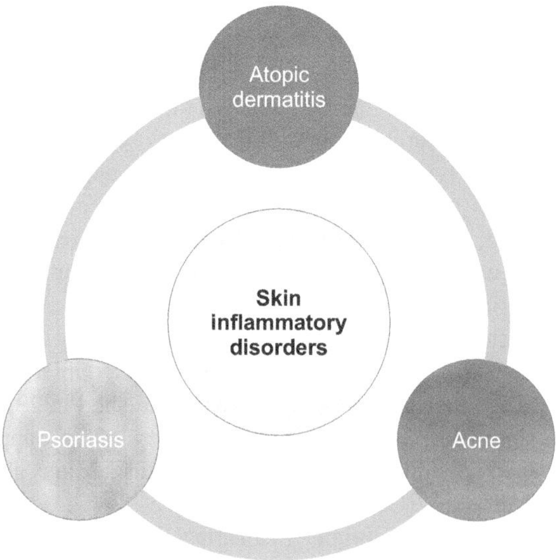

Fig. 1 Skin inflammatory disorders.

The significance of ML and natural language processing in electronic health record (EHR)-based phenotyping was illustrated by Gustofson's team use of an ML-based phenotypic method to recognize patients with atopic dermatitis (AD) and its integration of code information with the collected EHRs to attain a high positive estimation value and sensitivity in 2017. An ANN technique was established, to assess the impact of air pollutants and weather fluctuations on AD patients. The result of the data demonstrated a significant correlation between the severity of AD symptoms and outdoor temperatures, relative humidity, precipitation, PM10, NO2, and O3 (Patella et al., 2020).

Yin Yang et al. created a new acne grading algorithm in 2021 that used DL to categorize facial acne severity in accordance with Chinese criteria. The model showed a high correlation with dermatologists. Ultimately, Liu et al. presented a novel overall pruning strategy in 2022 to use DL models for precise acne detection and classification. Several base models were trained using the suggested approach, and redundant models were removed based on diversity and performance. The system outperformed previous studies with an excellent forecasting accuracy of 85.82% on the acne dataset (Traini et al., 2025).

According to research by Shrivastava et al. (2016), psoriasis patients' skin photos may be classified as either healthy or sick with an accuracy of about 99% once color, texture, and redness are extracted from the photographs. Other study teams have focused on distinguishing psoriasis from pictures of other prevalent skin conditions, such as seborrheic dermatitis or atopic dermatitis, which are frequently confused with psoriasis (Shrivastava et al., 2016). For example, when tested on 100 fresh photos, Zhao et al. used CNNs to categorize 8,021 photographs of nine prevalent illnesses from patients in a Chinese hospital, outperforming 25 Chinese dermatologists. Similar to this, several scientists have investigated the use of DL models to apply dermatoscopic pictures, in addition to skin images, for AI-based diagnosis. In order to differentiate between seborrheic dermatitis and scalp psoriasis, a new diagnostic technique was created that was more accurate than dermatologists who had received dermoscopy training. For the purpose of studying psoriasis, several research teams have combined AI algorithms with skin CT scans and confocal laser scanning microscopy (Goessinger et al., 2024).

6. AI in the Creation of Cosmetics

Designing and optimizing individual cosmetic chemicals is now part of the application of AI and ML in cosmetic formulation, which goes beyond the creation of completed products. This comprises basic ingredients including perfumes, polymers, surfactants, and preservatives, all of which are essential to the safety, functionality, and appearance of cosmetic items (Di Guardo et al., 2025). Conventional techniques of developing ingredients are normally based on expert view and continuous testing. These techniques, however, are laborious, resource-intensive, and have a limited capacity to investigate large chemical regions. However, AI-powered approaches facilitate the virtual screening, estimation, and creation of novel compounds with precise characteristics, facilitating speedy invention while adhering to legal, safety, and sustainability necessities (Chen et al., 2023).

Tong and colleagues were the first to present a technique for modeling virtual makeup applications in 2007. This approach used a computer-based technology known as "cosmetic transfer", which replicated makeup impacts on an individual's face by utilizing the ratio of before and after makeup photographs. Three aligned images with the same 2D geometry were used to figure out these effects pixel-by-pixel. It was admitted that this technique failed to produce perfect results, even though it was successful in producing realistic cosmetic transfers. More complex AI-based algorithms have now been created to evaluate facial traits for cosmetic purposes (Di Guardo et al., 2025).

6.1 Robotic-Aided Plastic Surgery

Since the beginning of robotic-assisted surgery (RAS), the application of robots in plastic surgery has been intriguing. In a Minipig model, the da Vinci method was used to harvest and anastomose the very initial free flap in 2005. Van der Hulst employed the da Vinci technique for microsurgical anastomosis, and the first clinical studies were published in 2007. Despite stating that the robotic-assisted anastomosis took longer than a typical one, they admitted that there was a rapid learning curve (Aitzetmüller et al., 2022).

A mastectomy and rapid breast reconstruction using implants were performed in 2017 using the da Vinci system. Toesca et al. hence adopted a 2.5 cm axillary strategy. After connecting an insufflator for proper preparation, the mastectomy was carried out. The authors once more reported a drastic learning curve, which is consistent with earlier research. According to them, the first strategy took three times as long as the third. The final approach's surgical time was similar to that of a mastectomy performed without robotic support. Furthermore, RAS made it possible to simultaneously improve the cosmetic result and lessen adverse effects like bleeding and increased circulation (Lee et al., 2025).

Transoral techniques including tumor removal and regeneration using free or local flaps have also made use of the da Vinci technology. Therefore, by making access easier and enabling procedures in confined spaces, the robotic technology made the anastomosis easier. Transoral robotic surgery, or "TORS", is safe, according to a number of case studies and reports (Nehma et al., 2017).

7. Prospective Research Paths

7.1 Advanced Robotics for Detecting Skin Cancer

Skin cancer can be detected more accurately with the assistance of robots. Existing robots, such as the Vectra WB360, track melanoma and non-melanoma skin cancer non-invasively by combining 3D photographs with the matching sequential digital dermoscopic scans. The WB360's photographic analysis creates a body map to document the progression of the lesions and provides a worldwide perspective of the skin's surface. This function is highly helpful in quickly identifying any questionable developments (Melarkode et al., 2023).

7.2 *Using Wearable Technology to Diagnose Skin Cancer*

One paradigm that deals with the computation of human-wearable equipment is wearable technology. Wearable computers are any compact, data-processing devices that are portable and can be carried on the body. The recognition of malignancy has made use of wearable computers. The high level of fragile nature, bendability, non-cooperative form factor of the sensors utilized, unsuitable connectivity, clinical inertia, and, finally, the expense and awareness surrounding wearable technology are some of the obstacles that have prevented widespread clinical acceptance thus far. Future studies and businesses should focus on lowering costs while addressing the difficulties associated with wearable technology as a crucial substitute for cancer diagnosis (Dobbelstein, 2016).

Regarding computational efficacy, increased productivity, adaptability, power consumption, and enhanced real-time performance, these event-driven tools are advantageous. In order to improve performance, it might be advantageous to integrate these tools into wearable technology (Ghadi et al., 2025).

8. The Legal and Ethical Views

Despite the obvious benefits, there are also several ethical issues with the application of AI in clinical settings and healthcare. There is uncertainty surrounding the use of informed consent when using health AI, even if it is intended to change the patient-clinician interaction. It is unclear to the professionals under what conditions they should or should not disclose to the patient that AI is a part of their interaction (Farhud & Zokaei, 2021). Decisions made by AI are very important, and they present safety and transparency issues. Even though it is acknowledged that no AI model can be 100% accurate, making the wrong choice can be lethal and can also make the right choice seem risky. This raises questions about the bias and fairness of model algorithms.While there are many potential advantages of AI in healthcare, it must be understood that as the foundation of the whole framework, ethical and legal issues must be resolved before it can be used commercially (Melarkode et al., 2023).

Some unresolved issues in the detection of skin cancer using methods based on DL and ML are depicted in Figure 2.

9. Conclusion

Dermatologists are depending on AI for better analysis and image recognition of skin lesions. AI is rapidly developing in the dermatology profession. It might drastically change the way that patients are treated, particularly when it comes to increasing the sensitivity and precision of skin lesion detection, including for cancer. However, in order to conduct in-depth study, AI research needed clinical and images data of all skin kinds, which must be produced through enhanced international skin imaging cooperation. Unintentional bias in the model's prediction

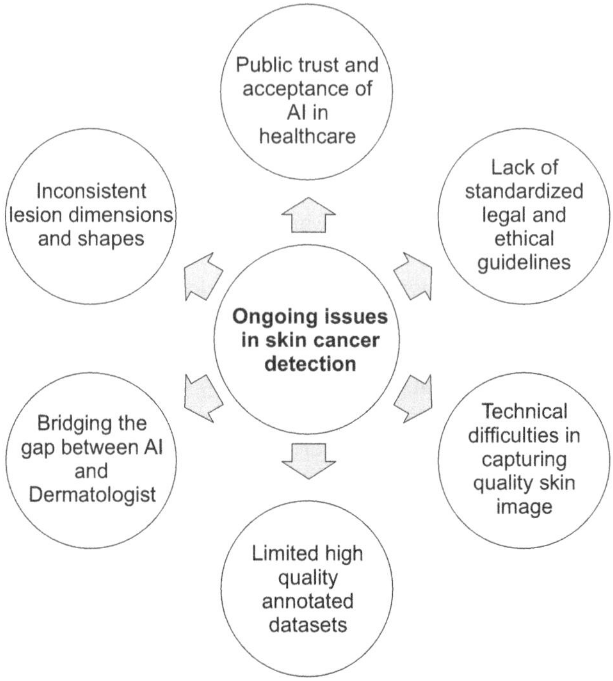

Fig. 2 Ongoing issues in skin cancer detection.

is caused by the ethical and legal difficulties in the AI study as well as the absence of clinical data on various skin types.

It is still unclear how robotic surgery will be used in clinical plastic and cosmetic surgeries. Although many plastic surgeons claim a lack of widespread adoption or exposure, practitioners are actively interested in the transferability of these prospective benefits into a specialty that collaborates with other surgical fields. As wearable technology and robots advance, AI healthcare can be integrated into these new developments to calm the tense market. There is potential to enhance automated skin cancer screening, even though the few data suggests that people who are enthusiastic about implementing AI healthcare are on level with those who are opposed to it. New techniques that fuse cutting-edge imaging with AI-powered analysis are opening up new avenues for continuous evaluation, real-time diagnosis, and efficient workflows. These developments demonstrate the increasing clinical maturity of AI in dermatology and reaffirm its value as a valuable tool for treatment and diagnostic decision-making, with real advantages for both patients and healthcare systems.

References

Aitzetmüller, M.M., Klietz, M.L., Dermietzel, A.F., Hirsch, T. and Kückelhaus M. (2022, Jun.). Robotic-Assisted Microsurgery and Its Future in Plastic Surgery. *J. Clin. Med., 11*(12): 3378. [Internet]. [cited 2025 Aug 13]. Available from: https://pmc.ncbi.nlm.nih.gov/articles/PMC9225011/.

Bajwa, J., Munir, U., Nori, A. and Williams B. (2021, Jul.). Artificial intelligence in healthcare: transforming the practice of medicine. *Futur. Healthc. J., 8*(2): e188–194. [Internet]. [cited 2025 Aug 13]. Available from: https://pmc.ncbi.nlm.nih.gov/articles/PMC8285156/.

Chen, W., Liu, X., Zhang, S., Chen S. (2023, Mar.). Artificial intelligence for drug discovery: Resources, methods, and applications. *Mol. Ther. Nucleic Acids, 31*: 691–702. [Internet]. [cited 2025 Aug 13]. Available from: https://www.sciencedirect.com/science/article/pii/S2162253123000392.

De, A., Sarda, A., Gupta, S. and Das S. (2020). Use of artificial intelligence in dermatology. *Indian J. Dermatol., 65*(5): 352. [Internet]. [cited 2025 Aug 13]. Available from: https://pmc.ncbi.nlm.nih.gov/articles/PMC7640800/.

Di Guardo, A., Trovato, F., Cantisani, C., Dattola, A., Nisticò, S.P., Pellacani, G., et al. (2025, Jul.). Artificial Intelligence in Cosmetic Formulation: Predictive Modeling for Safety, Tolerability, and Regulatory Perspectives. *Cosmetics, 12*(4): 157. [Internet]. [cited 2025 Aug 13]. Available from: https://www.mdpi.com/2079-9284/12/4/157/htm.

Dobbelstein D. (2016, May). Unobtrusive interaction for wearable computing. In: *Conf. Hum. Factors Comput. Syst.- Proc.* (pp. 203–207). [Internet]. [cited 2025 Aug 13]. Available from: https://dl.acm.org/doi/10.1145/2851581.2859016.

Farhud, D.D. and Zokaei S. (2021, Oct.). Ethical Issues of Artificial Intelligence in Medicine and Healthcare. *Iran J. Public Health, 50*(11): i. [Internet]. [cited 2025 Aug 13]. Available from: https://pmc.ncbi.nlm.nih.gov/articles/PMC8826344/.

Ghadi, Y.Y., Shah, S.F.A., Waheed, W., Mazhar, T., Ahmad, W., Saeed, M.M., et al. (2025, Dec.). Integration of wearable technology and artificial intelligence in digital health for remote patient care. *J. Cloud Comput., 14*(1): 1–25. [Internet]. [cited 2025 Aug 13]. Available from: https://journalofcloudcomputing.springeropen.com/articles/10.1186/s13677-025-00759-4.

Goessinger, E.V., Gottfrois, P., Muelle, A.M., Cerminara, S.E. and Navarini, A.A. (2024, Nov.). Image-Based Artificial Intelligence in Psoriasis Assessment: The Beginning of a New Diagnostic Era? *Am. J. Clin. Dermatol., 25*(6): 861–872. [Internet]. [cited 2025 Aug 13]. Available from: https://pmc.ncbi.nlm.nih.gov/articles/PMC11511687/.

Gomolin, A., Netchiporouk, E., Gniadecki, R. and Litvinov, I. V. (2020, Mar.). Artificial Intelligence Applications in Dermatology: Where Do We Stand? *Front. Med., 7*: 100. [Internet]. [cited 2025 Aug 13]. Available from: https://pmc.ncbi.nlm.nih.gov/articles/PMC7136423/.

Gustafson, E., Pacheco, J., Wehbe, F., Silverberg, J. and Thompson, W. (2017, Sep.). A Machine Learning Algorithm for Identifying Atopic Dermatitis in Adults from Electronic Health Records. In: *Proceedings - 2017 IEEE Int. Conf. Healthc. Informatics (ICHI)* (pp. 83–90). [Internet]. [cited 2025 Aug 13]. Available from: https://pmc.ncbi.nlm.nih.gov/articles/PMC5664951/.

Kantidakis, G., Hazewinkel, A.D. and Fiocco, M. (2022). Neural Networks for Survival Prediction in Medicine Using Prognostic Factors: A Review and Critical Appraisal. *Comput. Math Methods Med., 2022*: 1176060. [Internet]. [cited 2025 Aug 13]. Available from: https://pmc.ncbi.nlm.nih.gov/articles/PMC9553343/.

Kufel, J., Bargieł-Łączek, K., Kocot, S., Koźlik, M., Bartnikowska, W., Janik, M., et al. (2023, Aug.). What Is Machine Learning, Artificial Neural Networks and Deep Learning?: Examples of Practical Applications in Medicine. *Diagnostics, 13*(15): 2582. [Internet]. [cited 2025 Aug 13]. Available from: https://pmc.ncbi.nlm.nih.gov/articles/PMC10417718/.

Lee, S.B., Kim, J., Chung, I.Y., Kim, H.J., Lee, J.W., Son, B.H., et al. (2025, Dec.). Use of the Da Vinci SP surgical system in robot-assisted nipple-sparing mastectomy: A single-center, retrospective study. *Sci. Rep.*, *15*(1): 12. [Internet]. [cited 2025 Aug 13]. Available from: https://pmc.ncbi.nlm.nih.gov/articles/PMC11696119/.

Li, Z., Koban, K.C., Schenck, T.L., Giunta, R.E., Li, Q. and Sun, Y. (2022, Nov.). Artificial Intelligence in Dermatology Image Analysis: Current Developments and Future Trends. *J. Clin. Med.*, *11*(22): 6826. [Internet]. [cited 2025 Aug 13]. Available from: https://pmc.ncbi.nlm.nih.gov/articles/PMC9693628/.

Liu S, Fan Y, Duan M, Wang Y, Su G, Ren Y, Huang L, Zhou F. AcneGrader: An ensemble pruning of the deep learning base models to grade acne. Skin Res Technol. 2022 Sep;28(5):677-688. doi: 10.1111/srt.13166.

Manakitsa, N., Maraslidis, G.S., Moysis, L. and Fragulis, G.F. (2024, Jan.). A Review of Machine Learning and Deep Learning for Object Detection, Semantic Segmentation, and Human Action Recognition in Machine and Robotic Vision. *Technologies*, *12*(2): 15. [Internet]. [cited 2025 Aug 13]. Available from: https://www.mdpi.com/2227-7080/12/2/15/htm.

Melarkode, N., Srinivasan, K., Qaisar, S.M. and Plawiak, P. (2023, Feb.). AI-Powered Diagnosis of Skin Cancer: A Contemporary Review, Open Challenges, and Future Research Directions. *Cancers* (*Basel*), *15*(4): 1183. [Internet]. [cited 2025 Aug 13]. Available from: https://pmc.ncbi.nlm.nih.gov/articles/PMC9953963/.

Nehme, J., Neville, J.J. and Bahsoun, A.N. (2017, Sep.). The use of robotics in plastic and reconstructive surgery: A systematic review. *JPRAS Open*, *13*: 1–10. [Internet]. [cited 2025 Aug 13]. Available from: https://www.sciencedirect.com/science/article/pii/S2352587817300219.

Pinto-Coelho, L. (2023, Dec.). How Artificial Intelligence is Shaping Medical Imaging Technology: A Survey of Innovations and Applications. *Bioengineering*, *10*(12): 1435. [Internet]. [cited 2025 Aug 13]. Available from: https://www.mdpi.com/2306-5354/10/12/1435/htm.

Safran T, Viezel-Mathieu A, Corban J, Kanevsky A, Thibaudeau S, Kanevsky J. Machine learning and melanoma: the future of screening. J Am Acad Dermatol. (2018) 78:620–1. 10.1016/j.jaad.2017.09.055.

Sengupta D. (2023, Nov.). Artificial intelligence in diagnostic dermatology: Challenges and the way forward. *Indian Dermatol. Online J.*, *14*(6): 782–787. [Internet]. [cited 2025 Aug 13]. Available from: https://pmc.ncbi.nlm.nih.gov/articles/PMC10718130/.

Shrivastava, V.K., Londhe, N.D., Sonawane, R.S. and Suri, J.S. (2016, Apr.). Computer-aided diagnosis of psoriasis skin images with HOS, texture and color features: A first comparative study of its kind. *Comput. Methods Programs Biomed.*, *126*: 98–109. [Internet]. [cited 2025 Aug 13]. Available from: https://www.researchgate.net/publication/291386628_Computer-Aided_Diagnosis_of_Psoriasis_Skin_Images_with_HOS_Texture_and_Color_Features_A_First_Comparative_Study_of_Its_Kind.

Spyridonos P, Gaitanis G, Likas A, Bassukas ID. Automatic discrimination of actinic keratoses from clinical photographs. Comput Biol Med. (2017) 88:50–9. 10.1016/j.compbiomed.2017.07.001.

Sufyan, M., Shokat, Z. and Ashfaq, U.A. (2023, Oct.). Artificial intelligence in cancer diagnosis and therapy: Current status and future perspective. *Comput. Biol. Med.*, *1*: 165.

Tan E, Lin F, Sheck L, Salmon P, Ng S. A practical decision-tree model to predict complexity of reconstructive surgery after periocular basal cell carcinoma excision. JEADV. (2017) 31:717–23. 10.1111/jdv.14012.

Taye MM. (2023, Apr.). Understanding of Machine Learning with Deep Learning: Architectures, Workflow, Applications and Future Directions. *Comput.*, *12*(5): 91. [Internet]. 5 [cited 2025 Aug 13]. Available from: https://www.mdpi.com/2073-431X/12/5/91/htm.

Toesca A, Peradze N, Manconi A, Galimberti V, Intra M, Colleoni M, Bonanni B, Curigliano G, Rietjens M, Viale G, Sacchini V, Veronesi P. Robotic nipple-sparing mastectomy for the treatment of breast cancer: Feasibility and safety study. Breast. 2017 Feb;31:51-56. doi: 10.1016/j.breast.2016.10.009.

Traini, D.O., Palmisano, G., Guerriero, C. and Peris K. (2025, Jun.). Artificial Intelligence in the Assessment and Grading of Acne Vulgaris: A Systematic Review. *J. Pers. Med.*, *15*(6): 238. [Internet]. [cited 2025 Aug 13]. Available from: https://pmc.ncbi.nlm.nih.gov/articles/PMC12194645/.

Patella V, Florio G, Palmieri M, Bousquet J, Tonacci A, Giuliano A, et al. Atopic dermatitis severity during exposure to air pollutants and weather changes with an Artificial Neural Network (ANN) analysis. Pediatr Allergy Immunol [Internet]. 2020 Nov 1 [cited 2026 Feb 24];31(8):938–45. Available from: /doi/pdf/10.1111/pai.13314

Xu, Y., Liu, X., Cao, X., Huang, C., Liu, E., Qian, S., et al. (2021, Nov.). Artificial intelligence: A powerful paradigm for scientific research. *Innovation*, *2*(4): 100179. [Internet]. [cited 2025 Aug 13]. Available from: https://pmc.ncbi.nlm.nih.gov/articles/PMC8633405/.

Yang Y, Guo L, Wu Q, Zhang M, Zeng R, Ding H, Zheng H, Xie J, Li Y, Ge Y, Li M, Lin T. Construction and Evaluation of a Deep Learning Model for Assessing Acne Vulgaris Using Clinical Images. Dermatol Ther (Heidelb). 2021 Aug;11(4):1239-1248. doi: 10.1007/s13555-021-00541-9.

Yazici, İ., Shayea, I. and Din J. (2023, Aug..). A survey of applications of artificial intelligence and machine learning in future mobile networks-enabled systems. *Eng. Sci. Technol. and Int. J.*, *44*: 101455. [Internet]. [cited 2025 Aug 13]. Available from: https://www.sciencedirect.com/science/article/pii/S2215098623001337.

Zhao S, Xie B, Li Y, Zhao X, Kuang Y, Su J, et al. Smart identification of psoriasis by images using convolutional neural networks: a case study in China. J Eur Acad Dermatol Venereol [Internet]. 2020;34:518–24. 10.1111/jdv.15965.

10 Enhancing Medical Competence Using AR and VR Techniques

Chugh, Pinki[1*], Bhowmick Sangita[2], Sinha, Rahul[3] and Quazi Taif Sadat[4]

Surgical education is under pressure from increased complexity of procedures, limitations on working hours, and the need for patient safety. Traditional apprenticeship models alone are not sufficient to overcome these challenges. This systematic review explores how the use of Augmented Reality (AR) and Virtual Reality (VR) technologies in surgical training reshapes the training, by reviewing seven core studies and fifty peer-reviewed articles in various surgical specialties.

AR and VR technologies are extremely advantageous to surgical procedures in preoperative planning, intraoperative guidance, and technical skill acquisition. In research, procedural accuracy, efficiency, and confidence of the trainee are reported to be enhanced. However, there are still significant challenges: the haptic feedback is not very realistic, the image quality is still not up to the mark, and there is inconsistency in the integration of the curriculum. Moreover, the platforms currently available are not very helpful in terms of upgrading skills in communication, decision-making, and other such non-technical areas. Also, the question of whether these technologies are cost-efficient is still unanswered, and the sector is without standard validation protocols.

Innovations that are coming include sophisticated haptic devices, AI-based personalized learning, and remote-mentoring platforms for collaborative learning. This paper, by combining technical and pedagogical analyses of recent publications, is different in a way. We put forward the two most urgent tasks: constructing standardized validation frameworks and designing non-technical skill training modules for AR/VR platforms.

1. Introduction

Surgical training has typically been centred around the apprenticeship method of learning which was innovatively introduced by William Halsted, and is most

[1] Department of Computer Science, Uttaranchal Institute of Technology, Uttaranchal University, Dehradun, India.

[2] Director, Bangladesh University, Bangladesh.

[3] Student, UIT, Uttaranchal University Dehradun, India.
Email: taif@bu.edu.bd[4]

* Corresponding author: pinki.haridwar@gmail.com

DOI: 10.1201/9781003655121-10

simply described as "see one, do one, teach one". This model is heavily focused on the direct experiential learning of an activity under the guidance of a specialist, wherein the trainee slowly but surely takes on more autonomy. It was the main instrument of surgical education and skill enhancement for a time span of many years. Nevertheless, the challenges of surgical training which are of a nature and scale never before seen, render this model less and less adequate.

While case complexity goes up, technology advances, trainees are limited in the number of hours they can work, and patient safety concerns are raised, there is an urgent need to find new educational methods. On top of that, ethical concerns about patient outcomes are forcing trainees and staff surgeons to master skills in nonclinical settings before applying them to live patients. Though the cadaver model has been the most favoured one because of its closeness to real life, it also has some drawbacks, like different tissue fidelity, being single-use, difficult to obtain, and having expensive limits on replacement.

Among the most groundbreaking changes in medical education over the past ten years is simulation-based education. Simulation is any form of controlled activity that imitates a system or environment for the purpose of evaluating, educating, or changing the behaviour of the participants. It is necessary for the simulation to be able to offer a safe, repeatable, efficient, and affordable learning experience (from the point of view of patient risk and costly resources). As a result of providing immersive and interactive learning environments, XR (extended reality) technologies—which encompass VR (virtual reality), AR (augmented reality), and MR (mixed reality)—will still have that evaluative function and, consequently, will challenge surgical training to evolve further.

(VR) crafts complete computer-generated environments that the users get to experience personally and where they can interact through visual, auditory, and haptic feedback, while they are cut off from any external distractions. AR, however, follows a different path: it superimposes digital information—such as text, 3D objects, or annotations—onto real-world views taken from cameras or screens. MR is a step further, as it enables digital and real-world components to interact with each other continuously and in real-time. Some of the recent innovations in smartphone technology have resulted in making these "extended reality" (XR) devices simple and lifelike enough to be used in medical training at a much quicker pace

Presently, surgeons resort to these technological advances in various specialties. In general surgery, they facilitate laparoscopic methods and liver-related operations. Neurosurgeons employ them for tumor location. Maxillofacial surgeons to the utilization in dental implants and the creation of the jaw reconstruction plan. Orthopedic techniques that involve the use of the hardware include the fixation of the fracture as well as the positioning of the implant. Furthermore, the cardiovascular, thoracic, and ear-nose-throat surgeries are likewise able to take advantage of both the training simulations and the real-time intraoperative guidance.

This article focuses on how VR and AR have become the main factors in reshaping surgical-education routines. We base our arguments on seven pivotal studies and around 50 more peer-reviewed articles, evaluating the present implementations, the influence on skills and performance of the trainees, and probing into the future of these technologies. While the existing literature substantiates the AR/VR benefits, very few papers have systematically discussed as a review the development of technical and non-technical skills, documented the changes in learning outcomes due to device upgrading, or evaluated validation methods in different medical specializations. We respond to these quandaries by integrating technical analysis with education theory and the practical side of implementation, thus, producing the correct understanding of the future training programmes for the community of the researchers and educators.

2. Technological Foundations of Extended Reality in Surgical Contexts

XR technologies to train the surgical skills of medical students are dependent on three interrelated factors: the devices, the haptic feedback systems, and the software. Knowledge of these parts not only explains the potential of AR/VR in training but also their present ceilings.

2.1 The Extended Reality Spectrum

VR is a technology that completely takes the users into a world generated by the computer. It's generally done via devices that are mounted on the head and, to strengthen the feeling of being there, the sounds and touches are also made to correspond with the virtual environment. On the contrary, augmented reality is an alternative that is less invasive, as it simply superimposes the digital data like 3D anatomical models, measurements, and annotations onto the live videos of the real world that are taken by the camera. MR is a concept which is in between these two, as it allows the digital and the physical objects to interact with each other dynamically and, therefore, making it more difficult to separate the real from the virtual.

The first VR and AR devices had to be connected to an external computer and they could only produce limited graphics. Today "Phase 2" devices take advantage of the innovations that have been made in the field of smartphones: displays with very high resolutions, mobile processors with great computing power, and very sensitive motion sensors. These changes have contributed in lowering the prices significantly and thus, making the technology available to a larger number of training programmes have dramatically lowered costs and made the technology accessible to more training programmes.

2.2 Hardware: Head-Mounted Displays

VR and AR systems are fundamentally reliant on the use of head-mounted (HMD) displays. Examples of VR headsets like Oculus Rift, HTC Vive, and Google Daydream completely block out the user's view of the real world, thus creating full immersion. On the other hand, AR gadgets including Microsoft HoloLens, Magic

Leap One, and Vuzix M300 have transparent displays that superimpose the digital content over the direct view.

The HMD sector is still very much a battle ground. It is hard for universities to standardize their equipment or maintain long-term research when companies such as ODG R7, for instance, close their operations and therefore frequently disappear from the market. Besides these issues, there are also some problems that are still waiting for a solution: the users report that the eyestrain, nausea, and headaches (usually known as "cybersickness") which are caused by the use of such devices, while device weight, battery life, and wireless connectivity are the factors that limit the duration of training sessions.

2.3 Haptic Feedback

Haptic systems provide tactile feedback that simulate the physical things that happen—tissue resistance, texture differences, the feeling of instruments cutting or suturing. However, these machines are still struggling from a technical point of view to reproduce very subtle sensations such as a scalpel slicing through skin layers or a saw engaging bone while they enhance the surgical realities.

2.4 Software and Tracking

Essentially, advanced software is required for the operation of AR/VR. These programmes transform the raw data of medical imaging provided by CT (computed tomography) scan, MRI (magnetic resonance imaging), or laser scanning into 3D anatomical models. In order to align these models with the real patient in real- time, which is a crucial process for surgical guidance, image registration algorithms are used for AR applications.

The problem of tracking precision has remained. In general, it is easier to follow stiff anatomical parts such as bone and brain, but soft tissues like liver, intestines, heart, that are breathing, beating, and being surgically manipulated are hard to be figured out. Precisely recording such a dynamic movement still accounts for the biggest challenge. Besides that, tracking systems are far from being flawless: optical sensors require an unobstructed line-of-sight and cease functioning when it is blocked, while electromagnetic sensors suffer from the presence of metal surgical instruments.

3. Applications of AR/VR across Surgical Specialities

AR and VR technologies are changing surgical practice in three major areas: preoperative planning, intraoperative guidance, and skills training.

3.1 Preoperative Planning and Patient-Specific Modelling

Traditional 2D scans are confined to how surgeons visualize complicated anatomy. VR and AR technologies change CT, MRI, and cone-beam imaging into interactive

3D patient models, thus enabling surgeons to look through anatomy and plan their procedures in great detail before they can be at the operating room.

To decide the best dental implant size, place, and angle, the jaw, head, and face surgeons utilize these models. Apart from that, they also practice jaw realignment operations and plan facial reconstruction.VR for liver surgery is a far cry from that as it segments complex vascular and tumour anatomy automatically, thus giving surgeons a guide for resection boundaries.

Orthopedic surgeons have recourse to VR for joint replacement planning, implant position-testing virtually, and mechanical conflicts checking that could limit the range of motion. The virtual rehearsal method, in this case, allows surgeons to try different approaches and anticipate the complications even if they have not yet made their first cut.

3.2 Intraoperative Navigation and Image Guidance

AR offers direct real-time "x-ray vision" by vividly overlaying preoperative plans or non-visible anatomical structures right on the surgical area. Surgeons get to see subsurface anatomy without depending on the mental 3D reconstruction of the flat images.

Dental surgeons are using AR systems like Image-Guided Implantology (IGI) for implant placements with navigation errors that are around 0.35mm. Neurosurgeons utilize AR for tumour localization and the training of residents in procedures, such as ventriculostomy catheter insertion. The orthopedic field features applications such as hip and knee replacement alignment, pedicle screw insertion in spine surgery, and fracture reduction. The AR-KNEE system is very close to achieving the precision needed for joint replacement with a margin of error within 1–2mm. But, these advantages are accompanied by some sacrifices: the process of setting up and using AR navigation can be time-consuming and as a result, surgeons have to decide whether the gain in precision is worth the loss of their working time.

3.3 Simulation-Base Training for Technical Skills

VR and AR simulators provide standardized, risk-free practice settings that allow trainees to repeat procedures and get instant feedback. Numerous studies reveal tangible improvements: trainees get faster, more precise, and acquire better hand-eye coordination, as well as bimanual dexterity. Simulators, as opposed to conventional training which relies on the availability of patients and access to the operating room, offer regular practice that can be done at any time.

- **OMFS:** Voxel Man Simulator for virtual apicoectomy, VR-MFS system for Le Fort 1 maxillary surgery with haptic feedback, and haptic-enabled digital cephalometric analysis.
- **Neurosurgery:** AR for ventriculostomy training and ImmersiveTouch system for accelerating learning curves.

- **Orthopedics:** Immersive VR simulators are used in orthopedic training to help residents visually and practically align implants, place pedicle screws, and repair fractures. Research indicates that these simulators lead to higher skill results than conventional old training models.
- **Other Specialties:** Such innovations have been used in the areas of urology (inflatable penile prosthesis, ureteroscopy), gynaecology (myoma localization, uterosacral ligament suspension), general surgery (liver models, breast cancer), otolaryngology (temporal bone dissection), and vascular surgery (vascular access).

4. Pedagogical Impact of AR/VR in Surgical Training

AR and VR technologies have a major impact on surgical education far beyond their sheer technical usage. They basically dictate how trainees acquire skills, develop self-assurance, and retain information over time—the key elements that ultimately determine whether learning can be applied to actual clinical settings.

Nevertheless, existing systems concentrate almost solely on technical skills. The following generation of AR/VR training should be non-technical competences: situational awareness, communication under pressure, stress tolerance, and being efficient members of a team. The developers should focus on scenario-based learning modules and multi-user environments that necessitate real collaboration. There is a need for more studies on how teams perform in VR settings and using the analytics to that way of skills which are difficult to quantify.

4.1 Evidence for Accelerated Skill Development

Literature is consistent in showing that VR and AR technologies expedite the learning process at the initial stage. VR trainees are reported to be able to do the same operations as usually trained ones in 18–43% less time and with fewer mistakes. In one of the studies, it was found that after only 10 times of practice, laparoscopic procedures performed by AR-trained residents were 30.9% faster and the number of mistakes was significantly lower. Senior orthopedic residents who engaged with an IVR system demonstrated over 570% learning efficiency improvement in comparison with the traditional paper-based method.

Moreover, it should be pointed out that the difference in performance may become smaller over time as learners who are trained in the traditional way will get to the same level. Nevertheless, the initial learning curve advantage is still very significant and can have an impact on clinical practice.

4.2 Cognitive and Affective Outcomes

These are only some of the benefits that come from VR training in the clinic. Clinical reasoning, diagnostic skills, and patient assessment capabilities are all improved through VR training. A very common feedback from the trainees is that they feel more confident and that they are able to better evaluate their own performance, which is an important metacognitive skill, by means of self-reflection. Moreover, AR-enhanced curricula have resulted in a 40% increase in self-assessed preparedness as well as a clear rise in knowledge-based testing.

4.3 Retention and Real-World Application

Unexpectedly, VR training seems to be a variable that contributes to skill retention that is more prolonged as compared to skills gained through a traditional training method even though the evidence for this is quite sparse. Studies on transfer-of-training, which only focus on the testing of skills obtained through VR to lead to enhanced performance in actual surgery, have, in fact, been mostly positive. The issue, however, is the methodological problem: most of the studies have very short follow-up periods of only weeks or months. Therefore, we do not have enough evidence of the skills being at the same level over several years which is a time period that is important for clinical practice.

4.4 The Non-Technical Skills Deficit

There is a significant drawback in the current AR and VR platforms for the training of technical skills, which is the major factor. However, a surgical operation needs more than just hand skills. Clinical judgment, talking to patients and colleagues, being a good team player, and handling the situation under acute stress are the factors that are of the same level of importance to the medical practice. A single research team has even gone so far as to describe surgery as the use of "expert anatomical knowledge, spatial visualization, judgement, and inter-professional teamwork" whereas the present simulators come close to addressing only about one-fourth of that".

5. Validation Studies and Comparative Effectiveness

Surgical simulators need continuous validation to prove that they actually improve real-world performance. The field has standard frameworks for this, but implementation has been inconsistent at best.

5.1 The Validation Landscape

There are four core types of validity that are most often considered by researchers. Face validity queries if the simulator appears and behaves in a way that is believable to the users—basically a subjective check of realism. Content validity looks at whether the device actually teaches the skills that were the goal of the programme, again relying on feedback from the users. Construct validity offers objective evidence that a device can differentiate between a novice and an expert. Transfer validity, which can be considered the most important one, is a test of whether the skills learned in a simulation lead to improvements in the actual performance of an operation.

Messick proposed a more in-depth framework which included content representation, cognitive processes during training, internal structure, relationships with external variables, and real-world consequences. Despite these established standards, the literature is characterized by what the researchers have termed a "validation deficit". In many studies, only face and construct validity are considered, whereas the authors neglect response processes and downstream consequences. It is not a small methodological point that this greatly limits the extent to which we can make conclusions about whether these costly technologies have any effect.

5.2 How VR/AR Stacks Up

Comparative data is mostly in favour of virtual training, at least for the first time. Trainees using VR or AR are able to acquire skills faster, they make fewer mistakes, and they also have a higher level of confidence than those who are using traditional methods. The advantage seems to be the strongest one in the early learning curve; with more practice, students who have been trained in the conventional way are often able to catch up.

It is an interesting fact that user preference does not always correspond with the results of learning. Some studies indicated that trainees preferred cadaveric models because of their better tactile feedback, thus revealing a very obvious weakness in the current haptic simulation. However, VR has been at least as good as video-based training and has been, in general, better than box trainers for specific procedural tasks. Immersive VR seems to be especially efficient for the education of residents when compared to bench models or synthetic alternatives.

5.3 The Translational Evidence Gap

McGaghie's translational outcomes framework is a reality check of sorts. It hierarchically classifies the educational impact starting from mere acquisition of basic knowledge (Level 1) through change in behaviour in clinical environments (Level 3) to quantifiable patient benefit (Level 4) and effects at the system level like cost reduction or sustained competency (Level 5).

VR and AR in surgical training have been found in a recent systematic review to very rarely have a Level 3 effectiveness that is beyond behavioural changes. Behavioural changes have been demonstrated—residents trained in VR are different in the OR. But direct patient outcomes? Cost-effectiveness? Skill retention over time? The data are simply not available yet.

The current investment in AR/VR development has been driven primarily by the perceived ability to teach discrete psychomotor skills. However, establishing actual value to healthcare systems—and, significantly, to patient outcomes—requires a paradigm change toward rigorous, long-term, outcomes-focused research.

6. Data Sources and Study Selection

Our evaluation is conceptually founded in seven fundamental studies that jointly established the technological landscape and initial efficacy data for AR/VR surgical training.

We then chose about 50 peer-reviewed articles from a corpus of more than 100 references to guarantee a thorough evidence base. The following were given priority in the selection criteria:

- Empirical studies with quantitative performance outcomes
- Systematic reviews and meta-analyses
- Research employing established validity frameworks (Messick, McGaghie)
- Multi-institutional or high-impact studies
- Work addressing technology stacks, implementation barriers, pedagogical outcomes, validation methods, ethics, and future developments

This two-tiered approach balanced foundational understanding with current empirical evidence.

6.1 Data Extraction and Thematic Synthesis

Each study's design, participant demographics, AR/VR technology utilized, surgical specialty, control conditions, outcome measures, and major findings were all collected.

Through an iterative evaluation of the literature, the retrieved data underwent theme synthesis. After identifying recurrent ideas, approaches, and conclusions, we categorized them thematically:

- Technological Foundations (hardware, software, haptics, tracking).
- Applications across Surgical Specialties (e.g., orthopedics, neurosurgery, laparoscopy).
- Pedagogical Impact (skill acquisition, confidence, retention, transferability).
- Validation Studies (face, content, construct, transfer validity, Levels of Effectiveness).
- Comparisons with Traditional Training Modalities.
- Cost, Scalability, and Curriculum Integration Challenges.
- Ethical, Legal, and Patient Safety Implications.
- Emerging Innovations and Future Directions.

This thematic organization facilitated the identification of consistent patterns, contradictory evidence, and significant research gaps. We critically analysed findings to explain their implications rather than simply summarizing results.

7. Results and Discussion

The entire field has changed as a result of the usage of AR and VR in surgical education. Preoperative planning, intraoperative guiding, and skill acquisition have already begun to be impacted by these technologies in ways that were not even feasible ten years ago. This part of the study is about the literature review on their effectiveness, educational value, and the practical problems of implementation.

When compared to traditional training methods, AR/VR has nearly always been associated with performance gains. The warning here is that the majority of the evidence is derived from small groups of participants in one location, frequently with follow-ups lasting only a few weeks or months. The issue remains uncertain as regards the retention of skills over years or the training improvements being transferred into better patient outcomes. Frustratingly, the data on both concerns is still inconsistent.

What we need, but do not yet have, are extensive multicentre trials with common outcome metrics and reasonable timescales. Until then, the most we can say is that pricey curriculum selections are being founded on suggestive yet incomplete evidence.

8. Effectiveness of AR/VR in Surgical Skill Acquisition in and Knowledge Retention

Researchers consistently find that AR and VR increase surgical skill learning. VR training helps surgeons finish treatments 18–43% faster and make fewer mistakes than conventional training. According to meta-analyses, standardized means differ by 0.5–1.5. Compared with standard training cohorts, VR trainees make 3–9 times fewer errors and achieve 20–50% greater instrument placement accuracy.

For anatomically complex procedures, AR applications excel at spatial visualization and real-time guidance. Navigation errors in dental implant placement can be as low as 0.35mm with angular deviations under 4 degrees. The accuracy of AR-guided drilling and screw fixation is significantly better than freehand techniques. There are some AR procedures that take longer initially, but this is because trainees achieve submillimetre accuracy. Training purposes justify this trade-off.

These technologies enhance cognitive and emotive outcomes in addition to technical proficiency. VR promotes clinical reasoning, patient evaluation skills, and knowledge retention. Trainees report more confidence and develop higher self-assessment capabilities—crucial for independent skill enhancement. AR programmes enhance objective knowledge scores by around 40% in certain studies, with matching gains in self-perceived preparation. During preoperative planning, Microsoft HoloLens users demonstrated enhanced affective states, less cognitive load, and quicker reaction times.

8.1 Validation Types Reported and Comparative Performance Outcomes

Rigorous evaluation of AR/VR surgical simulators depends on recognized validity frameworks: face, content, construct, and transfer validity.

According to scholars, the field suffers from a "validation deficit". Numerous research only looked at a few aspects of validity, mainly ignoring the effects of response processes. Even worse, some continue to use antiquated metrics like face validity, which are essentially assessments of subjective reality with no quantitative rigour. This weakens their conclusions greatly. Even well-known systems exhibit this pattern: Google Glass and Perk Station have low ratings despite favourable user reviews, whereas Microsoft HoloLens performs well across validity measures.

AR and VR are often favored by comparative performance data. Compared to traditional approaches, these technologies increase student confidence, improve accuracy, and speed up initial skill learning. Early in training, the advantage seems to be greatest; with more practice, group performance frequently converges.

9. Technological Challenges: Latency, Fidelity, and Haptics

Various technologies and technical limitations have and still are the main causes why the use of AR/VR for educational purposes in the medical field is not yet very popular and widespread. A less than very realistic haptic feedback is and will be for a long time the biggest reason why it will be hard to get doctors to use VR/AR for learning the touch-related specialties. Getting the touch of a tissue cutting understandably or a bone being sawed, with enough accuracy, is almost impossible—users frequently point out that non-sufficient haptics is the factor that disappoints them most in a digital learning environment.

Better visual capabilities might pose new issues as well. The differences in resolution, refresh rates that are not stable, and even the extent of the fields of view are all factors that diminish the experience of a user. Cone-beam CT y is quite effective for the replication of the structure of bones, however, it does not allow for a clear picture of soft tissues and also produces some artefacts that can confuse the user when it comes to the degree of realism of the anatomy. Real-time registration of flexible organs such as the liver and intestines that are not only moving due to breathing but also changing in shape because of surgical manipulation, as well as their simulation, is a tough problem that has not yet been resolved by the research team. For this reason, AR applications for the bone and brain can be more effectively used than for soft tissues.

There are certain weaknesses, which are the limitations of the tracking systems, they were not able to be eliminated totally. It is possible that detectors become blocked by a process worker, as well as antioxidants that cannot find a beam of sight get into a failure situation and electromagnetic machines are disturbed by metals. In addition, the HMD human business sector's uncertainty makes these problems worse. To put it shortly, the HMD sector is not stable in general and the problems related to it are not easy to overcome in addition to the ones arising from the tracking systems. Research and curriculum developments experience difficulties due to these inconveniences as companies that have long been around like ODG R7 shut their doors (one example). When the support of the community for a particular type of hardware fades, hardware gets orphaned, platforms lose support, and academic programmes remain with costly obsolete equipment.

The ergonomic issues are a further reason for the hesitation of some people towards wearing an HMD for a long period of time. If the HMD is used for an extended period of time, then the phenomenon that the researchers in the respective fields call "cybersickness" will most likely occur, which means that the user will be affected by eyestrain, nausea, and headaches. The weight of the device as well as the way in which it is put on are the reasons why it cannot be used comfortably for a prolonged period of time. The use of a wireless connection along with limited batteries might bring about the interruption of a procedure even at its most crucial moment.

9.1 Logistical Barriers: Cost, Standardization, and Faculty Training

An important, yet mostly unaddressed, question is how hardware and software integration can be economically viable. The costs of hardware have gone down—there are now some functional VR systems that cost less than $2,000—but software licensing and updates are still costly. Despite of the frequent proclamations of cost-effectiveness, rigorous quantitative analyses are almost completely missing. Economic benefit is most of the time taken for granted without showing the real evidence especially when it comes to long-term follow-up like retention of skills or decrease in complication rates.

The muddle of methods in research papers makes it impossible to draw significant conclusions. The designs of studies as well as the selection of participants, interventions, and measures of outcomes differ drastically among studies, so it is not possible to carry out meta-analysis. This heterogeneity results from non-standardization because the field is not at a stage where it can agree on research protocols, validated outcome measures, or educational standards for simulators.

The requirements for the installation of the system further increase the obstacles. To implement AR/VR, secure networks, high-performance computing, and sophisticated data management are needed. Apart from that, curriculum redesign and faculty training are some more logistical problems that the institutions, in most cases, take for granted.

10. Future Directions: AI Tutors, Telementoring, and Long-Term Outcome Validation

AR/VR surgical training is globally set to improve significantly as innovations to the technologies that support it are being developed to remove the limitations that have been identified so far.

AI Integration: Artificial intelligence integration can be deemed the next step after AR/VR systems are already capable of monitoring performance and providing objective feedback, that is, a base for AI integration. AI-driven instruments can evaluate motor skills, foresee the level of proficiency, and furnish momentarily personalized feedback that suits the particular learner. This move from the use of general simulations to a customized training regimen may have a tremendous impact on the time it takes for a person to be trained.

Advanced Haptics: In order for the work to move forward, it depends largely on the haptic technology that is able to reproduce the sensations of the interaction of the tissues. The issue of closing the "reality gap" is still the most important one for successful transfer of skills from the simulation to the actual practice.

Remote Mentoring: AR permits telementoring, whereby an expert surgeon can give a newly qualified doctor directions through visual and auditory signals, even if these two are not in the same place, and this in real-time. This could be the way to opening the gate to the general public for advanced surgical skills, by the means of the underprivileged or distant areas. The multi-user platforms will support the training of the teams who, through the exercises, will become not only better at this, but will develop skills of communication and coordination, etc.

Next-Generation Systems: Further enhancements in quality of the image, the resolution, and the field of view will help the user be more immersed and feel as if he is really present in the place when wearing the HMD. As tracking and spatial registration become more efficient, AR/VR systems might also turn out to be the less cumbersome and expensive alternatives to traditional surgical navigation methods. The hybrid programs comprising AR/VR and conventionally used training methods are likely to benefit from the advantages that each of them possess.

Above importantly, the field needs to develop a worldwide consensus on uniform research processes and frameworks for validation. In the lack of similar, high-quality studies, claims about the long-term clinical and economic value of AR/VR should be considered speculative presumptions.

11. Conclusion and Future Directions

This extensive research investigated the application of AR and VR in surgical education by thoroughly examining a large body of scholarly work. We sought to clarify the technological foundation, educational applications, proven effectiveness, and future potential of immersive simulation while thoroughly analysing current challenges. The study shows that offering surgical education via secure, consistent, and unbiased platforms has significantly enhanced skill acquisition, procedural precision, and confidence in various specialties using AR/VR technology

There are significant learning benefits. Studies consistently show reduced error rates and shorter operation times; AR/VR enhances precision and decreases the learning curve (Mao et al., Gurusamy et al., Pulijala et al., 2019; Vera et al., Logishetty et al.). These platforms enable focused practice without adverse effects, reducing patient risk during training and enhancing clinical safety (Suresh et al.,

McKnight et al., 2020). They also facilitate consistent instruction, allowing for a data-driven method of evaluating competencies and presenting students with complex situations at an equivalent level (Suresh et al., Goh et al., 2023)

However, there are significant barriers to wider adoption. Inconsistent methodology and inadequate use of thorough validity frameworks, particularly in relation to long-term retention and patient outcomes, are the causes of a persistent "validation deficit" (Suresh et al., Williams et al., 2022).

Cadaveric models are frequently chosen for tactile realism due to unresolved technical issues, such as insufficient haptic feedback and unrealistic simulation of deformable anatomy (McKnight et al., 2020; Goh et al., 2023). The majority of AR/VR tools prioritize technical skills over non-technical ones, undervaluing clinical judgement, teamwork, and situational awareness (Ayoub & Pulijala, 2019; Suresh et al.). Adoption is further complicated by high costs, unclear long-term cost-effectiveness, and challenges with integration within strict curricula (McKnight et al., 2020; Sheik-Ali et al., 2019; Goh et al. 2023).

It is a clear ethical requirement that surgeons receive training in secure, simulated settings prior to providing patient care. This obligation calls for AR/VR platforms to become rigorously validated, pedagogically integrated parts of surgical education as their next stage of development.

Many of the innovations will probably influence the field's trajectory. Incorporating AI will allow training to be more custom-made through the use of smart tutoring, real-time analytics, and skill prediction modeling (Sheik-Ali et al., 2019; Suresh et al.). The use of tele-mentoring and multi-user platforms can help to remove geographical barriers that limit access to expert surgical advice, increase global training potential, and facilitate non-technical skill development through the use of simulated team-based activities (Sheik-Ali et al., 2019; Goh et al., 2023; McKnight et al., 2020).

In order for AR/VR to be used at the highest level, there needs to be a shift in research focus. Nowadays, the goal of the research is level 3 outcomes—changes in behaviour, however, the field should show level 4 and 5 effects: better patient outcomes and benefits to the health sector such as cost savings (Suresh et al., Goh et al., 2023). This involves bigger sample sizes, follow-up over a long period, and varied types of outcome measures. Standards at the international level concerning validation, cost-effectiveness reporting, and research methodology will help create policy, attract institutional funding, and obtain regulatory approval (Williams et al., 2022; Suresh et al., Goh et al., 2023).

AR/VR is evolving from a simple experiment to an increasingly important component of surgical training because of the continuous interdisciplinary collaboration, strict validation, and careful integration into the curriculum, these devices may be the means to not only create surgeons who are technically skilled but also holistically competent—ready to handle the complexities of contemporary healthcare with safety, confidence, and skill.

References

Andersen, D., Popescu, V., Mullis, B., Cabrera, M.E., Rojas Muñoz, E., Lin, C. (2018). Augmented visual instruction for surgical practice and training. In: *2018 IEEE International Symposium on Mixed and Augmented Reality Adjunct* (*ISMAR-Adjunct*) (pp. 61–66). IEEE. https://doi.org/10.1109/ISMAR-Adjunct.2018.00033.

Ashraf, A. and Pulijala, Y. (2019). The application of virtual reality and augmented reality in oral and maxillofacial surgery. *BMC Oral Health*, *19*, 238. https://doi.org/10.1186/s12903-019-0937-8.

Barteit, S., Dell, S., Schaefer, F., Ng, V.S.T., Greuel, R.M., Plange, D. and Njouom, R. (2023). The role of augmented reality in surgical training. *Journal of Medical Internet Research*, *25*(6), e45123. https://doi.org/10.2196/45123.

Caleb, T. (2024). Augmented reality and virtual reality applications in medical education and training: A systematic review. *Journal of Health and Medical Informatics*, *15*(2).

Dhivya, S., Aydin, A., James, S., Ahmed, K. and Dasgupta, P. (2021). The Role of Augmented Reality in Surgical Training: A systematic review. In: *Surgical Education: Training for the Future* (pp. 145–159). Sage Publications. https://journals.sagepub.com/doi/pdf/10.1177/15533506221140506.

Goh, G.S., Lohre, R., Parvizi, J. and Goel, D.P. (2023). Virtual and augmented reality for surgical training and simulation in knee arthroplasty. *Archives of Orthopaedic and Trauma Surgery*, *143*, 1–9.

Gurusamy, K., Aggarwal, R., Palanivelu, L. and Davidson, B.R. (2008). Systematic review of randomized controlled trials on the effectiveness of virtual reality training for laparoscopic surgery. The British journal of surgery, 95(9), 1088–1097. https://doi.org/10.1002/bjs.6344.

Jung, S.M., Kang, J.W., Kim, J.Y., Choi, J. and Moon, I.S. (2024). Surgical training using augmented reality-based optical head-mounted displays: A pilot study. *Ear, Nose, and Throat Journal*, *103*(2), 110–116.

Kim, H.Y., Lee, H., Park, K., Kim, T., Kim, K., Kim, S. and Kim, S. (2023). Effects of medical education program using virtual reality: A systematic review and meta-analysis. *International Journal of Environmental Research and Public Health*, *20*(2), 1373. https://doi.org/10.3390/ijerph20021373.

Mao, R.Q., Lan, L., Kay, J., Lohre, R., Ayeni, O.R., Goel, D.P. and Sa, D. (2021). Immersive Virtual Reality for Surgical Training: A Systematic Review. The Journal of surgical research, 268, 40–58. https://doi.org/10.1016/j.jss.2021.06.045

McKnight, R.R., Pean, C.A., Buck, J.S., Hwang, J.S., Hsu, J.R. and Pierrie, S.N. (2020). Virtual reality and augmented reality: Translating surgical training into surgical technique. *Current Reviews in Musculoskeletal Medicine*, *13*, 698–708.

Osso, V.R. (2023). VR surgical training and assessment platform. https://ossovr.com/.

Seymour, N.E., Gallagher, A.G., Roman, S.A., O'Brien, M.K., Bansal, V.K., Andersen, D.K. and Satava, R. M. (2002). Virtual reality training improves operating room performance: Results of a randomized, double-blinded study. *Annals of Surgery*, *236*(4), 458–464.

Sheik-Ali, S., Edgcombe, H. and Paton, C. (2019). Next-generation Virtual and Augmented Reality in Surgical Education: A narrative review. *Surgical Technology International*, *35*, 27–35. https://ora.ox.ac.uk/objects/uuid:c116032a-907f-4ac1-93ef-112901d159c1/files/mf5a62026561e3e39e6bceba5e9a7da0d.

Shuhaiber, J.H. (2010). Augmented reality in surgery. *Archives of Surgery*, *145*(12), 1239.

Ström, P., Hedman, L., Sarrafzadeh, O., Hedman, M., Kjellin, A. and Felländer-Tsai, L. (2006). Early exposure to haptic feedback enhances performance in surgical simulator training. *Surgical Endoscopy*, *20*, 1383–1388.

Sutherland, L.M., Middleton, P.F., Anthony, A., Hamdorf, J., Cregan, P., Scott, D. and Maddern, G.J. (2006). Surgical simulation: A systematic review. *Annals of Surgery*, *243*(3), 291–300. https://doi.org/10.1097/01.sla.0000200839.93965.26.

Suresh D, Aydin A, James S, Ahmed K, Dasgupta P. The Role of Augmented Reality in Surgical Training: A Systematic Review. Surgical Innovation. 2022;30(3):366-382. doi:https://doi.org/10.1177/15533506221140506.

Vera, A.M., Russo, M., Mohsin, A. and Tsuda, S. (2014). Augmented reality telementoring (ART) platform: a randomized controlled trial to assess the efficacy of a new surgical education technology. Surgical endoscopy, 28(12), 3467–3472. https://doi.org/10.1007/s00464-014-3625-4.

Williams, M.A., McVeigh, J., Handa, A.I. and Lee, R. (2022). Augmented reality in surgical training: A systematic review. *Postgraduate Medical Journal*. Advance online publication.

11 Smart Surgical Tools
Sensor-Integrated Instruments in Robotic Surgery

Arpit Goel[1*], Anuradha Brijwal[2] and Gaurav Kumar Rajput[3]

The incorporation of advanced sensors into robotic surgical devices has been marked as the beginning of a transformative phase in surgery, especially in procedures requiring minimal invasiveness and high precision. These sensor-integrated tools, referred to as intelligent surgical devices, are equipped with force, torque, pressure, and tactile sensors (as well as visual or motion detectors), enabling the restoration of critical sensory feedback that had been lost in robot-assisted operations and introducing capabilities previously unattainable with purely mechanical tools. Intraoperative navigation is improved by these devices through the provision of real-time data on tool–tissue interaction, ad hoc clinical decisions are supported, and gentle manipulation of delicate anatomical structures is facilitated. A comprehensive framework for the development of intelligent instruments is outlined in this chapter, including considerations for downsizing, material compatibility with biological systems, sterilizability, and ergonomic optimization. Key sensor technologies such as strain sensors, fiber Bragg gratings, piezoelectric transducers, and soft biologically inspired methodologies are examined, as they allow for the creation of highly sensitive and MRI-compatible systems. Challenges concerning signal accuracy, instantaneous data processing, and sensor integration are discussed along with their significance in delivering tactile feedback and enabling AI-supported surgical automation. Clinical relevance is demonstrated through case examples in laparoscopic suturing, neurosurgery, prostate surgery, and endovascular interventions, where real-time force and tactile feedback have been shown to reduce tissue damage and improve clinical outcomes. Moreover, intelligent tools are changing the landscape of surgical training by offering quantifiable performance feedback based on simulations. In the future, developed components such as 'soft' electronics, autonomous and surgical robotics, and personalized toolkits will continue to expand the impact of sensor

[1, 2] Uttaranchal Institute of Technology, Uttaranchal University, Dehradun (INDIA).
[3] College of Computing Sciences & Information Technology, Teerthanker Mahaveer University, Moradabad (INDIA).
Email: anuradhabrijwalgrd@gmail.com[2]; gauravrajput31@gmail.com[3]
* Corresponding author: arpitgoel29@gmail.com

DOI: 10.1201/9781003655121-11

augmented systems in the operating room. In summary, this chapter illustrates how the sensor-equipped instruments are revolutionizing surgical practice, enhancing not only what surgeons can see but also the safety, efficiency, and precision of operative care.

1. Introduction

Over the past few decades, surgery has undergone a revolution. Conventional open surgery has given way to less invasive and robotic surgery. These novelties improve accuracy, increase efficiency, and ensure safety (Okamura, 2009). Robotic surgery supports quicker patient recovery. Furthermore, they improve optical enlargement during operation. Regardless of all these improvements, there remains an area of improvement. Surgeons are limited by the instant touch-based response (Tavakoli et al., 2007). They typically trust an open operation. Discussing these challenges is key to developing the novelty of surgical tools. A major development has been the combination of a sensor into surgical instruments (Clevenger et al., 2018). Smart instruments use multiple sensors. These sensors can respond to touch-based responses for surgeons (Kim et al., 2020).

Figure 1 describes the surgical evolution. The development of the surgical practice starts with conventional surgery (Rosen et al., 2011). The current growth contains smart instruments equipped with sensors. Each progression gives a key enhancement in accuracy, safety, and patient recovery (Kim et al., 2020).

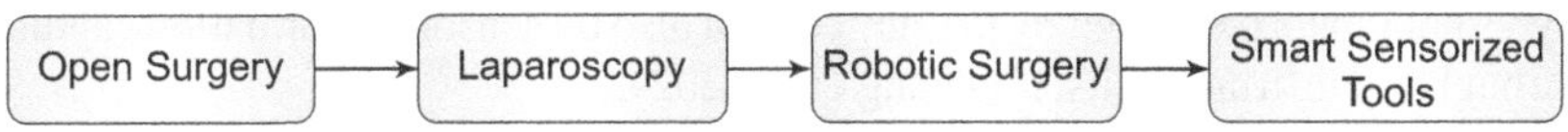

Fig. 1 Evolution of Surgical Methods.

The innovation of robotic tools is part of a major step toward healthcare systems. These tools combine physical modules, sensors, software, and connectivity. With smart tools, this integration permits not only automatically managed instruments but also tools that recognize their neighbourhood (Talasaz & Patel, 2021). For example, neurosurgery, heart surgery, and fetal surgery. In these conditions, accuracy and alertness can be an issue of survival.

The increasing growth shows the evolution in international demand for low-disruption, high-accuracy interference. This emphasis on the trend demonstrates the growing need for further research into intelligent surgical tools as a part of contemporary healthcare systems (Zhang et al., 2021).

Early robotic surgical systems primarily functioned in open-loop configurations, in which visual feedback provided by endoscopic cameras was the sole source of guidance (Tavakoli et al., 2007). Sole dependence was placed by surgeons on their visual interpretation and clinical expertise to deduce the magnitude of force exerted on tissues or to identify variations in tissue compliance (Tholey et al., 2005). This dependence on indirect indicators was associated with increased cognitive

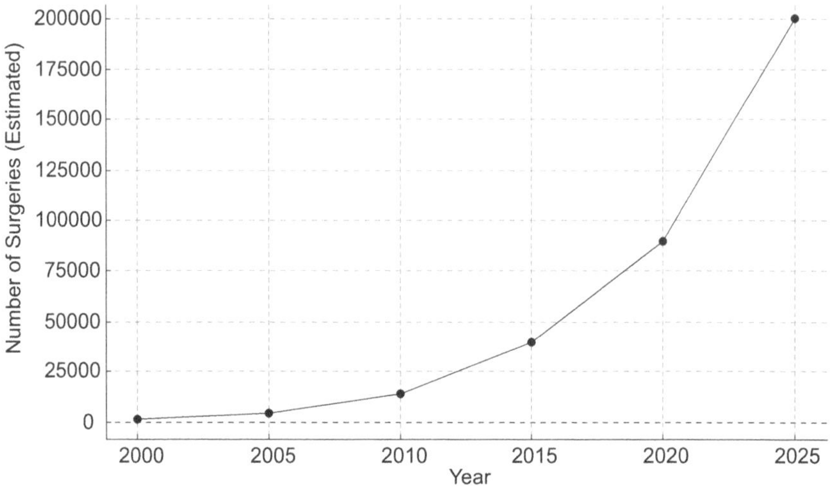

Fig. 2 Growth of Robotic Surgery Adoption (2000–2025).

demand on the surgeon and was accompanied by potential threats, including inadvertent tissue injury, excessive force application, or overlooked pathological abnormalities. This progression is characterized by a transition from a tool-oriented to a data-oriented surgical paradigm, wherein clinical decisions are guided not only by visual inputs perceived by the surgeon but also by sensory information captured through the instrument itself (Zhang et al., 2021).

Force and torque sensors, for instance, are employed to quantify grip pressure and tool–tissue interaction forces, assisting in the prevention of suture overtightening or unintended perforation of delicate organs (Hollis et al., 2022). Distributed pressure maps are delivered by tactile sensors, allowing the identification of texture and stiffness, which can be utilized for tumour detection or vascular palpation (Yip & Howe, 2016). Tool dynamics are precisely monitored by motion sensors—such as accelerometers and gyroscopes—making possible the evaluation of surgeon performance and the guidance of autonomous instrument movements (Ortmaier et al., 2002). When integrated with visual inputs, these sensors contribute to a comprehensive, multi modal data stream that can be processed through artificial intelligence and machine learning algorithms. As a result, intraoperative decision-making can be optimized, surgical subtasks automated, and both teleoperated and remote procedures facilitated (Zhang et al., 2021).

The importance of sensor-integrated instruments lies in highly precise, image-guided actions. In the operation of neurosurgery, accuracy is important. Minor variations in force, like millimetres, may result in major nervous system damage (Runciman et al., 2019). Motion and force sensor response is a crucial factor. It helps decrease accidental damage and increases targeting precision. Actual data collected from smart tools can be used to plan surgery (Mattos et al., 2014).

In addition to their clinical advantages, smart instruments play a crucial role in surgical education and training. Recent surgical simulators include actual tracking of force and movement. Still, ongoing advances in materials science, miniaturized electronics, wireless tech, and artificial intelligence are gradually overcoming these obstacles. This progress is helping sensor-integrated instruments move closer to widespread use in clinical care (Seneci et al., 2013).

This chapter is intended to offer a comprehensive overview of intelligent surgical instruments—emphasizing their design principles, categories of integrated sensors, data processing methodologies, clinical applications, and the challenges associated with their deployment. An in-depth discussion is first presented on the various types of sensors utilized in robotic surgery, including force/torque, tactile, motion, and imaging sensors. Subsequently, the engineering obstacles and integration techniques required for embedding these sensors into robotic instruments are examined. In the following sections, data fusion frameworks and haptic feedback mechanisms are explored in detail, along with real-world clinical and experimental use cases, as well as emerging trends in the development of smart surgical tools. The chapter is concluded with a set of recommendations pertaining to research priorities, clinical practice, and policy measures that can support the safe, effective, and accelerated integration of these transformative technologies into the surgical environment (Talasaz & Patel, 2021).

By highlighting the role of sensor integration in robotic surgery, this work is used to emphasize the increasing convergence of robotics, sensing technologies, and intelligent systems within contemporary healthcare. The innovation of smart tools is not only a hardware improvement. It shows an important move in the way surgery is conducted. This advancement shows a future where the association between humans and machinery is realized more closely.

2. Sensor Modalities in Smart Surgical Tools

The major novelty behind robotic tools is the use of multiple sensors. These smart tools detect and respond to their situation with greater accuracy (Rosen et al., 2011). Physical connections like force, pressure, movement, and tissue properties are converted into digital signals by the sensors. These signals are then processed by robotic systems or sent back to the surgeon through haptic feedback (Okamura, 2009). Each type of sensor captures a specific aspect of the surgical setting. When combined, they provide a clearer understanding of tool–tissue interaction. This enhances safety, precision, and overall performance during procedures (Clevenger et al., 2018).

2.1 Force and Torque Sensors

Force and torque sensors provide precise measurements of the linear and rotational forces surgical tools apply to tissue (Tholey et al., 2005). These sensors are crucial for restoring the sense of touch in robotic and minimally invasive surgeries, where surgeons cannot directly feel the tissue. Common technologies used include strain gauges, piezoelectric elements, capacitive sensors, and Fiber Bragg Gratings (FBGs). These sensors are embedded in tool tips, joints, or shafts. This allows monitoring of grip force during suturing, insertion force in catheterization, or torque in orthopedic drilling (Tavakoli et al., 2007).

2.2 Tactile and Pressure Sensors

Tactile and pressure sensors provide detailed, localized feedback about how surgical tools interact with tissue. They are especially useful for detecting small changes in texture or stiffness (Yip & Howe, 2016). This helps surgeons distinguish between healthy and abnormal areas. Tactile sensor arrays are usually based on resistive, capacitive, or piezoresistive technology. These arrays are placed on the surfaces of tools like grasper jaws, endoscope tips, or palpation instruments. They produce high-resolution pressure maps, mimicking the sensitivity and detail of human touch. For example, a tactile array on a laparoscopic grasper can help identify if a vessel is pulsatile, stiff, or calcified.

2.3 Pressure Sensors

Tactile sensors track how contact forces are spread across a surface (Dario et al., 2005). In contrast, pressure sensors are used to measure fluid or gas pressure inside the body or within surgical tools. In robotic instruments, pressure sensors help control and monitor gas pressure during laparoscopy. They are also used to check blood flow or detect blocked vessels in vascular procedures. Tiny pressure transducers placed inside catheters or endoscopic tools can measure pressure inside blood vessels or body cavities. This supports procedures like angioplasty or draining cerebrospinal fluid. Smart catheters with built-in pressure sensors can also identify narrowed vessels or bulging areas. They do this by detecting pressure changes along different segments of the vessel (Talasaz & Patel, 2021).

2.4 Motion and Position Sensors

Motion sensing is critical for both manual and autonomous surgical tools. Instruments embedded with accelerometers, gyroscopes, or magnetometers can detect linear and angular velocity, orientation, and acceleration (Ortmaier et al., 2002). This data supports precise control of tool trajectory, real-time pose estimation, and motion tracking in dynamic surgical fields. In robotic systems, motion sensors play an essential role in measuring the relative displacement between the instrument and patient anatomy, especially when visual line-of-sight is compromised. Combined with kinematic models, motion sensors also help in reconstructing tool paths for performance analysis, surgical training, and autonomous navigation tasks.

Some systems extend motion sensing through electromagnetic (EM) tracking or optical tracking technologies. EM tracking systems, which embed coils in the tool and use field generators for localization, are well-suited for confined spaces and MRI-incompatible environments. Optical tracking, including stereo cameras or structured light sensors, supports 3D pose estimation with sub-millimetre accuracy. These modalities are particularly valuable in neurosurgical navigation and image-guided interventions where instrument localization is paramount (Li et al., 2017).

2.5 Optical and Imaging Sensors

Optical sensors—including fibre-optic cameras, stereo endoscopes, and near-infrared (NIR) detectors—play a dual role in smart surgical tools: providing vision for the surgeon and acting as sensing elements for diagnostic tasks (Abiri et al., 2017). Advances in miniaturization have enabled the integration of high-resolution imaging sensors at the distal ends of laparoscopes, catheters, and needles (Zhang et al., 2021).

Smart tools with built-in optical coherence tomography (OCT) or fluorescence imaging capabilities can provide real-time visualization of subsurface tissue structures or metabolic activity. For example, tools embedded with fluorescence sensors can differentiate malignant from benign tissues based on their uptake of fluorescent dyes (Misra et al., 2008).

Table 1 Comparison of Sensor Modalities Used in Robotic Surgery.

Sensor Type	*Measured Parameter*	*Advantages*	*Limitations*	*Applications*
Strain Gauge	Force/Torque	Compact, cost-effective	Sensitive to temperature, drift	Graspers, suturing tools
FBG	Force/Strain	MRI-safe, high sensitivity	Complex integration	Neurosurgery, MRI-compatible tools
Capacitive	Tactile Pressure	High resolution, scalable	Affected by humidity	Tactile arrays, skin sensors
Piezoelectric	Dynamic Force	Fast response, high frequency	No static force measurement	Ultrasonic tools, orthopedic drills
Optical	Imaging/ Displacement	High resolution, depth data	Requires line of sight	Endoscopy, navigation

Table 1 highlights the diverse range of sensor modalities employed in robotic surgery, each tailored to specific measurement needs and surgical applications (Rosen et al., 2011). Strain gauge sensors are among the most widely used due to their compact size and cost-effectiveness, allowing accurate measurement of applied forces and torques in tasks such as grasping and suturing; however, they are sensitive to temperature variations and signal drift. FBG sensors offer high sensitivity and are inherently magnetic resonance imaging (MRI)-compatible, making them highly suitable for neurosurgery and image-guided interventions, though their integration remains technically complex (Tholey et al., 2005). Capacitive sensors provide high-resolution tactile pressure sensing and can be scaled into arrays that mimic human skin, but their accuracy can be compromised under humid surgical environments (Gerboni et al., 2017). Piezoelectric sensors are valuable for capturing dynamic forces and high-frequency responses in ultrasonic tools and orthopedic drilling, though their brittleness and inability to measure static loads limit their versatility (King et al., 2019). Finally, optical sensors deliver high-resolution imaging and displacement data critical for endoscopy and navigation but are constrained by line-of-sight requirements (Abiri et al., 2017). Collectively, the table demonstrates how each sensor type balances unique strengths with inherent limitations, underscoring the importance of modality selection based on the surgical context.

This breakdown highlights the key role of force and tactile sensing in safe tissue handling. It also points to the increasing use of vision-based systems for navigation. While advanced sensor types are widely used, the chart suggests there is still potential to combine multiple sensing methods. Doing so could further improve surgical accuracy and performance (Zhang et al., 2021) (Figure 3).

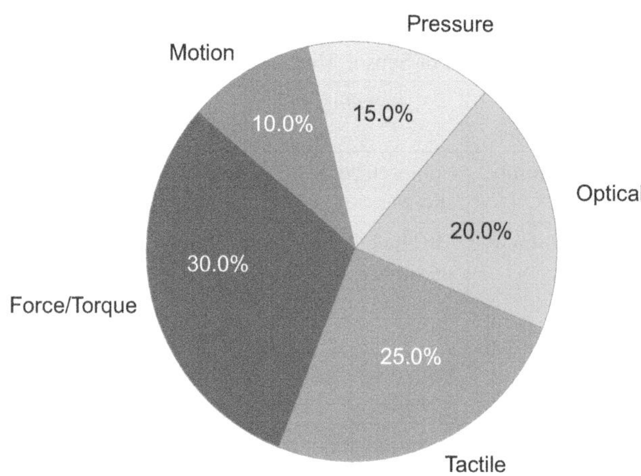

Fig. 3 Distribution of Sensor Modalities in Surgical Robotics.

3. Design and Integration Challenges

The development and adoption of sensor-enhanced instruments into the robotic surgical suite is a complex engineering challenge that must balance issues of functionality, safety, ergonomics, sterility, and integration into the surgical workflow (Misra et al., 2008). Although sensor technologies (force transducers, tactile arrays, and accelerometers) promise accurate and reactive tools, their application in real operating theatres is a challenging task (Hollis et al., 2022). The natural complexity of surgical environments—lack of space with high sterilization constraints and tissue dynamics, forcing dynamic performance *in vivo*—makes challenging the preliminary steps of smart tool development.

These restrictions are practical hurdles to allow cleaned tools in clinical practice. The proof recommends that engineering solutions should emphasize dependable, sterilizable, reduced, and biocompatible designs that do not lose performance. Figure 4 serves as a notice of the challenge in growing laboratory prototypes into clinically validated applications (Hollis et al., 2022).

The most interesting task is the mechanical incorporation and reduction. Surgical instruments, particularly those for minimally invasive surgery, on the other hand, are required to function in an extremely limited space (Mattos et al., 2014). Laparoscopic instruments, for example, often have outer diameters of 5–10 mm and must accommodate articulation joints, lighting elements, and occasionally channels for suction or irrigation (Gerboni et al., 2017).

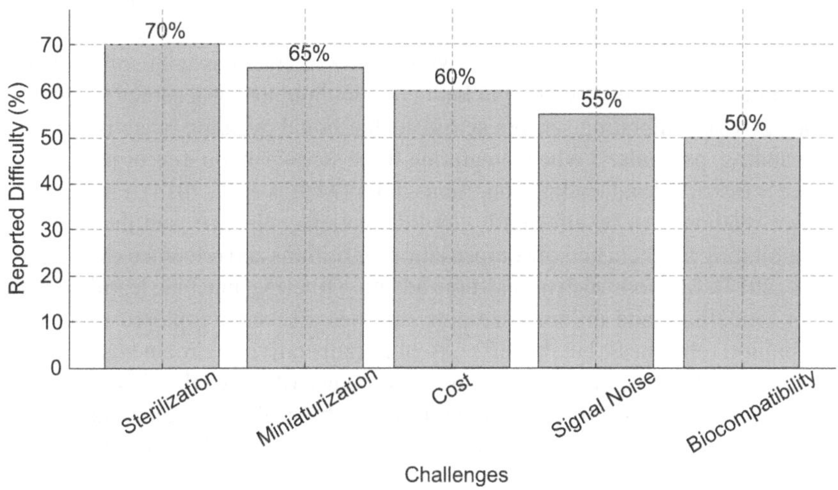

Fig. 4 Challenges in Sensor Integration.

Embedding several sensors, for example, strain gauges, fibre optic sensors, or piezo-resistive films, within these instruments demands innovative form factor engineering. Different conventional customer instruments, where sensor placement can be more flexible, surgical tools must preserve their mechanical integrity, toughness, and manoeuvrability despite the inclusion of sensor hardware. Completing this level of compactness without negotiating the tool's primary purpose often requires custom sensor packaging, flexible printed circuits, and the co-design of tool structures with sensor support frames.

Strictly linked to mechanical concerns are material compatibility and sterilization encounters (Dario et al., 2005). All surgical instruments must withstand repeated exposure to harsh sterilization environments, as well as autoclaving (high temperature and pressure), ethylene oxide (EtO) gas, or hydrogen peroxide plasma. These procedures can worsen sensor coatings, delaminate adhesive layers, or alter sensor calibration due to thermal expansion mismatches. For example, polymer-based tactile sensors may lose elasticity or suffer from hysteresis after several autoclave cycles (Gerboni et al., 2017). Furthermore, materials must be biocompatible and resistant to bodily fluids and chemicals without leaching harmful compounds. The need for non-ferromagnetic materials in MRI-compatible settings further restricts sensor and housing selections (Wurster et al., 2019). Inventions in bioinert polymers, medical-grade silicones, and hermetically sealed microelectromechanical systems (MEMS) have helped to address some of these concerns, but completing long-term robustness across diverse sterilization protocols remains a persistent challenge (Hollis et al., 2022).

An additional major design limitation is sensor calibration and sensitivity optimization. Surgical situations involve dynamic, non-linear connections between tool and tissue (Tavakoli et al., 2007). Sensors must be superbly tuned to detect a wide range of forces from sub-Newton tactile interactions with soft tissues to higher loads during bone cutting or knot tying without losing accuracy (Clevenger et al., 2018). Calibrating sensors across such a broad dynamic range is precisely demanding, particularly when integrating force sensors at tool tips or jaws, where space is restricted and loading conditions differ (Mattos et al., 2014). Furthermore, sensor readings can be affected by tool deflections, slippage, and thermal drift, necessitating the inclusion of compensation algorithms and reference channels (Li et al., 2017). Methods such as real-time adaptive filtering, machine learning-based error modelling, and on-board zeroing routines are being explored to advance calibration robustness, but the difficulty of intraoperative environments remains a challenge to the consistency of sensor performance (Abiri et al., 2017).

Additionally, electromagnetic interference from electrosurgical instruments or imaging devices can corrupt sensor signals unless robust shielding and filtering techniques are applied (Boctor et al., 2005).

From a system architecture perspective, software integration and real-time data computation represent another critical challenge (Okamura, 2009). Sensorized tools must interact seamlessly with robotic controllers, haptic interfaces, user displays, and safety systems. This requires high-speed data acquisition, synchronization across multiple sensor channels, and the integration of software modules into the broader surgical platform. Ensuring real-time performance with minimal latency is essential, particularly for force feedback loops and autonomous control algorithms. Depending on the system, data must be processed on edge devices (within the tool or arm), on centralized robotic controllers, or streamed to external AI inference engines. Achieving deterministic timing, especially under networked or wireless conditions, demands careful attention to protocol selection (e.g., CAN, SPI, BLE), priority handling, and buffering strategies. Furthermore, redundant safety checks must be built into the software to detect anomalies such as sensor failure, out-of-range values, or communication loss, thereby ensuring patient safety and regulatory compliance (Runciman et al., 2019).

An overarching challenge that affects the entire development process is cost and manufacturability. Many sensor technologies, especially fibre -optic or MEMS-based systems, are expensive to prototype and scale. Attaching them to surgical instruments can lead to a significant increase in unit cost. The impact is greater when the tool is intended for single-use. Even limited reuse can contribute to higher costs. Hospitals may hesitate to adopt high-cost instruments. To justify the expense, the instruments must demonstrate a clear return on investment. This could be through improved surgical outcomes, greater workflow efficiency, or fewer complications. As a result, developers must strike a balance between functionality, durability, and economic feasibility. New approaches like hybrid tool designs are gaining interest. These designs separate components based on reuse potential. The core instruments are reusable, but the sensor parts are intended to be disposable. In addition, Additive manufacturing and flexible electronics are gaining attention. Their adoption may open new pathways for upcoming designs. These technologies can reduce costs and enhance integration density (Polygerinos et al., 2015).

In conclusion, regulatory and interoperability challenges cannot be overlooked. Sensor-integrated tools must comply with strict medical device regulations. These regulations require thorough testing across multiple areas. This includes biocompatibility, mechanical reliability, electromagnetic compatibility, and software safety. Procurement regulatory approval typically involves extensive validation studies. These studies are time-consuming and resource-intensive. As a result, they can delay market entry and increase development costs. Also, these tools must work seamlessly with current robotic systems, surgical displays, and hospital IT infrastructure. To achieve this, they must comply with established interoperability standards. Examples include ISO 11073, DICOM, and HL7 (Wurster et al., 2019). Standardized interfaces and communication protocols are essential for integration. Without them, smart tools are difficult to implement across varied clinical settings. This challenge limits scalability and slows adoption (Misra et al., 2008).

4. Data Fusion and Haptic Systems

Surgical instruments with built-in sensors depend deeply on the precise insight of dynamic instrument tissue connections to safeguard, ensure efficient, and intuitive performance (Tholey et al., 2005). To achieve this, robotic surgical platforms integrate a variety of sensors, with force-torque sensors, accelerometers, tactile arrays, pressure transducers, and visual cameras. To deliver an actionable and unified response to the surgeon, the data from these varied sources must be intelligently combined. This process, known as multi sensor data fusion. This is fundamental to creating reliable haptic feedback systems. From this process, a surgeon "feels" the operative situation in robotic surgery (Okamura, 2009).

The line graph shows how growing the number of sensor-equipped instrument modalities significantly reduces surgical error rates. Using a single modality results in an error rate of about 20%. whereas combining four modalities reduces the error rate to as low as 6% (Tavakoli et al., 2007). This trend validates the control of sensor-equipped instruments in providing robust and accurate feedback to surgeons. By combining force, tactile, optical, and motion data, smart instruments achieve more reliable performance, especially in complex operative situations (Talasaz & Patel, 2021).

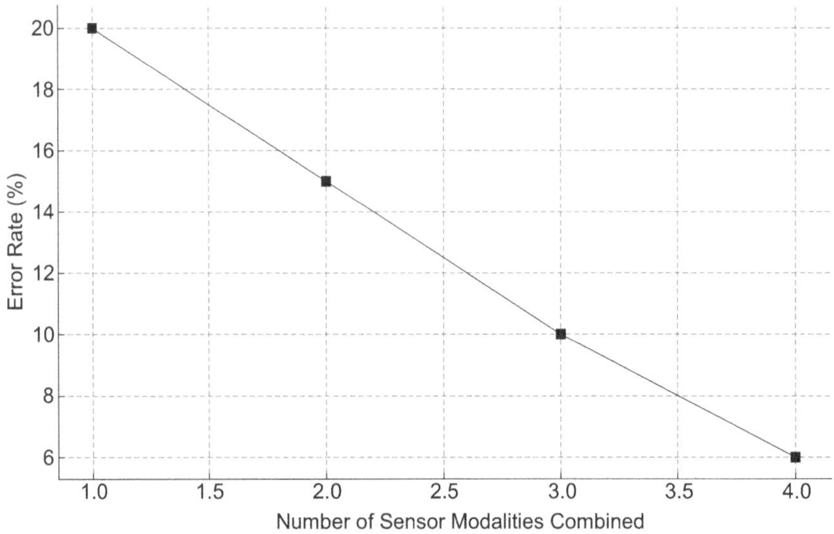

Fig. 5 Error Rate Reduction with Multi-sensor Fusion.

Data fusion refers to the method of combining sensor inputs. Data fusion combines various modalities to form a united, high-fidelity interpretation of the surgical context (Tavakoli et al., 2007). In robotic systems, force and motion sensors provide mechanical information such as grip strength, torque, and instrument trajectory. The tactile arrays deliver distributed pressure data. The electromagnetic systems contribute to spatial and contextual awareness (Tholey et al., 2005). The primary goal of data fusion is to compensate for the individual limitations of each sensor type by enhancing overall system robustness (Rosen et al., 2011). This increases spatial resolution and enables real-time responsiveness. For example, a force sensor may detect the magnitude of contact with tissue. But it cannot reveal whether the contact is localized or distributed.

There are three levels of data fusion in surgical robotics architecture (Zhang et al., 2021). First is the low level, also called sensor level. Second is the mid-level, also called feature level. Third is the high level, also called decision level. At the low level, raw data from different sensors are synchronized and pre processed for noise reduction and alignment. At the mid-level, features such as contact location, surface roughness, or force gradients are extracted and analysed to understand mechanical events like tissue rupture, slippage, or puncture. At the high level, this information is combined with instrument kinematics and patient anatomy to make real-time decisions (Hollis et al., 2022).

The fused data serve as the major role for haptic interfaces. This data is essential for restoring tactile sensation in sensor-supported surgery (Abiri et al., 2017). In traditional open surgery, a surgeon depends on direct contact with tissues. However, this natural haptic feedback is lost in minimally invasive or teleoperated procedures. Haptic systems recreate this sensation by translating sensor data into tactile. For instance, if a smart instrument detects a sudden increase in resistance while gripping tissue, the haptic interface might generate a vibration on the surgeon's hand to simulate the sensation of a firm structure (Tholey et al., 2005).

There are two major types of haptic feedback systems in robotic surgery: force feedback and tactile feedback. Force feedback systems use actuators to simulate mechanical resistance against a surgeon's movements (Abiri et al., 2017). These are often applied in the form of motorized arms that apply counter-forces. Tactile feedback systems provide pressure, vibration on the skin surface, typically through actuators embedded in finger gloves. When used together, these systems can replicate a wide range of surgical sensations, including soft-tissue compliance, tendon tension, or bone hardness (Gerboni et al., 2017).

Haptic systems go further by utilizing multimodal feedback. In a multimodal feedback system, force, tactile, and even visual information are presented simultaneously to enhance perception. For example, a surgeon may feel increasing resistance through the force feedback. A surgeon observes a color-coded force magnitude bar on the monitor (visual feedback). A surgeon senses a pulsating vibration on the thumb (tactile feedback) when approaching a force threshold. Multi modal interfaces can significantly reduce cognitive load and improve task performance (Abiri et al., 2017).

Artificial Intelligence also plays an important role in enhancing data fusion and haptic response. By training models on historical tool, tissue interaction data, systems can predict user intent, identify anomalies, or even modulate feedback based on tissue classification (He et al., 2022). For example, convolutional neural networks (CNNs) trained on fused force-vision data have been labelled tissue types with over 90% accuracy. In haptic feedback, to dynamically adapt to the procedural context, offering stiffer feedback in fibrotic zones or softer cues near vascular structures. Furthermore, predictive control models can simulate upcoming force profiles based on current motion trajectories. This enables feedforward haptics that inform the surgeon not only of what is being touched, but also of what lies ahead (Hollis et al., 2022).

Latency in data transmission is the biggest issue in the implementation of haptic systems. The second major issue is instability in feedback loops. Other issues, like mechanical compliance mismatches between instruments and the interface, can degrade the quality of haptic perception (Runciman et al., 2019). To address these challenges, many systems incorporate calibration routines, feedback from users, and sensor redundancy to maintain reliability.

Innovative technologies continue to push the limits of what haptic systems and data fusion can achieve. Soft robotic haptic gloves, bio-inspired tactile skins, and neuromorphic sensor arrays capable of spiking-based signal encoding are being explored to mimic the complex sensory integration seen in human hands (Polygerinos et al., 2015). Edge AI chips embedded in tools allow real-time fusion and decision-making at the instrument tip. It reduces the need for central processing and minimizes response latency. Integrated with AR/VR interfaces and immersive control environments, these technologies establish the foundation for a new approach in surgical instruments (Kim et al., 2020).

The workflow of sensor-enabled robotic tools can be defined as a series of individual phases that convert interactions into actionable intelligence and response for the surgeon. In this sensor layer, we use multiple sensors for sensing purposes. Combined, these sensors act as the sensing module of the robotic tools (Rosen et al., 2011).

The following tier in the design is the data processing layer. This layer enables these data to be accurate, stable, and suitable for processing. This layer amplifies and filters weak sensor signals. After finding, convert them from analog to digital form. At last, apply calibration routines and noise reduction strategies.

The output of the above layer enters as an input into the edge processing layer. This phase shows the first stage of intelligent computation. Microcontrollers execute real-time filtering and multi sensor fusion algorithms. This phase also enforces safety through log timers and limit checks that can trigger instant action or alarms in case of abnormal forces (Hollis et al., 2022).

The next layer is the AI layer, known as the system's brain. The high-speed system integrates multiple sensors and runs machine learning algorithms. This phase also performs data logging and analytics (Talasaz & Patel, 2021) (Figure 6).

The outcomes of this computation are delivered to the surgeon as a result. The outermost layer is the application layer, where the design displays its main value. It improved patient safety and also advanced the educational system.

5. Clinical and Lab Applications

Sensor-enabled surgical tools have transformed from experimental prototypes to clinically authorized instruments (Misra et al., 2008). These tools are progressively used in actual operating rooms. These inventions are not only valuable in laboratory situations but also represent benefits in patient outcomes and surgical precision.

The addition of force and tactile sensors to laparoscopic instruments significantly decreases the risk of accidental tissue perforation and increases procedural control. These tools calculate gripping forces in real time. Tactile sensors installed on a laparoscopic instrument allow actual assessment of tissue

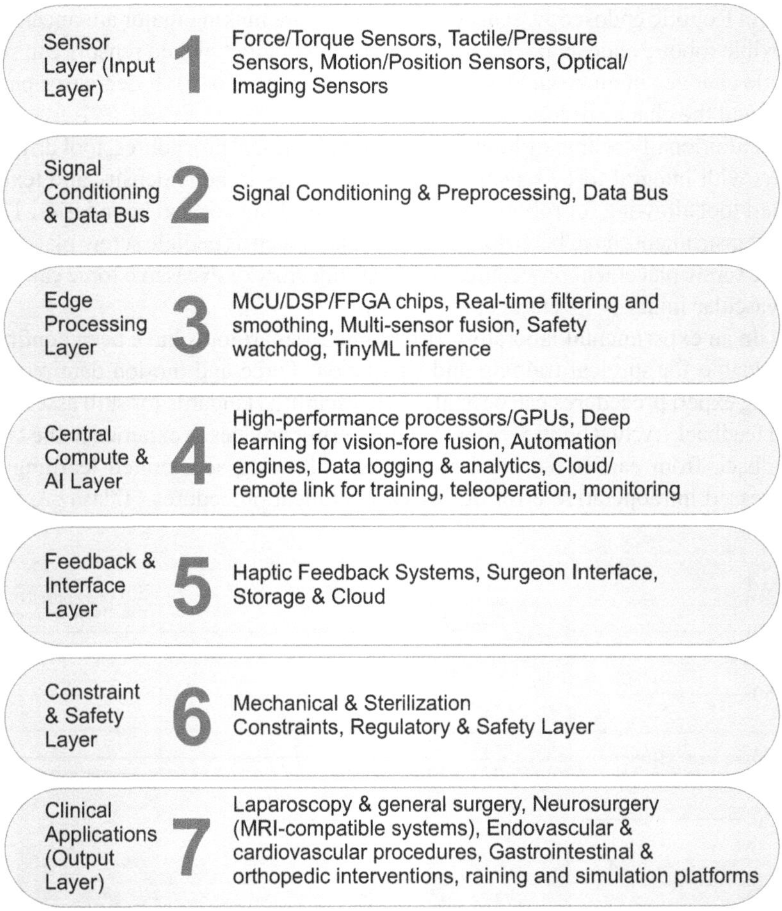
Sensor Layer (Input Layer)
1
Force/Torque Sensors, Tactile/Pressure Sensors, Motion/Position Sensors, Optical/ Imaging Sensors
Signal Conditioning & Data Bus
2
Signal Conditioning & Preprocessing, Data Bus
Edge Processing Layer
3
MCU/DSP/FPGA chips, Real-time filtering and smoothing, Multi-sensor fusion, Safety watchdog, TinyML inference
Central Compute & AI Layer
4
High-performance processors/GPUs, Deep learning for vision-fore fusion, Automation engines, Data logging & analytics, Cloud/ remote link for training, teleoperation, monitoring
Feedback & Interface Layer
5
Haptic Feedback Systems, Surgeon Interface, Storage & Cloud
Constraint & Safety Layer
6
Mechanical & Sterilization Constraints, Regulatory & Safety Layer
Clinical Applications (Output Layer)
7
Laparoscopy & general surgery, Neurosurgery (MRI-compatible systems), Endovascular & cardiovascular procedures, Gastrointestinal & orthopedic interventions, raining and simulation platforms

Fig. 6 Architecture of smart surgical instruments

stiffness. This assessment can be useful for distinguishing between healthy and pathological tissues, such as cysts and tumors (Gerboni et al., 2017).

Across Neurosurgery, it requires excellent precision and negligible tolerance for error. Introduction of smart surgical instruments has greatly benefited the field of Neurosurgery (Hollis et al., 2022).

In Cardiac and Vascular Interventions, the change of tubes and wires has been revolutionary. These tools are equipped with pressure, force, and sensors that allow operation within blood vessels (Boctor et al., 2005). Smart catheters with sensors provide an actual response during vascular dilation. This avoids excessive effort against blood vessel walls, a primary cause of vessel tear. Furthermore, incorporating haptic feedback into the catheter module allows for sensing vascular resistance (Abiri et al., 2017).

In Robotic endoscopy, sensor-enabled tools are making major advancements. Flexible robotic endoscope tips fixed with magnetically touched sensors can sense subtle changes in mucosal elasticity (Runciman et al., 2019). It decreases patient pain and the chance of mucosal harm.

Additionally, within orthopaedic and spinal surgical procedures, tool drills and burrs with integral force sensors can detect changes in bone density and texture. Smart tool allowing for robotic drilling upon breaching cortical boundaries. These smart instruments have been useful in procedures such as pedicle screw placement. In the screw placement procedure, improper trajectory or excessive force can result in vascular injury (Clevenger et al., 2018).

In an experimental laboratory environment, smart tools have been confirmed invaluable for surgical training and simulation. Force and motion data received during expert procedures can be analysed to establish standards for skill assessment and feedback. Actual haptic replay systems permit novices to experience the tactile feedback from earlier recorded procedures, allowing accelerated learning and decreased intraoperative error during early clinical procedures (Talasaz & Patel, 2021).

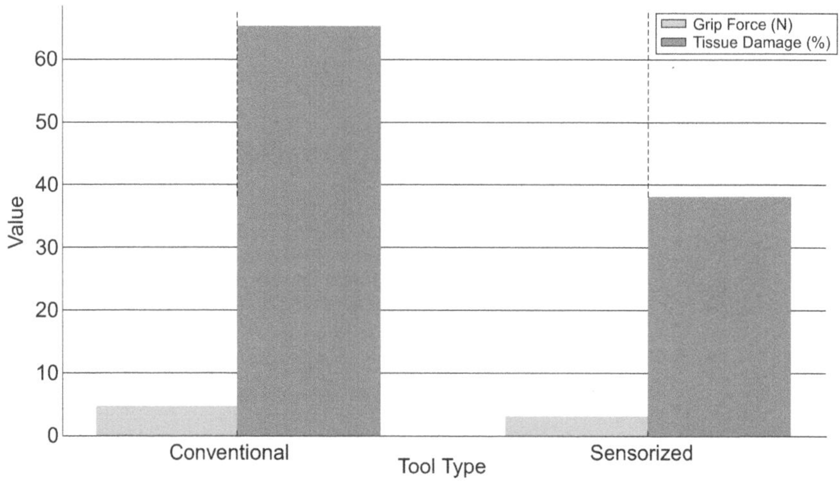

Fig. 7 Comparison of Grip Force and Tissue Damage Using Sensorized Tools.

Figure 7 illustrates the comparative performance of conventional surgical instruments and sensorized tools in terms of grip force exerted on tissue and the resulting tissue damage. Conventional tools typically require higher grip forces, averaging around 4.8 N, due to the lack of real-time feedback, which often leads to unintentional over-compression of delicate tissues (Tholey et al., 2005). This excessive force correlates with higher tissue trauma, with damage levels reaching nearly 65% in experimental evaluations. In contrast, sensorized instruments equipped with force and tactile feedback mechanisms allow surgeons to apply more controlled grip forces, averaging 3.1 N, which significantly reduces tissue trauma to approximately 38%. The figure highlights how sensor integration not only enhances precision but also directly improves patient safety by minimizing iatrogenic injury. This proof underscores the clinical value of feedback-integrated smart instruments. These tools demonstrate that even minor reductions in grip force can make extensive improvements in surgical outcomes.

The use of sensor-enabled surgical instruments is also used in minimally invasive fetal surgery. In this procedure, precise control and feedback are essential due to the fragility of fetal tissues and the confined intrauterine space (Hollis et al., 2022).

Table 2 Summary of Clinical Outcomes with Smart Surgical Tools.

Procedure	*Sensor Type*	*Key Outcome*	*Improvement (%)*	*Reference Study*
Laparoscopic Suturing	Force Sensor	Knot tension control	34%	Kim et al., 2020
Neurosurgery	FBG	Reduced tissue trauma	22%	He et al., 2022
Endoscopy	Tactile Array	Lesion localization accuracy	92%	
Catheterization	Pressure Sensor	Reduced wall rupture	45%	Chen et al. (2021)

Figure 8 illustrates a comparison of error rates between conventional and smart instruments across multiple operations. For example, like endoscopy,

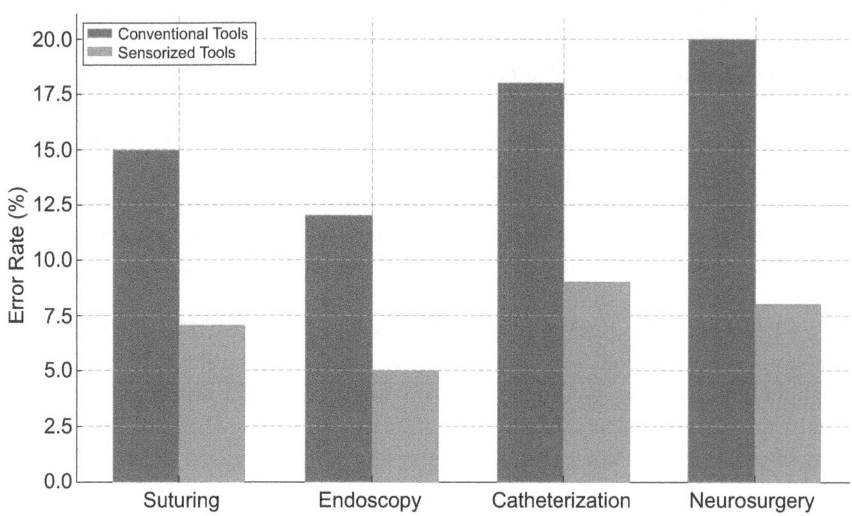

Fig. 8 Error Reduction with Smart Surgical Tools.

catheterization, and neurosurgery. The results show that smart instruments consistently decrease error rates by 40–50% relative to conventional tools.

6. Future Trends and Innovations

The innovation of smart surgical instruments is a major evolution period of smart and artificial intelligence systems. Keyhole surgery becomes more and more reliant on intelligent techniques.

The development of flexible and elastic sensors is known as a drastic transition in surgical tools. These sensors are engineered for flexibility and adaptability. These sensors are made from materials such as flexible polymers, magnetic material, or graphene-coated films. They also provide touch response, enhance sensing accuracy. Such tools not only result in high spatial resolution for actual body tissue analysis but also provide enhanced safety in sensitive surgical environments. Additionally, soft sensors can be integrated into robotic graspers to detect slip, shear forces, and surface compliance during dynamic surgical interactions

Traditional wired sensors are associated with physical encumbrance, sterilization challenges, and increased points of mechanical failure. The design trajectory for future smart tools is expected to favor untethered, miniaturized systems, powered through inductive wireless power transfer (WPT) and capable of transmitting data via Bluetooth Low Energy (BLE) or other low-latency wireless communication protocols. Successful wireless power delivery across sterilizable instrument housings—with stable operation at power levels below 20 mW—has been demonstrated in recent studies. In addition, modular sensor sleeves and interchangeable sensor cartridges are being introduced to facilitate rapid instrument replacement and improve maintenance efficiency—both of which are critical requirements in high-throughput clinical environments (Boctor et al., 2005).

The development of edge computing within surgical tools. In conventional systems, sensor data is typically sent to a centralized processor for analysis. Edge-integrated sensors are now being developed with onboard microcontrollers. These microcontrollers use local data preprocessing to reduce the need for centralized processing. By this development, latency and bandwidth requirements are effectively decreased. Moreover, distributed intelligence is enabled by edge AI, allowing smart tools to scale without dependence on centralized computing systems (Hollis et al., 2022).

MRI-adapted sensor tools are progressively being used as intraoperative imaging. Conventional sensors frequently contain metallic or ferromagnetic components that are incompatible with high-field MRI environments. This challenge is being addressed through innovations in Fibre Bragg grating (FBG) sensors, ceramic piezoelectric elements, and polymer-based electronics. The NeuroArm platform exemplifies this transition; it integrates non-metallic force sensors and operates safely inside MRI suites, providing surgeons with continuous feedback during real-time imaging-guided brain procedures. MRI-compatible robotic systems are especially vital for procedures requiring ultra-precise targeting, such as glioma resection and deep brain stimulation.

Looking further ahead, the integration of augmented reality (AR) and virtual reality (VR) with sensor data streams will redefine how surgeons perceive and interact with operative environments. Immersive platforms that combine visual, haptic, and auditory cues can simulate real tissue interaction and improve both training and telepresence applications. For instance, VR-based robotic surgery simulators with real-time haptic overlays have been shown to enhance learning curves by over 25% compared to visual-only training environments. In teleoperated setups, surgeons can experience force feedback through wearable exoskeletons or wristband haptics, allowing precise remote manipulation of instruments with enhanced control and reduced cognitive load.

Additionally, important technical, governing, and ethical encounters are also covered by these developments. Cybersecurity is seriously important for wireless and AI-driven surgical tools. The need becomes more important in telesurgery applications. In these cases, real-time data must be transmitted securely over networks. This is especially true for systems that employ predictive AI algorithms or perform partially autonomous functions. As a result, this lack of regulation creates a bottleneck to clinical implementation. Finally, Ethical issues related to decision-making authority, accountability for errors, and surgeon-robot collaboration must be addressed. This requires multidisciplinary dialogue involving clinicians, engineers, ethicists, and policymakers.

7. Conclusions and Recommendations

Sensor technology is increasingly being integrated into robotic surgical instruments. This development represents a major innovation in medical technology. Many consider it one of the most groundbreaking inventions in modern medicine. Smart surgical tools now incorporate sensors for force, tactile feedback, pressure, motion, and vision. This integration has transformed robotic platforms from simple mechanical devices into intelligent systems. These systems can interact with biological tissues in a context-aware, responsive, and minimally invasive way. Perceptual feedback to surgeons is not only augmented by these smart surgical instruments, but precision is also enhanced, complications are reduced, and new modalities of human-machine collaboration, previously confined to experimental environments, are now enabled.

Over the past 20 years, the field has progressed from rudimentary tactile sensing experiments to the development of advanced, multi-modal sensor arrays that are capable of producing haptic feedback, estimating interaction forces, and being synchronized with imaging systems in real time. Tools equipped with strain gauges, Fibre Bragg gratings (FBGs), piezoelectric elements, and soft sensor composites have been successfully deployed in diverse clinical environments ranging from laparoscopy and neurosurgery to interventional cardiology and robotic endoscopy. Clinical trials and laboratory validations consistently demonstrate reduced tissue damage, enhanced manoeuvrability, and increased success rates when sensor feedback is available. Moreover, the integration of these tools into master slave teleoperation systems or autonomous robotic platforms has improved procedural reproducibility and extended the applicability of robotic surgery to complex, anatomically sensitive interventions.

Despite these advancements, several challenges persist in the design, implementation, and standardization of sensor-integrated surgical tools. Embedding sensors without compromising the sterility, flexibility, and miniaturization of the tool remains a non-trivial engineering task. Many force sensors suffer from limited dynamic range, susceptibility to temperature and sterilization-related drift, or inconsistent performance across tool batches. In addition, the addition of sensing modules often increases the size, weight, or wiring complexity of the instrument, potentially counteracting the very benefits of robotic minimalism. The development of wireless and edge-based solutions capable of local signal processing and modular data transmission will be key to overcoming these physical constraints and unlocking new levels of design flexibility and scalability.

Beyond hardware, the interpretation of sensor data presents another critical frontier. Real-time force data, tactile maps, and motion trajectories must be converted into meaningful, actionable insights for surgeons. This requires the integration of high-performance computing, data fusion algorithms, and, increasingly, AI-driven inference models capable of anticipating tool tissue interactions and adapting behavior accordingly. The emergence of deep learning models that can learn from video, force, and kinematic inputs has opened the door to semi-autonomous and even fully autonomous surgical subtasks, such as suturing, dissection, and palpation. However, these systems must be carefully validated against clinical outcomes and safety benchmarks to ensure that the benefits of automation do not come at the cost of surgical judgement or patient safety.

Looking ahead, the future of sensor-integrated robotic surgery is likely to be shaped by a convergence of several technological and clinical trends. MRI-compatible sensors and tools will become essential for image-guided interventions in oncology and neurosurgery. Soft robotic end-effectors embedded with e-skin and conformal pressure sensors will enable safer and more adaptive manipulation of fragile tissues. Wireless, modular sensing platforms will facilitate faster tool exchange, easier maintenance, and compatibility with sterilization protocols. AR overlays will translate raw sensor data into intuitive visual and haptic cues, providing surgeons with real-time feedback on tool tissue forces, anatomical boundaries, and motion trajectories. Cloud-connected robotic systems will allow for remote diagnostics, data logging, and AI-assisted coaching in surgical education. Furthermore, edge-AI and closed-loop feedback architectures will facilitate true cyber-physical surgical systems tools that not only perceive their environment but also respond intelligently and autonomously within it.

In parallel, regulatory frameworks and medical device standards must evolve to accommodate these innovations. The inclusion of AI modules in surgical tools, for instance, requires clear definitions of accountability, interpretability, and post-deployment monitoring. Sterilization-resistant sensor designs must pass rigorous biocompatibility and fatigue testing. Data privacy, particularly in the context of remote surgery and cloud analytics, will become increasingly critical. Training programmes will need to be updated to teach not only tool operation but also sensor interpretation, system diagnostics, and collaborative decision-making with robotic agents.

Figure 9 presents the projected market growth of sensorized surgical tools from 2023 to 2035, with an expected rise from USD 2.1 billion to over USD 8.5 billion. The upward trajectory reflects increasing hospital adoption, expanding applications, and technological innovation in bio-inspired sensors and AI-based systems. The projection highlights that sensor incorporation is not only a clinical requirement but also a rapidly rising commercial sector. It highlights how upcoming inventions will drive broader availability and improved accessibility of robotic surgical solutions.

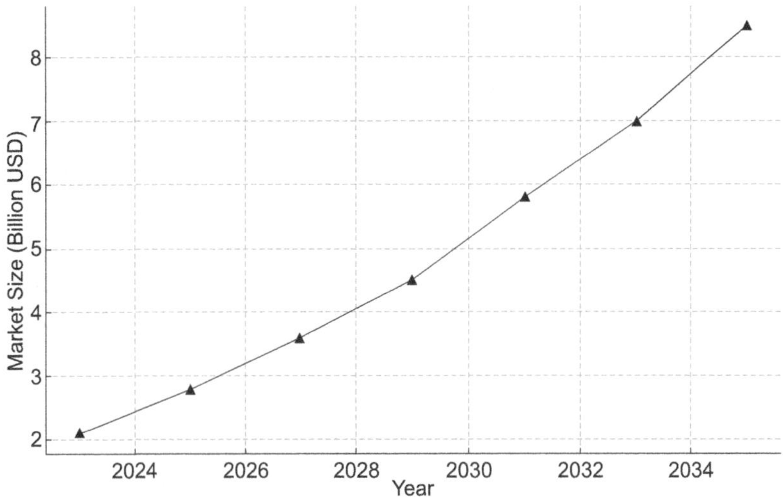

Fig. 9 Projected Market Growth of Sensorized Surgical Tools (2023-2035).

Based on the insights gained throughout this chapter, some recommendations can be made. These recommendations are intended to accelerate the safe and effective incorporation of sensor-enabled tools in robotic surgery:

1. **Foster Interdisciplinary Collaboration in Sensor Design:** Sensor development must be strongly combined with mechanical design, sterilization protocols, and clinical usability. The association between engineers, surgeons, and material scientists is critical.
2. **Create Common Metrics for Sensor Performance:** The development of common performance metrics and standardization protocols for force and tactile sensors will allow more consistent assessments across vendors and systems.

3. **Focus on Scalable and Modular Sensor Solutions:** Tools should be designed with sensor packages that can be replaced, upgraded, or sterilized independently of the tool body.
4. **Integrate On-Device Processing to Enhance Performance:** Embedding real-time signal processing capabilities in the tool will reduce latency. It will also improve safety and pave the way for semi-autonomous functions.
5. **Leverage Sensor Feedback in Surgical Education and Simulation:** Sensor-enabled tools should be used not only in the operating room but also in surgical education. In this setting, real-time feedback can improve learning and credentialing.
6. **Maintain Surgeon Control with Transparent Robotic Actions:** As AI and robotics increase in importance, surgical robots must offer interpretable, auditable actions. Surgeons must remain in control and understand the rationale behind machine-assisted decisions.

References

Abiri, K.M., Tao, A., Ma, J. and Bisley, J. (2017). Multi-modal haptic feedback for robotic-assisted surgery. *IEEE Transactions on Biomedical Engineering, 64*(2), 296–306. https://doi.org/10.1109/TBME.2016.2550638.

Boctor, F., Fichtinger, G. and Taylor, R.H. (2005). A novel MRI-compatible robot for transperineal prostate interventions: Preliminary experiments. *IEEE Transactions on Biomedical Engineering, 52*(2), 306–313. https://doi.org/10.1109/TBME.2004.840473.

Clevenger, M.C., Kim, Y., Morrell, J. and Hannaford, B. (2018). Design and validation of a force-sensing instrument for robotic surgery. *IEEE Transactions on Biomedical Engineering, 65*(3), 553–561. https://doi.org/10.1109/TBME.2017.2719438.

Dario, P., Hannaford, B. and Menciassi, A. (2005). Micromechatronics in minimally invasive surgery. *IEEE/ASME Transactions on Mechatronics, 10*(2), 261–270. https://doi.org/10.1109/TMECH.2005.844715.

Davies, B.M. (2018). A review of robotics in spinal surgery. *Surgical Technology International, 32*, 284–291.

Gerboni, G., Diodato, A., Ciuti, G., Menciassi, A. and Cianchetti, M. (2017). A soft and smart modular robot for minimally invasive surgery. *IEEE Robotics and Automation Magazine, 24*(3), 66–76. https://doi.org/10.1109/MRA.2017.2700320.

He, H., Wang, J., Zhang, X. and Li, Y. (2022). High-sensitivity FBG-based force sensor for robot-assisted minimally invasive surgery. *IEEE Sensors Journal, 22*(5), 4560–4569. https://doi.org/10.1109/JSEN.2022.3142925.

Hollis, R.G., Howell, L.L. and Webster, R.J. (2022). Force and torque sensors for surgical applications: A review. *IEEE/ASME Transactions on Mechatronics, 27*(3), 1349–1362. https://doi.org/10.1109/TMECH.2021.3107541./

Hunt, T.R., Lee, D. and Park, S. (2020). Low-cost optical force sensors for surgical applications. *IEEE Sensors Journal, 20*(4), 2175–2183. https://doi.org/10.1109/JSEN.2019.2945380.

Kim, Y., Murphy, R.J. and Hannaford, B. (2005). Tissue property identification and modeling for surgical simulation. *Studies in Health Technology and Informatics, 111*, 203–209. https://doi.org/10.3233/978-1-60750-929-5-203.

Kim, K., Park, J., Lee, S. and Choi, H. (2020). Smart surgical tool with force/tactile sensors and deep learning-based tissue classification. *IEEE Access, 8*, 104905–104914. https://doi.org/10.1109/ACCESS.2020.2999938.

King, H., Bianchi, G. and Long, J. (2019). Instrumented surgical tools for skill assessment and force feedback in robotic surgery. *IEEE Transactions on Biomedical Engineering, 66*(10), 2827–2836. https://doi.org/10.1109/TBME.2019.2901772.

Klatzky, R.L. and Lederman, S.J. (2013). Multisensory integration during manual object recognition. *Current Opinion in Neurobiology, 23*(2), 187–193. https://doi.org/10.1016/j.conb.2012.10.011.

Li, Y., Gao, H. and Chen, X. (2017). Machine learning for haptics: Classification and control. *IEEE Robotics and Automation Letters, 2*(2), 927–934. https://doi.org/10.1109/LRA.2017.2658547.

Mattos, L.S., Deguet, A., Vagvolgyi, B., Taylor, R.H. and Hager, G.D. (2014). Miniaturized force sensors for minimally invasive surgery. *IEEE Sensors Journal, 14*(7), 2307–2315. https://doi.org/10.1109/JSEN.2014.2305473.

Menciassi, A. and Dario, P. (2012). Bio-inspired solutions for locomotion in the gastrointestinal tract: Background and perspectives. *Philosophical Transactions of the Royal Society A, 370*(1965), 2427–2441. https://doi.org/10.1098/rsta.2011.0421.

Misra, S., Macura, K., Taylor, R.P. and Okamura, A.M. (2008). Medical robotics for interventions. *Annual Review of Biomedical Engineering, 10*, 59–89. https://doi.org/10.1146/annurev.bioeng.10.061807.160523.

Mohareri, A., Tavakoli, M. and del Pobil, A.P. (2021). Recent advances in haptics for teleoperated and autonomous robotic surgery. *IEEE Access, 9*, 98077–98095. https://doi.org/10.1109/ACCESS.2021.3096867.

Netter, F.H. (2018). *Atlas of Human Anatomy* (7th Edn.). Elsevier.

Okamura, A. M. (2009). Haptic feedback in robot-assisted minimally invasive surgery. *Current Opinion in Urology, 19*(1), 102–107. https://doi.org/10.1097/MOU.0b013e32831a478c.

Ortmaier, T., Groger, M. and Hirzinger, H. (2002). Motion estimation in minimally invasive surgery. *IEEE Transactions on Biomedical Engineering, 49*(6), 642–651. https://doi.org/10.1109/TBME.2002.1001971.

Pacchierotti, C., Prattichizzo, D. and Kuchenbecker, K.J. (2015). Cutaneous haptic feedback to ensure correct grasping in robot-assisted surgery. *IEEE/ASME Transactions on Mechatronics, 20*(1), 95–106. https://doi.org/10.1109/TMECH.2014.2305844.

Polygerinos, P., Lyne, S., Wang, Z., Nicolini, L.F., Mosadegh, B. and Walsh, C.J. (2015). Soft robotic glove for combined assistance and at-home rehabilitation. *Robotics and Autonomous Systems, 73*, 135–143. https://doi.org/10.1016/j.robot.2014.08.014.

Prattichizzo, D., Chinello, F., Pacchierotti, C. and Malvezzi, M. (2013). Towards wearability in fingertip haptics: A 3-DoF wearable device for cutaneous force feedback. *IEEE Transactions on Haptics, 6*(4), 506–516. https://doi.org/10.1109/TOH.2013.53.

Rosen, J., Lum, M.N., Sinanan, M.L. and Hannaford, B. (2011). Sensing and force feedback for surgery. In: *Surgical Robotics* (pp. 361–389). Springer. https://doi.org/10.1007/978-1-4419-1126-2_14.

Okamura, A.M. (2004). Methods for haptic feedback in teleoperated robot-assisted surgery. *Industrial Robot, 31*(6), 499–508. https://doi.org/10.1108/01439910410566260.

Runciman, M., Darzi, A. and Mylonas, G.P. (2019). Body-mounted robotic instruments for laparoscopic surgery. *Surgical Endoscopy, 33*(10), 3437–3445. https://doi.org/10.1007/s00464-019-06957-2.

Seneci, G.T., Deguet, A. and Davies, B.L. (2013). A review of sensing technologies for minimally invasive surgery. *Surgical Innovation, 20*(3), 255–272. https://doi.org/10.1177/1553350612458544.

Simaan, N., Taylor, R.H. and Flint, P. (2005). Design and integration of a telerobotic system for minimally invasive surgery. *IEEE Engineering in Medicine and Biology Magazine, 24*(1), 66–73. https://doi.org/10.1109/MEMB.2005.1384164.

Talasaz, A. and Patel, R.V. (2021). Force sensing and control in robot-assisted surgery. In: *Medical Robotics*. Springer. https://doi.org/10.1007/978-3-030-52625-1.

Tavakoli, M., Howe, R. D. and Liu, Y.M. (2007). Haptic feedback and sensor fusion for improved laparoscopic force sensing. *IEEE Transactions on Robotics, 23*(4), 722–730. https://doi.org/10.1109/TRO.2007.900810.

Tholey, S., Desai, A.M. and Castellanos, A.M. (2005). Force feedback plays a significant role in minimally invasive surgery. *Annals of Surgery, 241*(1), 102–109. https://doi.org/10.1097/01.sla.0000149306.97370.c1.

Wurster, D., Kahn, R., Maier-Hein, L. and Raczkowsky, J. (2019). MRI-compatible robotics: A review. *IEEE Transactions on Medical Robotics and Bionics, 1*(4), 311–321. https://doi.org/10.1109/TMRB.2019.2952558.

Yang, S., Ottensmeyer, M.P. and Howe, R.D. (2008). A tactile sensor for minimally invasive surgery based on fiber Bragg grating. *IEEE Transactions on Biomedical Engineering, 55*(10), 2329–2338. https://doi.org/10.1109/TBME.2008.919138.

Yip, D. and Howe, R.D. (2016). A neural network-based tactile sensing system for robotic surgery. *IEEE Transactions on Robotics, 32*(6), 1360–1371. https://doi.org/10.1109/TRO.2016.2609388.

Zhang, T., Wang, J. and Yang, M. (2021). Sensor fusion for robot-assisted minimally invasive surgery: A review. *IEEE Access, 9*, 101542–101558. https://doi.org/10.1109/ACCESS.2021.3095897.

12 Surgical Robots
Principles, Technologies and Clinical Application

Sakshi Koli[1*], Gopal Krishna[2], Kapil Sharma[3] and Quazi Taif Sadat[4]

Robots are changing many surgical specialties by enhancing accuracy and dexterity and providing minimally invasive procedures. Much of this progress is enabled by robotics platforms that unify high quality sensors, real-time imaging devices, user-friendly human–machine interfaces, and intelligent machine controllers. Although advancements have occurred, there are still several enduring obstacles that hinder the ubiquity and productivity of robotic surgical systems like cost, complexities of technical hurdles as autonomy in robotics is being challenged, time spent training surgeons, and regulatory ambiguity. As robotics and artificial intelligence (AI) become more routine in clinical practice, and during procedures that are mechanically driven, ethical considerations about patients' consent for interventions that are 'long in the tooth' become relevant. In theory, robotic surgery may be utilized in key areas of clinical practice such as urology, cardiothoracic surgery, neurosurgery, and perhaps orthopedics, which also can have a limiting effect on the external research context of surgery for robotics. The research also presents promising future directions that have the potential to revolutionize robotic-assisted surgery practices, such as advances in artificial intelligence, augmented reality, autonomous robots, and artificial haptics. The critical problem of safety, cost, and equitable international access has yet to be addressed, so strides must be made towards creating low-cost type systems, limiting the size of the systems, for many different uses, improving the surgical human capacity with simulation training, and building collaboration on internationally recognized ethical and regulatory issues.

[1,2] Uttaranchal Institute of Technology, Uttaranchal University, Dehradun, 248007, India.
[3] Department of Computer Science and Engineering, Accurate Institute of Engineering and Technology, Greater Noida, India.
[4] Director, Bangladesh University, Bangladesh.
Email: cse.gopalkrishna@gmail.com[2]; k.kapil.s@gmail.com[3]; taif@bu.edu.bd[4]
* Corresponding author: Kolisakshi84@gmail.com

DOI: 10.1201/9781003655121-12

1. Introduction

With the introduction of cutting-edge technologies targeted at increasing accuracy, reducing invasiveness, and improving patient outcomes, the discipline of surgery has undergone a paradigm shift in recent decades.

Surgical robots have been one of the most revolutionary of these technical breakthroughs, drastically altering the face of contemporary healthcare (Cleary & Nguyen, 2001). Surgical robotics, which includes computer-assisted and robotic-assisted surgical (CAS and RAS) systems, uses biomechanics, engineering, and artificial intelligence (AI) to enhance the surgeon's skills and provide more precision, improved dexterity, and improved visualization during intricate procedures (Zamorano et al., 2004). The capacity of surgical robots to overcome many of the drawbacks of traditional open and minimally invasive operations highlights their significance in modern medical practice. Although they provide less stress and a quicker recovery, traditional laparoscopic procedures frequently provide ergonomic difficulties and limit the surgeon's range of motion. However, robotic systems give surgeons the ability to execute complex procedures with previously unheard-of control and accuracy by providing articulated instruments with more degrees of freedom, high-definition 3D vision, and tremor filtration (Vitiello et al., 2013).

Numerous clinical disciplines, including urology, cardiothoracic surgery, neurology, and orthopedics, are among those that use surgical robotics (Reddy et al., 2023), among others. For example, the da Vinci Surgical System is now a well-known platform for urological and gynaecological robotic-assisted laparoscopic procedures. Similar to this, developments in image-guided systems and computer-assisted navigation have made it easier for robotic treatments to expand in fields like neurosurgery and orthopedics, where accuracy on a millimeter scale is crucial (Mavrogenis et al., 2013) More autonomy, miniaturization, and better surgical results are being driven by the field's ongoing advancements in robotics, artificial intelligence (AI), sensing technologies, and sophisticated materials. Ensuring the safe integration of robotic technology in clinical practice, issues of cost-benefit, surgeon training, patient welfare, and ethical consideration will have to be answered alongside these developments. This chapter provides coverage of the basic concepts, technological developments, and clinical uses in the field of surgical robotics. It considers the development of surgical robotics in regard to currently available systems, such as intelligent reconfigurable articulated part-man-sized manipulators, known here as collaborative robots. It also discusses previously developed systems, reconfigurable or not, with these improved capabilities.

2. Motivation for Robotic Surgery: Precision, Minimally Invasive Techniques, and Patient Outcomes

The primary motivation for exploring robotic devices, to address the shortfalls of traditional surgical methods and provide superior clinical outcomes with improved precision and less invasiveness while maintaining patient safety, is clear. Good alternatives exist with laparoscopic procedures in comparison to open surgery, though the laparoscopic option brings its own set of limitations, including greater recovery times, higher rates of infection, larger incisions, and further painful recovery in the short term. Additionally, traditional laparoscopic and minimally invasive approaches to many complex operations are limited by reduced instrument range of motion, lack of visualization, and surgeon fatigue. Robotic surgery addresses these limitations with the ability to complete complex operations using unmatched accuracy and precision with high-definition 3-D image quality (Blenda Johansson et al., 2021).

Robotic surgery is now valued for its ability to allow surgical treatment to be performed more easily and in a more minimally invasive manner. Robotic systems provide dexterous manipulation of articulated wristed end effectors, which can simulate or exceed the dexterity and range of motion of the human hand, while providing a degree of precision from the surgeon's perspective that is practical for secure execution in confined areas. This is particularly valuable in sensitive surgical procedures of the prostate, heart, brain, and spine, as damaging errors can create significant disasters for patient recovery and well-being. In addition to increased dexterity, motion scaling and tremor filtering capabilities can increase the accuracy of surgical techniques employed by a surgeon, further reducing the chances of unintentional inaccuracies during surgery (I. H. A. Chen et al., 2021).

Aside from the precision expected from surgical techniques, robotic-assisted approaches provide many benefits to patients, including decreased blood loss, decreased complications associated with surgery, shorter hospital stays (Khan et al., 2021), and decreased recovery times. The literature from various surgical specialties, including cardiothoracic, gynecological, urological, and other specialties, consistently shows that robotic surgery is linked to improved quality of life for patients, decreased morbidity, and improved functional outcomes. Additionally, the ergonomic benefit to the surgeon, in terms of decreased physical strain and improved visual feedback, can add to the consistency of the procedure and the decrease in surgical fatigue, both of which are important components of providing high levels of care for patients. All of this represents the greatest driving force for the creation and implementation of surgical robotics in operating rooms today. With continued upgrades to the systems, their impact in surgery will only improve as we become safer, more effective, and more patient-oriented surgical solutions.

3. Scope of the Review

This review's objective is to present a thorough and critical examination of the basic ideas, developments in technology, and clinical uses of surgical robotics, with a focus on how it might improve contemporary surgical procedures (Pal, 2024a). Researchers, physicians, biomedical engineers, and legislators who want to comprehend the clinical significance and technical foundations of RAS and CAS can use this paper as a comprehensive scientific resource.

Beginning with its historical context and following the technological turning points that have led to its current condition, the content methodically examines the development of surgical robots. A thorough examination of the basic engineering concepts guiding robotic systems and computer-assisted platforms, such as kinematics, control mechanisms, human-machine interfaces HMI), sensor technologies, and material advancements, is included in this review in addition to technological evolution. Along with a review of cutting-edge CAS tools like navigation systems and real-time imaging modalities, special attention is paid to commercially available robotic systems, like the da Vinci Surgical System (Bodner et al., n.d.), and other emerging platforms.

Furthermore, the review addresses the clinical translation of these technologies across various medical domains, including urology, cardiothoracic surgery, neurosurgery, and orthopaedic surgery, highlighting both the successes and the current limitations of robotic-assisted interventions (Pal, 2024b). Because this subject is interdisciplinary, it requires an integrated strategy that takes into account patient safety, surgical expertise, engineering innovations, regulatory considerations, and ethical implications all of which are addressed in this work. This review concludes by outlining current issues like high costs, technical complexity, and training needs, as well as predicting emerging trends like the incorporation of AI, greater system autonomy, and the creation of robotic platforms that are smaller and tailored to a single patient. The study is to enhance the field of surgical robots and their safe, efficient application in clinical practice by offering insightful information about the current state, new trends, and research directions. The study's organization and structure are depicted in Figure 1.

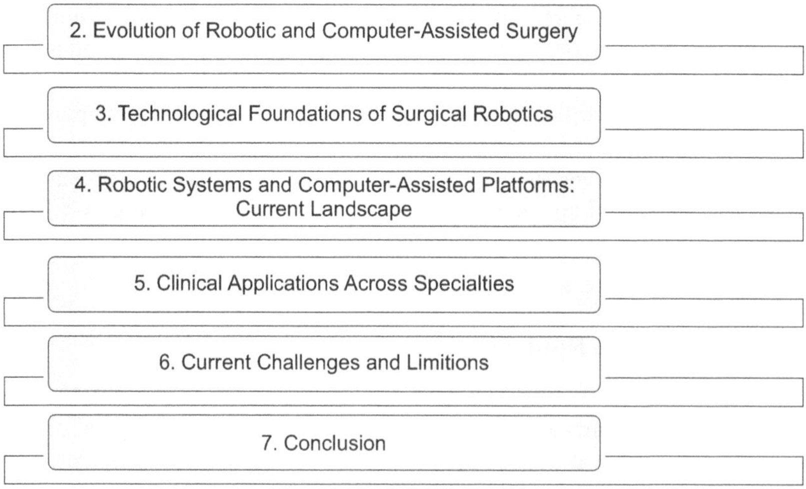

Fig. 1 Structure and Organization of the Study.

4. Evolution of Robotic and Computer-Assisted Surgery

4.1 Historical Background and Technological Evolution

At the nexus of engineering, medicine, and information technology, the development of RAS and CAS marks a critical turning point, propelled by the ongoing quest for better surgical accuracy, safety, and patient outcomes. The 1980s were when surgical robotics first began to take shape (Camarillo et al., 2004), with the early conceptualization and experimental use of robotic devices in medical procedures. One of the earliest recorded instances was the development of the PUMA 560 robotic arm, which was utilized in 1985 to perform a neurosurgical biopsy (Elsabeh et al., 2021), marking the first documented use of a robotic system in a clinical setting. This use case illustrated how robotics might improve surgical precision, especially in delicate and minimally invasive procedures. Significant progress was made in the 1990s as increasingly complex robotic systems created especially for surgical purposes were introduced. One of the first robotic platforms to be approved by the government was Computer Motion's AESOP (Automated Endoscopic System for Optimal Positioning), which allowed laparoscopic cameras to be positioned using voice commands (Pugin et al., 2011), providing voice-controlled positioning of laparoscopic cameras. Following this, the ZEUS Robotic Surgical System was developed, which offered improved control of instruments (Varghese et al., 2019a) and led the way for more complex, robot-assisted procedures. In 2000, the da Vinci Surgical System, developed by Intuitive Surgical and authorized by the U.S. Food and Drug Administration (FDA) (Ratnayaka et al., 2016), was an amazing technological achievement. The da Vinci system featured robotic arms that mimic-wristed movement, 3D high-definition visualization, and surgeon-controlled interfaces for a new alternative to minimally invasive surgery. Following the da Vinci system, many surgical fields have accepted this surgical platform as its popularity has grown, including urology and gynaecology, which demonstrate clinical benefits in surgery-associated complications, hospital length of stay, and functional recovery. Broadly, and outside the scope of robotics, surgical systems for computer-assisted surgery (CAS) have evolved to improve the accuracy of surgical techniques during the surgical procedure (Fan et al., 2016a). Likewise, imaging guided surgery, computer-assisted navigation, and the inline of additional imaging modalities, imaging such as MRI (magnetic resonance imaging) or CT (computed tomography), have coalesced into surgical techniques that further supplement more complicated surgical procedures (Despinoy et al., 2018a). The combination of robotic systems and CAS systems has merged into highly integrated surgical systems that not only allow for real-time input, but also provide for better viewing and the unparalleled precision of instrument manipulation.

Recent accomplishments include the development of next-generation robotics systems such as CMR Surgical's Versius® robotic system, Medtronic's Hugo TM RAS system, and custom platforms for neurosurgery and orthopaedics. These developments are evidence of a trend to make the surgical robot more compact and dexterous, and also better integrated with imaging and navigation technology.

More autonomous, intelligent, and patient-specific surgical systems have been developed in recent years thanks to the integration of AI, machine learning (ML) algorithms, tiny robotic equipment, and smart sensor technologies. Additionally, new opportunities for extending surgical care to underserved or geographically inaccessible areas have been made possible by the development of telesurgery and remote-controlled robotic operations. With the ultimate goal of improving surgical capabilities, lowering patient morbidity, and enhancing healthcare delivery, the historical trajectory of RAS and CAS thus reflects an ongoing cycle of innovation, propelled by interdisciplinary collaboration between engineers, medical professionals, and researchers. Key turning points in the evolution of RAS and CAS are compiled in Table 1, which also highlights significant technologies, innovators, and their long-term therapeutic effects.

Table 1 Historical Milestones in Robotic and Computer-Assisted Surgery.

Year	*Technology/System*	*Key Features*	*Significance/Application*
1985	PUMA 560	Robotic arm used for neurosurgical biopsy	First documented use of a robotic system in a clinical procedure
1994	AESOP	Voice-controlled laparoscopic camera positioning	First FDA-approved surgical robot; enhancesd camera control
Late 1990s	ZEUS Surgical System	Remote instrument control	Progress toward full robot-assisted surgery
2000	da Vinci Surgical System	3D-HD vision, wristed instruments, surgeon console	FDA-approved; revolutionized minimally invasive surgery
2000s+	CAS (Computer-Assisted Surgery)	CT/MRI integration, image-guided navigation	Improved surgical planning and intraoperative precision
2010s+	AI & ML Integration	Predictive analytics, decision support	Emergence of intelligent surgical systems
2010s+	Miniaturized Robotic Devices	Compact, flexible systems for MIS	Increased precision, less invasiveness
2010s+	Telesurgery	Remote-controlled robotic procedures	Enabled remote access to surgical expertise

5. Transition from Manual to Robotic-Assisted Procedures

The desire for more precision, less invasive techniques, and better patient outcomes has led to a major development in surgical practice with the shift from traditional manual surgery to robotic-assisted procedures (Heng et al., 2022a). Even though they work well for many problems, traditional open procedures are linked to significant tissue damage, more discomfort after the procedure, longer hospital stays, and a higher chance of complications. Despite the advent of laparoscopic procedures, surgeons still have to deal with steep learning curves, restricted instrument mobility, and ergonomic issues. By providing increased dexterity, better vision, and more control over surgical instruments, robotic-assisted surgery overcomes these drawbacks (Pal, 2024c). With a greater range of motion than the human hand, wristed tools in robotic systems allow surgeons to execute intricate procedures with more accuracy and less tremor. Robotic consoles' ergonomic designs also help surgeons operate consistently over long procedures by reducing tiredness. At first, people were skeptical of robotic-assisted operations because of worries about their expense, complexity, and training needs. However, universal adoption has been progressively aided by clinical evidence showing improved surgical outcomes, shorter recovery periods, lower complication rates, and less blood loss (Checcucci et al., 2023a) . Robotic prostatectomy, hysterectomy, and heart valve repair are just a few examples of the fields where robotic-assisted procedures have grown commonplace over time, demonstrating the effective incorporation of robots into everyday surgical workflows. Advances in CAS, such as image-guided interventions, real-time navigation, and AI integration, also aid in the transition by improving intraoperative decision-making, surgical planning, and execution. The distinction between manual and robotic-assisted treatments is anticipated to become increasingly hazy as robotic technology advances, with robotic systems eventually emerging as essential instruments in the contemporary operating room.

6. Global Trends in Adoption and Innovation

Over the past two decades, the global landscape of surgical robotics has experienced remarkable growth, driven by technological advancements, increased clinical acceptance, and evolving healthcare demands. The United States has led the adoption of RAS, particularly through the widespread use of the da Vinci Surgical System, which has performed over 10 million procedures globally (Varghese et al., 2019b). Europe, particularly in countries such as Germany, the United Kingdom, and France, has also witnessed significant growth in the use of robotic platforms, supported by favorable regulatory environments and investments in medical technology.

In recent years, several developing countries, including China, India, Brazil, and South Korea, have begun to embrace surgical robotics in light of the poor development of health infrastructure facilities and an increase in demand for advanced surgery. China, for example, is investing substantially in domestic robotic technology. Some companies are dedicating time and resources to creating surgical robots for Chinese contexts, perhaps suggesting a new era of locally adopted innovation and self-sufficiency (Smith et al., 2013a). Figure 2 shows further where the majority of surgical robotics applications are situated around the world, with the large majority being found within the United States. Most emerging and not necessarily first-world countries have made some foray into RAS, and interest is generating in many emerging healthcare regions, much like the global trend. These developments and interests go along with the developments in surgical technique, innovations, and techniques. In addition to the advancements within surgical robotics, there is also noting new and smaller lower-cost robotic systems, improvements in instrument design and imaging, and perhaps utilizing AI to potentially semi-automate some of the surgical procedures. Of course, within the four main companies that are racing to define and make a future system, which include companies like Medtronic, CMR Surgical, Johnson & Johnson, and a variety of start-ups, looking to consider how robots will manoeuvre in, around, and across the human body (Ratnayaka et al., 2017).

Additionally, the COVID-19 pandemic has stimulated interest in the use of technologies that are remote, or thinly intrusive, in a relatively non-physical medium, which has fostered research on robotic-assisted procedures that incorporate as little physical contact as possible (e.g., tele-surgical techniques), particularly also in the context of remote surgical education and simulation. Aspects of accessibility and real-time data, connectivity to the operating room, and surgeon-robot surgical collaboration continue to grow on the R&D (research and development) agenda. To summarize, trends of global acceptance and innovation predict a path for surgical robotic technology as an increasingly commonplace aspect of surgical practice worldwide, with a continued emphasis on cost-effective platforms, while enhancing accessibility, safety, and clinical effectiveness across practice settings more generally.

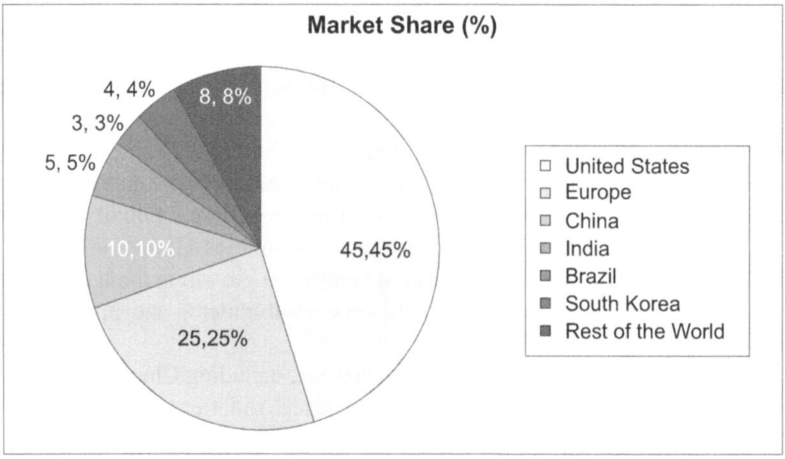

Fig. 2 Global Distribution of Surgical Robotics Usage by Region (Fan et al., 2016b).

7. Technological Foundations of Surgical Robotics

7.1 Principles of Robotics in Surgery

The impact of robotics-enabled integration in modern surgical practice is driven by the convergence of engineering disciplines, improvements in computing power, and changing clinical needs. Kinematics, automation, control theory, and HMI are fundamental topics that comprise surgical robotics, which enables the safe and accurate use of surgical instruments inside the body. These areas support robotic platforms that cannot just duplicate, but also often improve upon human hand performance, including improved dexterity, scalable motion, and repeatability in very complex procedures.

A. Basics of Robotic Systems: Kinematics, Control, and Automation

Kinematics, which is key in the design of the robotic system, refers to the mathematical descriptions of motion and the causes of the motion. There are two types of kinematics in regard to surgical robotics that we have identified: forward kinematics, which estimates position and orientation of the end-effector given angles of the robotic joints; and inverse kinematics, which determines a configuration of joints to create an end-effector position. Understanding these models is important to conduct proper instrument tracking and positioning, especially in the context of discussing minimally invasive surgery (Van Der Meijden & Schijven, 2009a). Other kinematics that we discuss refer to structural control systems that respond to our natural and unbiased hand movements, and convert these movements into robotic movements while operating in real-time. These systems respond to rapidly changing conditions in the surgical field by being supplied with high-resolution encoders, force sensors, and feedback loops, and thus feel stable and accurate while operating (Schneeberger & Michler, 2001).

Additional advanced control methods related to kinematics (e.g., impedance control, hybrid position/force control, haptic feedback) are being used more to provide intuitive operation for the user, especially when performing tasks that require fine motor control. By implementing these technologies, there is a reduced risk of unintentional injury to the patient due to the robotic systems ability to detect and modulate the firmness of the tissue. There exists a spectrum of automation in surgical robotics, from simple imitative motion to complex and partially autonomous task performance. Although most clinical systems are still run under the direction of the surgeon through teleoperation, current research is exploring how AI, ML, and real-time analysis of images can increase the robot's autonomy.

The application of robots to perform certain subtasks with minimal human assistance, such as suturing, retraction, and anatomical navigation, has the potential to enhance surgical efficiency and reduce the cognitive burden on the operator (Prata et al., 2023a). In summary, all contemporary robotic platforms are guided by core principles in surgery, including motion modeling, control theory, and adaptive automation, which ultimately afford the increased precision and control required for improved safety and outcomes, making robotic systems an extension of the surgeon's skill set, as more than just a set of tools. Three main areas characterize the principles of robotic surgery, illustrated in Figure 3, which are as follows: Automation (involving teleoperation, semi-autonomy, and AI/ML integration); Control Mechanisms (including hand-motion mapping, real-time feedback, and haptic feedback); and Kinematics (forward and inverse kinematics).

These principles of robotic surgery, when combined, provide increased accuracy, responsiveness, and improved decision-making to robotically assisted procedures. The successful adoption of robotics in the modern surgical ecosystem is driven by medical need, use of technology principles, and computer science advances. To design and effectively utilize surgical robotics, a basic comprehension of kinematics, control systems, computerized systems, and HMI is required. These principles are ensuring robotic platforms afford higher accuracy, dexterity, and reproducibility during complicated surgical procedures and not just replicate, but often exceed the capabilities of the human hand.

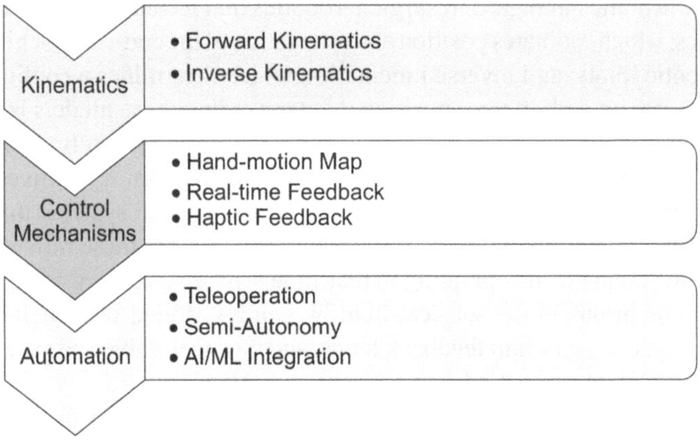

Fig. 3 Core principles of surgical robotics.

B. Human-Machine Synergy in Surgical Procedures

The smooth fusion of human skill and machine accuracy is a hallmark of surgical robotics. Surgical robots are designed to be the surgeon's partner as opposed to an independent machine like its industrial counterparts. At the heart of this synergy is the HMI that translates the surgeon's hand movements into scaled, filtered, and smoothed robotic instrument movements. Through ergonomic control consoles, high-definition 3D visualization, and intuitive instrument manipulation, surgical robots significantly reduce the cognitive and physical workload on surgeons (Despinoy et al., 2018b). Advanced robotic systems incorporate features such as motion scaling, which translates large hand movements into fine instrument movements, and tremor filtration, which eliminates unintentional hand tremors, thereby improving the overall precision of surgical procedures (Heng et al., 2022b). The design concept of human-machine synergy also applies to training and skill development, as virtual reality modules and simulation platforms are incorporated into robotic systems to support surgeon education and competency building. This cooperative strategy guarantees that robotic technology complements the surgeon's vital operational and decision-making abilities rather than takes their place.

C. Role of Computer-Assisted Surgery Platforms

Within the field of surgical robotics, the utilization of CAS systems is required as an additional layer of technological expertise that adds decision support, navigation, and visualization in the intra-operative environment. CAS systems rely on a combination of advanced imaging technologies, including CT, MRI, and real-time fluoroscopy, which are coupled with computer algorithms to develop multimodal 3D models of the anatomy to direct planning and performance of surgical procedures. CAS can also facilitate aspects such as accuracy aiming/trajectory planning and real-time feedback during increasingly complex procedures when used in conjunction with robotic systems.

One example of this is in neurosurgery and orthopedic surgery. Navigation systems provide the opportunity for clinicians to interactively and precisely place implants (Azari & Nikzad, 2008) or instruments based on patient-specific anatomy and uniquely track and minimize the chances of error. Second, image-guided robotic surgery permits for safe navigation of very sensitive anatomy, including but not limited to the brain and spinal cord. Recently, CAS has evolved to include AR (augmented reality) and VR (virtual reality), which is a development of CAS and a new technique used to assist in providing immersive and contextualized visualizations in the surgical context (Checcucci et al., 2023b). Moreover, there is a growing prevalence of data-driven algorithms and ML to analyze intraoperative data, estimate operative outcomes, and assist with clinical reasoning at the moment. With the use of robotic systems, computer-assisted platforms enhance the accuracy, efficiency, and safety with which surgical procedures can be performed, reinforcing the potential and value of technology partnerships in the operating room of today.

8. Human-Machine Interfaces

Another important element in surgical robotic systems is the HMI, which acts as a conduit for effective interaction between the surgeon and the robotic platform. HMIs that are effective afford real-time sensory feedback, which is necessary for safe and accurate surgical performance as well as transposing the surgeon's motor and cognitive intents into refined, stable, precise, and controlled operation of the robot interface. Ongoing advancement of HMI characteristics has dramatically improved the operation of RAS, ensuring that the surgeon remains in command while accessing machine-augmented capabilities, in an effort of ease of use, precision, and overall performance.

A. Surgeon Control Consoles and Feedback Systems

At the core of modern surgical robotic systems lies the surgeon control console, which functions as the primary interface through which the surgeon operates the robotic instruments (Smith et al., 2013b). Because of their ergonomic design, these consoles maximize comfort and minimize tiredness, enabling surgeons to carry out lengthy, intricate procedures with little physical strain. Hand controls on the console usually mimic the surgeon's movements and convert them into precise, scaled, and filtered movements of the robotic arms and instruments within the patient's body. Advanced robotic platforms incorporate high-definition, 3D visual displays within the control console, providing the surgeon with enhanced depth perception, spatial awareness, and magnified views of the surgical field. Such enhanced visualization is important in the process of locating anatomical structures, judging the integrity of some tissue, and executing fine manipulation tasks with a high degree of precision. Modern systems also include multimodal feedback such as audio (aural) cues, system alarms, and graphic displays of the instrument location, forces applied, and general system status (Freeman et al., 2017). These feedback mechanisms are critical to improve the awareness of the situation and avoid unintentional harmful tissue damage, thereby maintaining safe surgical performance.

B. Teleoperation and Real-Time Decision Support

Teleoperation is defined as the ability to control robotic surgical systems from a location physically apart from the robot by a surgeon. This concept not only provides for improved ergonomics in the operating room, but it also offers possibilities of telesurgery, where expert surgeons can remotely undertake procedures on patients based miles apart. Teleoperation is enabled by high-speed communication networks and low-latency data transmission to real-time robotic control systems, which execute the surgeon's commands without any noticeable delay (H. Chen & Liu, 2021)

The addition of real-time decision support to teleoperators and traditional robots further enhances the ability of the surgeon. Real-time decision support systems are designed to use intraoperative data such as imaging, instrument tracking, and physiological information to help surgeons maneuver through complex anatomy, plan surgical paths, and avoid critical areas. Moreover, AI and ML algorithms are being increasingly investigated to support predictive analytics, early recognition of potential complications, and to improve outcomes of the procedure at the time of surgery. This integration of teleoperation and real-time decision support is a new generation of surgical robotics, one that provides not only high precision but also brings expert surgical care to medically underserved areas through the use of remote or rural connectivity.

C. Advances in Haptic Feedback and User Experience

The most notable limitation of robotic surgery has been the absence of traditional tactile feedback, which delivers essential information to surgeons about tissue properties, force applied, and instrument interactions. In an effort to address this limitation, there has been a significant amount of research aimed at creating haptic systems in which the sensation of touch can be mimicked or simulated in RAS. Recent developments in haptic feedback systems have incorporated force sensors, tactile actuators, and haptic interfaces into the console or robotic instrument (Van Der Meijden & Schijven, 2009b).

These technologies enable the immediate transfer of touch and force cues from the surgical site to a surgeon's hands, thus enhancing their ability to feel tissue resistance, manipulate fragile structures, or lessen excessive forces that may cause tissue damage. In addition to enhancing safety in procedures, haptic feedback can create a more instinctive and natural user experience, reducing cognitive load on the surgeon and creating educational opportunities in training. Clinical studies (N = 100) have shown that the integration of haptic feedback in robotic surgery improves task performance, decreases error rates, and improves overall surgical efficiency. In addition to haptics, user experience has been enhanced through developments in augmented reality (AR)/virtual reality (VR) and simulation-based training platforms that engage users in a more interactive learning environment for both preoperative planning and intraoperative navigation. Collectively, these technologies have engendered relentless advancements in HMI such that robotics continues to be the future of surgery and the surgeon.

9. Robotic Systems and Computer-Assisted Platforms: Current Landscape

9.1 Commercial Surgical Robotic Systems

The commercial landscape of surgical robotic systems has changed substantially in the last 20 years, characterized by progress and clinical penetration of sophisticated robotic platforms that aim to improve precision, ergonomic, and patient outcomes in different surgical disciplines. A number of players have entered this market with companies offering surgical robotic systems with different levels of technical complexity, flexibility, and clinical usage. This section reviews some of the well-known commercial robotic systems and makes a critical comparison between them with respect to their characteristics, pros, and cons. While the da Vinci Surgical System (Intuitive Surgical Inc., Sunnyvale, Calif.) is maintaining its position as the most commonly used robotic platform in the world and has a proven and vast clinical experience, having been introduced earlier than other systems. The da Vinci system has undergone several phases of technological improvement, following its first introduction to the U.S. market in 2000 by the U.S. FDA. The system has automated robotic arms with wrists and is equipped with high-definition three-dimensional (HD 3D) visualizations, using an ergonomically designed surgeon console that enables the surgeon to perform telemanipulation accurately (Schneeherger & Michler, n.d.).

It could be used in various operative sites as urological, gynecological, general surgery, cardiothoracic, and head and neck surgeries. The da Vinci platform has been the turning point for introducing to all over the world robotic-assisted mini invasive surgery as a new form of performing surgery without opening up directly and not even laparoscopic instead. In recent years, Medtronic, the global leader in medical technology, has brought to market the Hugo™ RAS System (Prata et al., 2023b), Created to challenge the da Vinci system. The Hugo system's modularity, portability, and integration with capable data and analytics platforms support stand-alone robotic arms, 3D visualization, and cloud-based data storage, offering a less costly and scalable alternative that is particularly effective for budget-conscious and space-conscious settings such as hospitals. The Versius® Surgical Robotic System (CMR Surgical, Ltd., England) is a portable surgical robot specifically developed with a modular design for suitability with laparoscopic procedures (Brodie & Vasdev, 2018). "With independent access to every bedside unit in the Versius system, along with an open console environment, it allows some flexibility in the OR; we think it is a good solution for facilities operating in limited space or facilities that are required to do many procedures," said Nigel Wilson. Other relevant systems include the Senhance® Surgical Robotic System by Asensus Surgical, which emphasizes haptic feedback and eye-tracking camera control, or Robotic Orthopedic Platforms such as the MAKO® Robotic-Arm Assisted Surgery system by Stryker (Takai et al., 2018), which has a penetration rate established for joint replacement and orthopaedic procedures. Table 2 represents the comparison of leading robotics.

Table 2 Comparison of Leading Robotic Surgery Systems: Key Features, Advantages, and Limitations.

System	*Key Features*	*Advantages*	*Limitations*
da Vinci (Intuitive Surgical)	Multi-arm system, wristed instruments, 3D HD vision, intuitive console	Established clinical efficacy, broad specialty use, and advanced ergonomics	High acquisition and maintenance costs, limited haptic feedback
Hugo RAS (Medtronic)	Modular arms, 3D vision, data integration, cloud connectivity	Cost-effective, modular setup, advanced data analytics	Relatively new in the market, clinical adoption is still expanding
Versius (CMR Surgical)	Compact, modular design, open console, portability	Space-efficient, ergonomic design, suitable for diverse laparoscopic cases	Limited long-term clinical data compared to da Vinci
Senhance (Asensus Surgical)	Haptic feedback, eye-tracking camera control, reusable instruments	Real-time tactile feedback, lower operating costs	Smaller market presence, limited instrument dexterity compared to competitors
MAKO (Stryker)	Robotic-arm assistance for orthopedic procedures, CT-based preoperative planning	Enhanced precision in joint replacement, improved implant alignment	Application restricted to orthopedic surgeries

9.2 Role of Sensors: Force, Tactile, Position, and Imaging

The sensors are the fundamental sensory mechanism between the robotic surgical system, the surgeon, and the surgical environment. They also allow for the measurement of real-time data and increase surgical precision and the dynamic behavior resulting from procedures done intraoperatively.

- **Force Sensors:** These sensors measure the forces exerted by robotic end-effectors on tissue during manipulation, dissection, or suturing. The force sensation is an important awareness to prevent excess force application, making it less likely for tissue damage to occur and increasing the surgeon's safe performance, for example, at anatomically sensitive sites or conditions.
- **Tactile Sensors:** Tactile or pressure sensing provides information about tissue feel or contact forces and the surface quality. Tactile sensing is being incorporated with pressure sensing, partly to emulate the lost feeling when using RAS (Kang et al., 2016). The possible role for more tactile feedback has been defined in pilot investigations of soft sensors and flexible electronics.
- **Position Sensors:** Position sensors with high precision can identify and track actual real-time location, orientation, and motion in robotic arms and devices (Khoury & Kamat, 2009). Most of these sensors are optical, magnetic, or inertial-based sensors that ensure that the instruments are in the correct position along their intended trajectories, which are essential in cases requiring sub-millimeter precision (for example, neurosurgery or cardiovascular interventions).
- **Imaging Sensors:** Imaging sensors, including HD cameras, endoscopes, and intraoperative ultrasound, offer visual feedback to the surgeon. Imaging sensors and systems are progressively developing for 3D endoscopy and hyperspectral imaging that continue to improve visualization and tissue contrast.

The integration of these sensor technologies allows closed-loop control, performs real-time monitoring, and allows for improved haptic feedback which maximizes safety and efficiency of robotic-assisted procedures.

9.3 Advanced Materials for Surgical Instruments

The selection of the materials used is a vital component to robotic surgical instruments, and a fundamental component of their performance and tissue compatibility. Many advanced materials are used today in surgical instruments to withstand the harsh mechanical, chemical, and biological environments present in the operating room. Materials commonly employed include:

- **Stainless Steel and Titanium Alloys:** Known for their high strength, corrosion resistance, and biocompatibility, these materials are widely used in robotic surgical instruments, particularly for structural components requiring mechanical robustness.
- **Shape Memory Alloys (e.g., Nitinol):** These types of materials have tuneable properties, such as recovering to a defined shape after an elastic deformation, and these properties make them well-suited to steerable/flexible robotic tools with high dexterity.

- **Polymeric and Composite Materials:** Advanced polymers and fiber-reinforced composites are employed to reduce instrument weight, enhance flexibility, and improve electrical insulation. Certain polymeric materials also facilitate the development of disposable or semi-disposable instruments.
- **Bioinspired and Soft Materials:** Recent research focuses on the development of soft robotic instruments using bioinspired materials that mimic the compliance and adaptability of biological tissues. These materials offer enhanced safety when interacting with delicate or complex anatomical structures.

The integration of these advanced materials enables the development of instruments that are not only mechanically efficient but also compatible with sterilization protocols, imaging systems, and patient safety standards. Figure 4 illustrates the advanced materials used in robotic surgical instruments, categorized into metals (such as stainless steel and titanium alloys), polymers and composites, and emerging bioinspired materials.

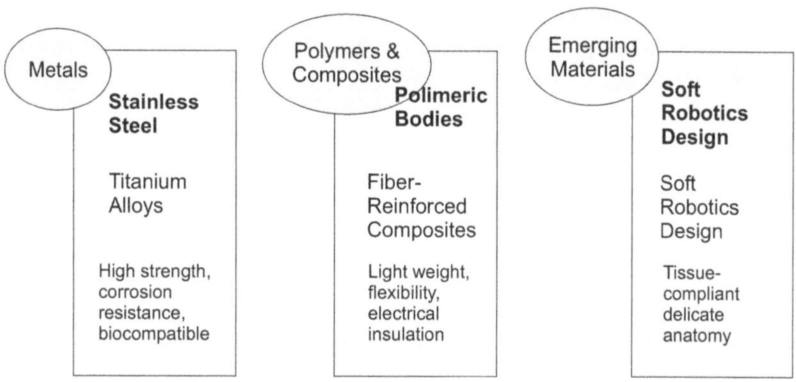

Fig. 4 Advanced Materials for Surgical Instruments.

The integration of these advanced materials enables the development of instruments that are not only mechanically efficient but also compatible with sterilization protocols, imaging systems, and patient safety standards.

10. Clinical Applications across Specialities

With more precision, less invasiveness, and better clinical results, the use of robotic-assisted surgical devices in a variety of medical disciplines has completely changed how complicated procedures are approached. Although urology was the primary use for surgical robotics, its uses have since grown to include orthopaedic procedures, neurology, and cardiothoracic surgery. An overview of the principal uses, supporting data from clinical trials, technological advantages, and difficulties of robotic surgery in different fields is given in this section.

10.1 Urology

Urology has led the way in robotic-assisted surgical techniques, including robotic-assisted partial or radical nephrectomy and robotic-assisted laparoscopic prostatectomy (RALP). The da Vinci Surgical System device allowed for precision with dissection and nerve sparing, and reconstruction, allowing RALP to become the treatment of choice for localized prostate cancer. In addition to having excellent long-term oncological control (Falagario et al., 2020), it translated into better functional outcomes when it comes to preservation of sexual function and urinary continence. Robotic-assisted nephrectomy has assured much to be happy about, as it also minimized blood loss, complication rates, preserved renal function and access to an anatomic complex site for tumors in patients with malignancy of the urinary tract, either partial or radical. Large clinical series have demonstrated less blood loss in the operating room, shorter hospital stay, and lower complication rates compared to traditional laparoscopic or open techniques. How appealing this advanced technique may be, it is still limited by many factors for general adoption, including the expense of the entire system and the unique demands of operating while still employed in health, along with restrictions.

10.2 Cardiothoracic Surgery

Robotic techniques are transforming thoracic surgery and extending the boundaries of minimally invasive surgery for complicated heart and lung resections. Robotic technology has allowed for the repair of the mitral valve, coronary artery bypass grafting (CABG) and pulmonary lobectomy using limited port access and enhanced visualization, precision, and freedom of movement in a complicated intrapleural/ intrapericardial space (Holmes et al., 2025). The development of robotic platforms in cardiac surgery has also enabled complex fine motor tasks, such as suturing and ultra-complex valve repair, using limited port access. This sometimes facilitates no sternal reconstruction and bypass treatment in select patients. In thoracic surgery, robotic-based approaches began with access to difficult anatomic areas, which led to precision resections in the mediastinum, lymph node dissections, and esophageal cases. In addition, these findings and the early and hereafter overwhelmingly established clinical benefits compared to traditional laparoscopy (less pain, shorter hospital stay, faster recovery time, better cosmetic repair 3–5) were generated while confronting operational challenges with the learning curve, longer initial operative time, and loss of haptic feedback. However, there are several studies that report robotic cardiothoracic surgery can be performed safely and efficaciously with, in many cases, improved outcomes, especially in high-volume centres of excellence.

10.3 Neurosurgery

The brain and spinal cord are two central organs of the body required for regular activities in our daily lives. These two bodies are also extremely complicated and critical organs in the body. Therefore, precision and safety are the most important considerations in the practice of neurosurgery. Recently, robotics-assisted in neurosurgery has made a significant difference between those two critical requirements. Robotic-assisted neurosurgery is more stable, provides sub-millimeter precision and repeatability of complicated surgical tasks, and minimizes human error to increase accuracy in the surgical procedure. Robotic assistance has been used in several settings, including stereotactic biopsy, deep-brain stimulation electrode placement, spinal instrumentation, and complex and tumor resections. Robotics assists in trajectory planning, instrument guidance, and real-time positioning, which greatly minimizes human error. Image-guided robotic systems make use of both preoperative and intraoperative robotic capabilities, such as MRI or CT, and have been shown to result in improved neurosurgical outcomes. Improved depth of determination and minimizing access to complex or previously treated anatomical spaces have been made possible. This is clinically supported by the advantages of robotic-assisted neurosurgery, such as lower complication rates, increased accuracy, and shorter operative times. However, barriers, including expensive equipment, infrastructure requirements, and the need for specialized training, still restrict the widespread use, especially in resource-limited settings.

10.4 Orthopedic Surgery

Robotic-assisted devices have gained attention in the field of orthopedic surgery, for example, joint arthroplasty and spinal manipulation. Owing to the accuracy of bone preparation, placement of implants, and alignment, the MAKO® Robotic-Arm Assisted Surgery System and other similar platforms are applied to perform procedures including THA, TKA, and UKA (Roche, 2021). In spine surgery, robot-assisted systems help improve the accuracy during pedicle screw insertion, spinal fusion, and deformity correction, which decreases the morbidity of the procedures among those performed with the freehand method. These technologies provide revolutionary preoperative planning using patient-specific imaging, thereby facilitating virtual reenactments for the selection and placement of the implants. Robotic platforms offer the benefit of instantaneous feedback, and they guide the instruments with greater accuracy, thus increasing the accuracy and reproducibility of bone cuts and hardware positioning at the time of surgery. Robot-assisted orthopaedic surgery is clinically proven to be effective with beneficial outcomes to include increased implant survival, favourably functional results, and reduced occurrences of malalignment and revision procedures. But, for all of its promise, access to the system currently remains limited due to the high relative costs, steep learning curves, and the requirement for seamless integration with the current surgical workflow.

11. Current Challenges and Limitations

Still, although great advances have been made both in surgical robotics and its adoption and adaptation for clinical contexts, several significant barriers and limitations remain that inhibit more widespread implementation of such technology and more effective usage of its capabilities. These obstacles are numerous and varied and include technical, clinical, regulatory, and ethical. Addressing these limitations is vital for the safe, equitable, and effective uptake of robotic devices into routine surgical practice.

- **Technical Constraints: Cost, Size, and Complexity:** One of the primary limitations regarding the more widespread adoption of robotic surgery remains the costs associated with the initial investment, the operational costs, and the consumables, particularly in resource-limited contexts. Additionally, robotic surgical systems are large, complex devices in need of physical space and substantial logistical demands on many centres; needing modifications of infrastructure, dedicated technicians, and perhaps, specialized staffing as well. As with any new technology, the miniaturization of the robotic system will still be a technical and practical challenge, most critically with the use of microsurgery or in conducting procedures in more minimal anatomical spaces. Changing the size of the robot will be an obstacle in the near term for engineers and researchers; however, balancing size constraints with the original performance of the robot is still also an engineering and performance problem.
- **Surgeon Training and Learning Curve:** When surgery is performed using robotics, there is a new system of training required for the surgeons as they are working with telemanipulation techniques and the configuration of 3D views, creating a significant learning curve. If early adopters of surgical robotics typically will experience longer surgeries and an increase in complications, they might want simulation-based training and/or VR platforms 29, 30, assuming that an institution of schools stores them securely through a proctoring service and other official sources, may make skills acquisition quicker; however, the conundrum of expanding and securing access to quality training among the many living in resource-limited situations that seems to be the same core challenge.
- **Regulatory and Standardization Issues:** The speed of advancement of surgical robotic systems is not matched by the orderly development of regulation and standardization–thus, approval, testing, and safety standards differ from one jurisdiction to another, limiting global use and applicability for clinical use. Other issues creating variability include a lack of universal training, certification, and reporting of outcome standards in the operating room, as limitations to patient safety and consequences.
- **Ethical Dilemmas in Robotic Autonomy:** The intertwining of AI and autonomy in surgery raises ethical concerns of accountability, informed consent, surgeon autonomy, and fairness of algorithms. As systems become more autonomous the responsibilities of error and means of transparency, and understanding of patients becomes more complicated. These dilemmas will require clinicians, engineers, ethicists, and policy makers to work together to establish ethical boundaries that are subject to regulation.

12. Conclusion

Surgical robots are transforming contemporary medicine, with minimally invasive applications spanning multiple specialties, as well as improving dexterity and accuracy to a level never before achieved. In this review, we demonstrate how advances in technology in robotic systems, smart sensors, imaging systems and ergonomic HMI have increased the quality of operations and patient safety. Robotically assisted procedures have shown increased accuracy, fewer complications, and improved recovery times in neurosurgery, orthopaedics, cardiothoracic surgery, and urology. High system costs, complexity, and the requirement for structured surgeon training are just a few of the technological, financial, and regulatory obstacles that continue to prevent widespread implementation. Careful consideration must also be given to the ethical issues of robotic autonomy and accountability. Future studies should concentrate on creating modular, inexpensive, and small robotic platforms to increase accessibility, especially in environments with limited resources. The combination of machine learning and artificial intelligence has the potential to improve semi-autonomous functions, surgical accuracy, and decision-making. Enhancing haptic feedback, integrating real-time imagery, and upgrading surgeon training with sophisticated simulation tools should also be prioritized. For robotic surgical technology to be used in routine clinical practice in a safe, efficient, and responsible manner, international regulatory frameworks and ethical standards must be established.

References

Azari, A. and Nikzad, S. (2008). Computer-assisted implantology: Historical background and potential outcomes: A review. *The International Journal of Medical Robotics and Computer Assisted Surgery*, *4*(2), 95–104. https://doi.org/10.1002/RCS.188.

Blenda Johansson, Elvira Eriksson, Nellie Berglund, & Ingrid Lindgren. (2021). Robotic Surgery: Review on Minimally Invasive Techniques. Fusion of Multidisciplinary Research. *An International Journal*, *2*(2), 201–210. https://doi.org/10.63995/gqnc2594.

Bodner, J., Augustin, F., Wykypiel, H., Fish, J., Muehlmann, G., Wetscher, G. and Schmid, T. (n.d.). The da Vinci robotic system for general surgical applications: A critical interim appraisal.

Brodie, A. and Vasdev, N. (2018). The future of robotic surgery. *Annals of the Royal College of Surgeons of England*, *100*, 4–13. https://doi.org/10.1308/rcsann.supp2.4.

Camarillo, D. B., Krummel, T. M. and Salisbury, J. K. (2004). Robotic technology in surgery: Past, present, and future. *American Journal of Surgery*, *188*(4 SUPPL. 1), 2–15. https://doi.org/10.1016/j.amjsurg.2004.08.025.

Checcucci, E., Verri, P., Amparore, D., Cacciamani, G.E., Rivas, J.G., Autorino, R., Mottrie, A., Breda, A. and Porpiglia, F. (2023a). The future of robotic surgery in urology: From augmented reality to the advent of metaverse. *Therapeutic Advances in Urology*, *15*. https://doi.org/10.1177/17562872231151853.

Checcucci, E., Verri, P., Amparore, D., Cacciamani, G.E., Rivas, J.G., Autorino, R., Mottrie, A., Breda, A. and Porpiglia, F. (2023b). The future of robotic surgery in urology: From augmented reality to the advent of metaverse. In: *Therapeutic Advances in Urology* (Vol. 15). SAGE Publications Inc. https://doi.org/10.1177/17562872231151853.

Chen, H. and Liu, Z. (2021). Time-delay prediction-based smith predictive control for space teleoperation. *Journal of Guidance, Control, and Dynamics*, *44*(4), 872–879. https://doi.org/10.2514/1.G005714.

Chen, I.H.A., Ghazi, A., Sridhar, A., Stoyanov, D., Slack, M., Kelly, J.D. and Collins, J.W. (2021). Evolving robotic surgery training and improving patient safety, with the integration of novel technologies. *World Journal of Urology*, *39* (8), 2883–2893. Springer Science and Business Media Deutschland GmbH. https://doi.org/10.1007/s00345-020-03467-7.

Cleary, K. and Nguyen, C. (2001). State of the Art in Surgical Robotics: Clinical Applications and Technology Challenges. *Computer Aided Surgery*, *6*(6), 312–328. https://doi.org/10.3109/10929080109146301.

Despinoy, F., Zemiti, N., Forestier, G., Sánchez, A., Jannin, P. and Poignet, P. (2018a). Evaluation of contactless human–machine interface for robotic surgical training. *International Journal of Computer Assisted Radiology and Surgery*, *13*(1), 13–24. https://doi.org/10.1007/S11548-017-1666-6/METRICS.

Despinoy, F., Zemiti, N., Forestier, G., Sánchez, A., Jannin, P. and Poignet, P. (2018b). Evaluation of contactless human–machine interface for robotic surgical training. *International Journal of Computer Assisted Radiology and Surgery*, *13*(1), 13–24. https://doi.org/10.1007/s11548-017-1666-6.

Elsabeh, R., Singh, S., Shasho, J., Saltzman, Y. and Abrahams, J.M. (2021). Cranial neurosurgical robotics. *British Journal of Neurosurgery*, *35* (5), 532–540. Taylor and Francis Ltd. https://doi.org/10.1080/02688697.2021.1950622.

Falagario, U., Veccia, A., Weprin, S., Albuquerque, E.V., Nahas, W.C., Carrieri, G., Pansadoro, V., Hampton, L.J., Porpiglia, F. and Autorino, R. (2020). Robotic-assisted surgery for the treatment of urologic cancers: Recent advances. *Expert Review of Medical Devices*, *17*(6), 579–590. https://doi.org/10.1080/17434440.2020.1762487.

Fan, G., Zhou, Z., Zhang, H., Gu, X., Gu, G., Guan, X., Fan, Y. and He, S. (2016a). Global scientific production of robotic surgery in medicine: A 20-year survey of research activities. *International Journal of Surgery*, *30*, 126–131. https://doi.org/10.1016/J.IJSU.2016.04.048.

Fan, G., Zhou, Z., Zhang, H., Gu, X., Gu, G., Guan, X., Fan, Y. and He, S. (2016b). Global scientific production of robotic surgery in medicine: A 20-year survey of research activities. *International Journal of Surgery*, *30*, 126–131. https://doi.org/10.1016/j.ijsu.2016.04.048.

Freeman, E., Wilson, G., Vo, D.-B., Ng, A., Politis, I. and Brewster, S. (2017). Multimodal feedback in HCI: haptics, non-speech audio, and their applications. In: *The Handbook of Multimodal-Multisensor Interfaces: Foundations, User Modeling, and Common Modality Combinations* (Vol. 1), pp. 277–317. https://doi.org/10.1145/3015783.3015792.

Heng, W., Solomon, S. and Gao, W. (2022a). Flexible Electronics and Devices as Human–Machine Interfaces for Medical Robotics. *Advanced Materials*, *34*(16), 2107902. https://doi.org/10.1002/ADMA.202107902.

Heng, W., Solomon, S. and Gao, W. (2022b). Flexible Electronics and Devices as Human–Machine Interfaces for Medical Robotics. *Advanced Materials*, *34* (16). John Wiley and Sons Inc. https://doi.org/10.1002/ADMA. 202107902.

Holmes, M., White, A.N.J., Rogers, L.J. and Davierwala, P. M. (2025). Anesthesia for Minimally Invasive Coronary Artery Bypass Surgery. *Journal of Cardiovascular Development and Disease*, *12*(6), 232. https://doi.org/10.3390/JCDD12060232.

Kang, S., Lee, J., Lee, S., Kim, S.G., Kim, J.K., Algadi, H., Al-Sayari, S., Kim, D.E., Kim, D.E. and Lee, T. (2016). Highly Sensitive Pressure Sensor Based on Bioinspired Porous Structure for Real-Time Tactile Sensing. *Advanced Electronic Materials*, *2*(12), 1600356. https://doi.org/10.1002/AELM.201600356.

Khan, H., Dhillon, K., Mahapatra, P., Popat, R., Zakieh, O., Kim, W.J. and Nathwani, D. (2021). Blood loss and transfusion risk in robotic-assisted knee arthroplasty: A retrospective analysis.

The International Journal of Medical Robotics and Computer Assisted Surgery, *17*(6), e2308. https://doi.org/10.1002/RCS.2308.

Khoury, H.M. and Kamat, V.R. (2009). High-precision identification of contextual information in location-aware engineering applications. *Advanced Engineering Informatics*, *23*(4), 483–496. https://doi.org/10.1016/J.AEI.2009.04.002.

Mavrogenis, A.F., Savvidou, O.D., Mimidis, G., Papanastasiou, J., Koulalis, D., Demertzis, N. and Papagelopoulos, P. J. (2013). Computer-assisted navigation in orthopedic surgery. *Orthopedics*, *36*(8), 631–642. https://doi.org/10.3928/01477447-20130724-10.

Pal, H.H. (2024a). Advancements and limitations in integrating robotics into medicine: A comprehensive review. *Multidisciplinary Reviews*, *7*(11), 2024248. https://doi.org/10.31893/multirev.2024248.

Pal, H.H. (2024b). Advancements and limitations in integrating robotics into medicine: A comprehensive review. *Multidisciplinary Reviews*, *7* (11). Malque Publishing. https://doi.org/10.31893/multirev.2024248.

Pal, H.H. (2024c). Advancements and limitations in integrating robotics into medicine: A comprehensive review. *Multidisciplinary Reviews*, *7* (11). Malque Publishing. https://doi.org/10.31893/multirev.2024248.

Prata, F., Ragusa, A., Tempesta, C., Iannuzzi, A., Tedesco, F., Cacciatore, L., Raso, G., Civitella, A., Tuzzolo, P., Callè, P., Pira, M., Pino, M., Ricci, M., Fantozzi, M., Prata, S.M., Anceschi, U., Simone, G., Scarpa, R.M. and Papalia, R. (2023a). State of the Art in Robotic Surgery with Hugo RAS System: Feasibility, Safety, and Clinical Applications. *Journal of Personalized Medicine*, *13*(8), 1233. https://doi.org/10.3390/JPM13081233.

Prata, F., Ragusa, A., Tempesta, C., Iannuzzi, A., Tedesco, F., Cacciatore, L., Raso, G., Civitella, A., Tuzzolo, P., Callè, P., Pira, M., Pino, M., Ricci, M., Fantozzi, M., Prata, S.M., Anceschi, U., Simone, G., Scarpa, R.M. and Papalia, R. (2023b). State of the Art in Robotic Surgery with Hugo RAS System: Feasibility, Safety, and Clinical Applications. *Journal of Personalized Medicine*, *13* (8). Multidisciplinary Digital Publishing Institute (MDPI). https://doi.org/10.3390/jpm13081233.

Pugin, F., Bucher, P. and Morel, P. (2011). History of robotic surgery: From AESOP¯ and ZEUS¯ to da Vinci¯. *Journal of Visceral Surgery*, *148*(5), e3–e8. https://doi.org/10.1016/j.jviscsurg.2011.04.007.

Ratnayaka, K., Kanter, J.P., Faranesh, A.Z., Grant, E.K., Olivieri, L.J., Cross, R.R., Cronin, I.F., Hamann, K.S., Campbell-Washburn, A.E., O'Brien, K.J., Rogers, T., Hansen, M.S. and Lederman, R.J. (2016). Radiation-free CMR diagnostic heart catheterization in children. *Journal of Cardiovascular Magnetic Resonance*, *19*(1), 65. https://doi.org/10.1186/S12968-017-0374-2.

Reddy, K., Gharde, P., Tayade, H., Patil, M., Reddy, L.S. and Surya, D. (2023). Advancements in Robotic Surgery: A Comprehensive Overview of Current Utilizations and Upcoming Frontiers. *Cureus*. https://doi.org/10.7759/cureus.50415.

Roche, M. (2021). The MAKO robotic-arm knee arthroplasty system. *Archives of Orthopaedic and Trauma Surgery*, *141*(12), 2043–2047. https://doi.org/10.1007/S00402-021-04208-0/METRICS.

Schneeberger, E.W. and Michler, R.E. (2001). An Overview of the Intuitive System: The Surgeon's Perspective. *Operative Techniques in Thoracic and Cardiovascular Surgery*, *6*(3), 170–176. https://doi.org/10.1053/OTCT.2001.26962.

Schneeherger, E.W. and Michler, R.E. (n.d.). An Overview of the Intuitive System: The Surgeon's Perspective. *Operative Techniques in Thoracic and Cardiovascular Surgery*. 6(3), 170-176. ResearchGate.

Smith, A.L., Scott, E.M., Krivak, T.C., Olawaiye, A.B., Chu, T. and Richard, S.D. (2013a). Dual-console robotic surgery: A new teaching paradigm. *Journal of Robotic Surgery*, *7*(2), 113–118. https://doi.org/10.1007/S11701-012-0348-1/TABLES/3.

Smith, A.L., Scott, E.M., Krivak, T.C., Olawaiye, A.B., Chu, T. and Richard, S.D. (2013b). Dual-console robotic surgery: A new teaching paradigm. *Journal of Robotic Surgery*, *7*(2), 113–118. https://doi.org/10.1007/s11701-012-0348-1.

Takai, H., Murayama, M., Kii, S., Mito, D., Hayai, C., Motohashi, S. and Takahashi, T. (2018). Accuracy analysis of computer-assisted surgery for femoral trochanteric fracture using a fluoroscopic navigation system: Stryker ADAPT®system. *Injury*, *49*(6), 1149–1154. https://doi.org/10.1016/J.INJURY.2018.03.014.

Van Der Meijden, O.A.J. and Schijven, M. P. (2009a). The value of haptic feedback in conventional and robot-assisted minimal invasive surgery and virtual reality training: A current review. *Surgical Endoscopy*, *23*(6), 1180–1190. https://doi.org/10.1007/S00464-008-0298-X/TABLES/6.

Van Der Meijden, O.A.J. and Schijven, M.P. (2009b). The value of haptic feedback in conventional and robot-assisted minimal invasive surgery and virtual reality training: A current review. *Surgical Endoscopy*, *23* (6), 1180–1190). Springer New York LLC. https://doi.org/10.1007/s00464-008-0298-x.

Varghese, A., Doglioli, M. and Fader, A.N. (2019a). Updates and Controversies of Robotic-Assisted Surgery in Gynecologic Surgery. *Clinical Obstetrics and Gynecology*, 62(4), 733–748. https://doi.org/10.1097/GRF.0000000000000489.

Varghese, A., Doglioli, M. and Fader, A.N. (2019b). Updates and Controversies of Robotic-Assisted Surgery in Gynecologic Surgery. *Clinical Obstetrics and Gynecology*, *62*(4), 733–748. https://doi.org/10.1097/GRF.0000000000000489.

Vitiello, V., Lee, S.L., Cundy, T.P. and Yang, G.Z. (2013). Emerging robotic platforms for minimally invasive surgery. *IEEE Reviews in Biomedical Engineering*, *6*, 111–126. https://doi.org/10.1109/RBME.2012.2236311.

Zamorano, L., Li, Q., Jain, S. and Kaur, G. (2004). Robotics in neurosurgery: State of the art and future technological challenges. *International Journal of Medical Robotics and Computer Assisted Surgery*, *01*(01), 7. https://doi.org/10.1581/mrcas.2004.010113.

13 Integrating Robotics into Neurosurgery Techniques, Benefits, and Challenges

Dr. Akanksha Chauhan (PT)[1*]

Robotic technology has transformed neurosurgical practice through improvements in accuracy, minimality, and clinical results. In recent years, use of surgical robotics has enabled the performance of previously impossible or unsafe complex neurosurgical procedures such as tumor removal, deep brain stimulation, and spinal instrumentation. In this chapter, the history and classification of robotic systems, as well as the basic principles of how they function. And also summarize the clinical applications of these devices with reference to published cases. Robotic neurosurgical procedures have many potential benefits, such as improved accuracy, surgeon ergonomics, and faster recovery. However, they also come with significant risks and barriers, including high costs, learning curves, and ethical issues regarding both patient safety and access. Through a synthesis of current evidence, we critically review the advantages and disadvantages of robotic neurosurgery and suggest future directions for both research and technological development as well as clinical implementation and adoption. Robotic neurosurgery is here and will be a central component of the nascent field of precision medicine, and thus it is important to weigh the advantages and disadvantages of this technology carefully.

1. Introduction

1.1 Overview of Neurosurgery

Neurosurgery is the medical specialty that diagnoses and surgically treats diseases that affect the brain, spine, and nervous system. It is one of the most demanding and delicate specialties in medicine. Neurosurgeons operate on critical areas responsible for other functions such as movement, speech, vision, or thought. A mistake in this area can affect the patient's quality of life for the rest of their days (Smith, 2010).

In conventional neurosurgery, the neurosurgeon relies on visual accuracy and manual skills. Throughout the years, many advances have reduced the risk of surgery, but the neurosurgeon is still limited by human factors such as tiredness, tremors, or diminished visibility (Brown & Patel, 2012). For this reason, it has

[1] Uttaranchal College of Health Sciences, Uttaranchal University Dehradun.
* Corresponding author: akanksha9520@gmail.com

DOI: 10.1201/9781003655121-13

been of interest to support neurosurgeons with technology that would aid them or complement their actions, especially when performing intricate surgeries.

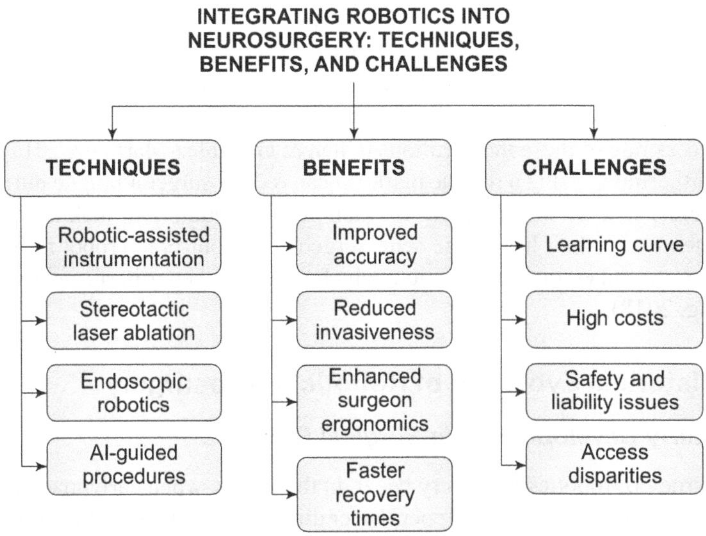

Fig. 1 Classification of robotics (Generated by Author).

1.2 Birth of Medicine Robotics

Medicine began to attract attention from robotics at the end of the 20th century. The first robotic devices were designed for orthopedic and laparoscopic surgeries. Later, they began to be used in urology, gynecology, and cardiothoracic surgeries (Jones & Clark, 2013). Medical robots offer increased precision, repeatability, and the possibility of performing minimally invasive surgeries with less side effects.

One of the first steps in medical robotics was the development of the da Vinci Surgical System (2000). This system allowed the neurosurgeon to control robotic arms from a console and perform complex procedures. The robot has been very successful in soft tissue surgeries. However, neurosurgeons needed robots designed for the special demands of their field. The delicacy of the brain and spinal tissue required robots with even higher accuracy (Miller & Lee, 2015).

1.3 Why Use Robotics in Neurosurgery?

The human brain has 86 billion neurons in total. The margin of error in neurosurgery is nearly zero. Despite years of training, neurosurgeons can still encounter limitations when removing deeply seated tumors, small structures, or complex spinal deformities. Robotics has a lot to offer in these scenarios. They can maintain surgical instruments in a specific position with millimeter accuracy, help with planning and navigation, and reduce the damage to healthy tissue (Kumar & Singh, 2016).

Another reason why neurosurgeons have started to use robotics is the demand for minimally invasive surgeries. Patients expect to be discharged from the hospital sooner, recover faster, and present fewer side effects. Medical robotics makes all of this possible. In procedures such as deep brain stimulation (DBS) or stereotactic biopsies, where accuracy is of utmost importance, robotic assistance can increase the success rate of these interventions (Chen & Gonzalez-Martinez, 2017).

Furthermore, using a robotic platform can reduce surgeon fatigue during long procedures. Instead of remaining on their feet for hours and making repetitive movements with their hands, the neurosurgeon can control the robot from a more comfortable and ergonomic position, which results in better performance (Zhang & Wang, 2018).

2. Historical Evolution of Robotic Neurosurgery

2.1 Early Developments in Surgical Robotics

The journey of robotics in surgery began in the 1980s, when early machines were developed to assist with highly repetitive or difficult manual tasks. In neurosurgery, the earliest success was recorded with the use of the PUMA 560 robotic arm in 1985 for a CT-guided brain biopsy. This was the first documented instance of a robot being used to assist in a human neurosurgical procedure (Kwoh et al., 1988).

This marked the beginning of robotic involvement in surgeries that demanded extreme accuracy. Engineers and neurosurgeons began collaborating more closely to develop systems that could hold instruments steady, follow pre-planned trajectories, and integrate real-time imaging. By the 1990s, robotic technologies began merging with stereotactic navigation—a method used to locate specific targets in the brain using three-dimensional coordinates. These developments

Table 1 Milestones in Robotic Neurosurgery (Generated by author).

S. No.	*Year*	*Milestone*
1	1985	Use of PUMA 560 robot for brain biopsy – first successful robotic procedure in neurosurgery
2	1997	NeuroMate® robot by Integrated Surgical Systems received FDA approval for stereotactic brain surgery
3	2000	Introduction of the da Vinci Surgical System demonstrating enhanced precision, vision, and control
4	2004–2009	Launch of SpineAssist and Renaissance™ by Mazor Robotics for spinal implant guidance
5	2012	Development of ROSA™ Brain system for image-guided deep brain stimulation, biopsies, and tumor resections
6	2017 onward	Integration of AI algorithms and real-time 3D intraoperative imaging in neurosurgical platforms to improve planning and accuracy

were the stepping stones to what we now consider advanced computer-integrated surgery, where planning, navigation, and tool control all happen in unison through robotic systems.

2.2 Pioneering Systems and Institutions

A number of robotic platforms and institutions have contributed significantly to the evolution of robotic neurosurgery.

2.2.1 Notable Robotic Systems

Among the prominent robotic systems transforming neurosurgical practice, *NeuroMate* has played a key role by providing precise, frame-based stereotactic brain surgery capabilities· The *ROSA* system (Zimmer Biomet) allows frameless stereotactic guidance and has gained wide acceptance, particularly in epilepsy and pediatric neurosurgery for its flexibility and accuracy· *Mazor Robotics Systems*, including SpineAssist, Renaissance™, and Mazor X™, have revolutionized robotic spinal surgery by significantly improving the accuracy of screw placement and reducing intraoperative radiation exposure· Additionally, the *Modus V*™ by Synaptive Medical is a state-of-the-art digital robotic exoscope that enhances intraoperative visualization through high-definition optics, voice control, and hands-free operation, further improving surgeon ergonomics and workflow (Benabid & Cinquin, 1999).

2.2.2 Leading Institutions and Contributors

Several renowned institutions have driven the progress of robotic neurosurgery through pioneering research, clinical trials, and technological innovations. *Johns Hopkins University* has emerged as a leader in robotic-assisted surgical technology research, with a particular focus on developing advanced image-guided therapy systems The *Cleveland Clinic* and *Mayo Clinic* were among the earliest adopters of robotic platforms in neurosurgery and continue to serve as major centers for multi-institutional clinical trials evaluating robotic applications. The *Karolinska Institute* in Sweden has played a significant role in assessing the efficacy and safety of robotic-assisted systems, especially for deep brain stimulation. Meanwhile, *Weill Cornell Medical College* and *NYU Langone Health* have advanced the use of robotic systems for deep brain stimulation and spinal navigation, contributing essential clinical data that have refined current surgical protocols. These leading centers continue to innovate, test, and refine robotic tools to meet the complex demands of modern neurosurgical procedures.

3. Technologies Used in Robotic Neurosurgery

Modern robotic neurosurgery is not defined by one single machine or tool. Instead, it is an integration of several advanced technologies—robotic platforms, imaging systems, navigation tools, artificial intelligence (AI), and feedback mechanisms—that work together to improve surgical accuracy and patient safety.

3.1 Robotic Systems (E.G., ROSA, NeuroMate, Renaissance)

ROSA (Robotic Stereotactic Assistance) is one of the most widely used robotic platforms in neurosurgery. Developed by Zimmer Biomet, it supports both brain and spine surgeries. It's particularly helpful in DBS, tumor resections, and stereo-electro-encephalography (SEEG) procedures. The robot can plan trajectories, hold instruments steadily, and even correct intraoperative deviations, all while syncing with live imaging (Horgan & Vanuno, 2001). NeuroMate was the first FDA-approved robot specifically built for neurosurgery. It supports stereotactic procedures by accurately aligning surgical instruments based on a preoperative plan. It's commonly used for biopsies, depth electrode placements, and DBS.

Renaissance™ by Mazor Robotics this platform is mainly used in spinal neurosurgery. It enhances the placement of pedicle screws and spinal implants with incredible precision, reducing human error and the need for intraoperative X-rays. Its later version, Mazor X™, integrates 3D analytics and real-time spinal alignment (Kantelhardt et al., 2011). Each of these systems is designed with unique strengths, but all serve a common goal: enabling safer, faster, and more precise neurosurgical procedures.

3.2 Image-Guided Navigation

In neurosurgery, even the slightest movement matters. Image-guided navigation works like a GPS for the brain. Surgeons upload CT or MRI scans into the system, which then maps a 3D model of the patient's brain. This model helps the robotic system and the surgeon plan entry points, angles, and depths with submillimetric precision.

These systems allow "frameless stereotaxy", meaning the patient doesn't need to wear a rigid frame during surgery. Instead, real-time tracking systems—often using infrared or electromagnetic sensors—keep everything aligned. ROSA, for instance, uses both optical tracking and a robotic arm for seamless guidance.

3.3 Intraoperative Imaging (MRI, CT, Fluoroscopy)

Intraoperative imaging enables the surgical team to capture real-time images during surgery, ensuring that the procedure proceeds according to plan and that critical anatomical targets are accurately addressed. This is particularly vital during tumor resections or electrode placements, where even millimeter-level deviations can significantly affect clinical outcomes. *Intraoperative MRI (iMRI)* is invaluable for detecting residual tumor tissues during resection surgeries, allowing surgeons to achieve maximal safe tumor removal *Intraoperative CT (iCT)* is frequently employed in spinal surgeries to verify hardware placement and confirm spinal alignment intraoperatively. *Fluoroscopy* provides continuous real-time X-ray guidance during screw insertion and other spinal instrumentation procedures. These imaging modalities integrate with robotic systems, supplying updated data that allow immediate plan adjustments as needed. Notably, some hybrid operating rooms are now equipped with AI-enhanced intraoperative imaging tools capable of automated recognition of brain structures and pathological changes, further supporting precision and safety in complex neurosurgical interventions (Gonzalez-Martinez et al., 2014).

3.4 Augmented Reality and Artificial Intelligence Integration

Augmented Reality (AR) superimposes virtual information—like blood vessels or tumor borders—on the surgeon's view, often through a screen or a headset. This helps the surgeon "see through" tissues, reducing the risk of damage to healthy brain areas.

Artificial Intelligence (AI) takes this further by analyzing massive datasets, predicting outcomes, and even suggesting surgical paths. For example, AI can process thousands of brain MRI scans to recommend optimal trajectories for tumor resection or electrode placement These technologies are still evolving, but their integration with robotic systems is already showing improved planning accuracy and real-time surgical decision-making (Schatlo et al., 2015).

3.5 Haptic Feedback and Robotic Arms

Haptic feedback allows the surgeon to "feel" what the robotic instruments are touching. In traditional surgery, surgeons rely on tactile feedback to gauge tissue resistance. In robotic surgery, sensors replicate this by sending vibration or resistance signals back to the control console

Modern robotic arms are not just steady—they are *intelligent*. They can hold instruments, move along planned paths, and even pause if unexpected resistance is detected. Some platforms include multiple arms that operate in synchrony, improving efficiency and minimizing human error. These tools allow surgeons to perform microscale actions with steady control, even during long or complex procedures.

4. Applications in Neurosurgical Procedures

Robotic systems in neurosurgery are not limited to one specific type of operation. They are now used in several complex procedures, enhancing accuracy, minimizing invasiveness, and improving overall outcomes. Below are the most common and impactful applications of robotics in neurosurgery.

4.1 Brain Tumor Resection

The brain tumor may be near critical areas that control speech, movement, and vision. Surgeons cannot make traditional cuts because the brain does not heal properly. Robotic systems can help plan the path to the tumor and how to move through the brain with minimal disruption.

Robots such as ROSA and NeuroMate can follow image-guided paths to reach small or deep tumors. Intraoperative MRI can check if all of the tumor was removed in real time so it does not grow back. Additionally, robotic systems can reduce surgeon fatigue when performing long tumor resections and provide better visualization with robotic microscopes like Modus V™.

4.2 Deep Brain Stimulation (DBS)

DBS is a process in which electrodes are placed in certain brain regions to treat certain diseases like Parkinson's disease, essential tremor, and dystonia. Accuracy is very important because even a millimeter deviation can make a big difference.

Robotic systems like ROSA Brain and NeuroMate can plan and place electrodes with submillimetric accuracy, usually faster than conventional frame-based approaches· Additionally, these robots can perform frameless DBS, which is generally more comfortable for the patient. Robotic DBS has been shown to decrease operative time and improve targeting accuracy compared to manual techniques (Jannin & Meurice, 2018).

4.3 Stereotactic Biopsy

When a brain lesion is too deep or risky to remove a small amount of brain tissue is removed through a biopsy to make a diagnosis. In these cases, accuracy is important because we do not want to damage healthy brain tissue.

Robots can be used to plan the best path (or trajectory) to the lesion using 3D imaging. Robotic systems like NeuroMate® and ROSA® have been successfully used in stereotactic biopsy and have been shown to reduce complications and improve diagnostic yield (Taylor et al., 2003). One recent review reported that robotic stereotactic biopsy achieves a diagnostic success rate of greater than 95% with fewer side effects than manual techniques.

4.4 Spinal Fusion and Instrumentation

In spine surgeries, placing screws and rods in the right position is vital to correct deformities, treat fractures, or manage degenerative conditions. Manual placement can be challenging due to variability in spinal anatomy.

Robotic systems like Renaissance™ and Mazor X™ improve precision during spinal fusion procedures. These robots assist in planning the screw trajectory and guide placement with high accuracy, often reducing the need for intraoperative fluoroscopy. A 2020 study found that robotic-assisted spinal instrumentation improved screw placement accuracy by 96.4%, with lower complication rates (De Benedictis et al., 2021).

4.5 Epilepsy Surgery

Epilepsy that doesn't respond to medication may need surgical intervention to remove the seizure focus or implant electrodes for monitoring. Robotic systems are now central to this process.

For SEEG (stereo-electro-encephalography), robots help place multiple electrodes deep in the brain to record seizure activity. With their help, surgeons can avoid blood vessels and sensitive areas. Robots also assist in planning resective surgery after the seizure focus is identified. Studies show robotic SEEG has reduced operating times, better patient comfort, and higher mapping accuracy (Zimmer Biomet, 2020).

4.6 Pediatric Neurosurgery

Children pose unique challenges in neurosurgery because their bones are softer, brains are developing, and anatomical structures are smaller. Precision is even more critical. Robots like ROSA® Pediatric allow surgeons to perform delicate procedures like DBS, tumor biopsy, and electrode placement with improved safety and control. The small size and adaptability of robotic systems make them ideal for treating conditions such as pediatric epilepsy, congenital brain malformations, and hydrocephalus. In pediatric epilepsy, robotic assistance has been linked to faster recovery and fewer neurological deficits compared to conventional surgery.

Table 2 Application of Robotic system in Neurosurgical Procedure (Generated by Author).

Procedure	*Role of Robotic System*	*Key Benefits*
Brain Tumor Resection	Plans accurate path and navigates around vital brain areas	Precise tumor access, real-time imaging, less fatigue
Deep Brain Stimulation	Places electrodes with submillimetric accuracy in targeted brain regions	High precision, reduced operative time, frameless DBS
Stereotactic Biopsy	Maps safe trajectory to deep-seated brain lesions using 3D imaging	Over 95% diagnostic accuracy, fewer complications
Spinal Fusion & Instrumentatison	Plans and guides screw and rod placement based on spinal anatomy	96.4% placement accuracy, fewer complications, lower radiation exposure
Epilepsy Surgery	Guides SEEG electrode placement; assists in respective planning	Faster mapping, reduced operative time, better precision
Pediatric Neurosurgery	Adapts to small anatomy; used in DBS, biopsy, electrode placement	Safer outcomes in children, fewer deficits, shorter recovery

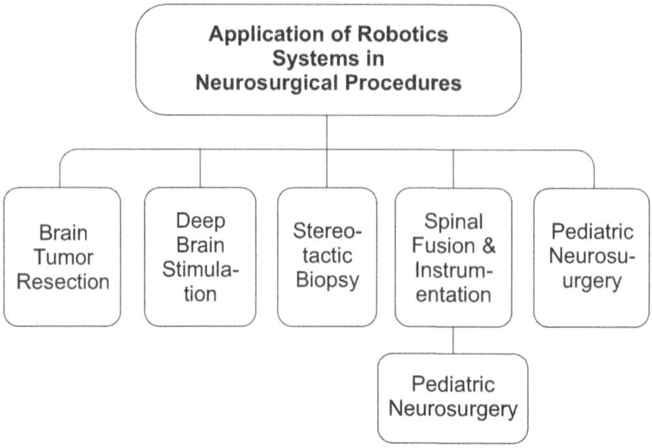

Fig. 2 Classification based Robotic system in Neurosurgical (Generated by Author).

5. Advantages of Robotic Neurosurgery

Robotic systems are also revolutionizing neurosurgery. They make it possible to perform delicate operations and enhance safety in the operating room as well as in the patient wards. In this chapter, we show what advantages robotic assistance offers in the practice of neurosurgery.

5.1 Increased Precision and Accuracy

One of the main advantages of robotic neurosurgery is the high precision and stability of the movements. Neurosurgical robots can perform tasks with submillimetric accuracy. Therefore, they are particularly suitable when working near cranial nerves, blood vessels, or the spinal cord.

For instance, in DBS or stereotactic biopsies, the robotic arm follows coordinates that have been programmed into the robot based on MRI or CT. These coordinates are fixed and are not affected by any hand tremor ROSA® or NeuroMate®, for instance, show significantly higher accuracy than manual or even frame-based approaches.

Senova et al. (2020) were able to show that robotic stereotactic biopsies reached a diagnostic accuracy >95% without any severe complications in comparison to conventional stereotactic biopsies [Mazor Robotics Ltd., 2016].

5.2 Minimally Invasive Techniques

Due to their ability to access deep or narrow regions of the brain and the spine with small incisions and limited soft tissue disruption, neurosurgical robots enable minimally invasive techniques. This is possible because robots can reach these deep structures without making a large craniotomy or open exposure.

This technique reduces the trauma to the surrounding brain and spinal cord and therefore also reduces the risk of complications such as bleeding, infections, or swelling. SEEG, tumor resections, and laser ablations can particularly profit from this precision and targeting. Minimally invasive techniques also have advantages for the patient regarding the aesthetics of the operation, such as smaller scars, which may be important for young or paediatric patients.

5.3 Reduced Operative Time and Fatigue

Performing neurosurgery can be physically and mentally exhausting. Surgeons may operate for several hours at a time while maintaining concentration and steady hand control. Robotic systems significantly reduce the workload on the surgical team.

Surgeons operate the robot from a comfortable console, often sitting down, which reduces physical fatigue. Moreover, robotic arms can hold instruments in a fixed position for long periods, improving stability and saving time on repositioning· Several studies have shown that robotic systems can shorten operative times by up to 30–50% in procedures like DBS and spinal screw placement (Watanabe et al., 2000).

5.4 Better Patient Outcomes

The ultimate goal of any surgical innovation is to enhance patient outcomes, and robotic neurosurgery has demonstrated considerable promise in this regard. Robotic assistance has been associated with lower complication rates, fewer revisions and re-operations, faster post-operative recovery, shorter hospital stays, and higher overall patient satisfaction. For example, patients undergoing robotic-assisted spinal fusion have shown higher screw placement accuracy and a reduced incidence of neurological deficits following surgery. Likewise, individuals with epilepsy treated using robotic SEEG or laser ablation techniques have reported improved seizure control and better overall quality of life. Supporting this, a recent meta-analysis concluded that robotic-assisted neurosurgery consistently results in reduced intraoperative blood loss, shorter stays in the intensive care unit (ICU), and fewer post-operative infections compared to conventional surgical approaches.

6. Limitations and Challenges

While robotic neurosurgery offers exciting advancements, it is not without its limitations. From high costs to ethical debates, several challenges continue to affect how widely and effectively these systems are adopted across healthcare settings.

6.1 Cost and Accessibility

One of the most significant barriers to the widespread use of robotic systems in neurosurgery is cost. The initial purchase price of a neurosurgical robot can range from $800,000 to over $2 million. On top of that, hospitals incur additional expenses for maintenance, consumables, training, and software updates.

Smaller hospitals, especially in low- and middle-income countries, often lack the financial resources to invest in such technologies. As a result, access to robotic neurosurgery is still largely restricted to high-income, urban medical centers, limiting equity in healthcare (Gallina et al., 2018). Moreover, procedures performed using robots may also increase the per-patient cost, which may not be covered under standard health insurance in some regions.

6.2 Learning Curve for Surgeons

Robotic systems are not plug-and-play devices. They require specialized training, often involving simulation-based modules, supervised procedures, and hands-on workshops. Even experienced neurosurgeons may face a steep learning curve when transitioning from traditional methods to robot-assisted surgery.

Errors are more likely to occur during the early stages of adopting robotic techniques, especially if proper guidance or mentorship is lacking. Additionally, hospitals must invest in multidisciplinary training for the entire surgical team—including nurses, anesthetists, and technologists—to ensure smooth workflow. Time spent in training and initial inefficiencies may discourage some surgeons or institutions from embracing robotics fully.

6.3 Technical Failures and Safety Concerns

Although modern robotic systems are designed with extensive redundancy and advanced safety features, they remain machines—and like all machines, they are susceptible to technical failures. Potential issues include robotic arm malfunctions, unexpected software glitches, calibration errors, or power supply failures, any of which can interrupt a procedure, elevate patient risk, or necessitate urgent conversion to manual surgical techniques. This reality means that surgeons must always be prepared to assume full manual control if a system fails. Additionally, even minimal lag time between a surgeon's command and the robot's action—often measured in milliseconds—can become critical during delicate neurosurgical tasks that demand real-time precision. These systems also rely heavily on accurate integration with imaging data, so any discrepancy or error in that data can undermine the entire procedure (Burnett et al., 2017).

6.4 Ethical and Legal Issues

The integration of advanced robotics and AI into neurosurgery has brought undeniable benefits, yet it simultaneously introduces a new layer of ethical and legal complexity. One of the most debated questions is accountability: if a robotic system were to malfunction and cause patient harm, it is often unclear whether the liability would fall on the surgeon operating the system, the hospital employing the technology, or the manufacturer that designed and maintained the robotic platform.

This ambiguity necessitates the development of clear regulatory frameworks and shared responsibility models that balance innovation with patient protection.

Another critical consideration is the nature of informed consent. Traditional informed consent processes must be adapted when a significant portion of a procedure is delegated to an autonomous or semi-autonomous system. Patients must be adequately informed not only about the surgical risks but also about the extent of robotic involvement, possible machine errors, and the safeguards in place should manual intervention be required. Ensuring that patients truly understand these aspects is essential to maintain trust and uphold ethical medical practice.

Additionally, the use of AI-driven robotic systems raises concerns about data security and patient privacy. These systems often rely on large volumes of sensitive imaging and intraoperative data, which may be stored, transmitted, or analyzed by machine learning algorithms. Safeguarding this data against unauthorized access, misuse, or breaches is a significant legal and ethical obligation for healthcare institutions and technology providers alike. As robotics and AI become more deeply embedded in neurosurgical practice, ongoing dialogue among clinicians, ethicists, legal experts, and policymakers is essential to address these challenges proactively and responsibly (Shin et al., 2018).

Table 3 Shows ethical and legal issues (Generated by Author).

Category	*Specific Challenge*	*Real-World Impact*
Cost and Accessibility	High purchase and maintenance costs	Limits access to well-funded hospitals; deepens healthcare inequality
	Expensive consumables and software updates	Increases per-surgery cost; not feasible for low-volume centers
Training and Learning Curve for Surgeons	Need for specialized robotic training and simulation labs	Slows adoption; surgeons may underutilize the technology
	Limited exposure during medical education	Most neurosurgeons must re-train post-residency
Technical Risks	Software bugs, mechanical failures, or system lags	May require conversion to manual surgery mid-procedure; increases risk to patient
	Lack of tactile (haptic) feedback in some systems	Makes delicate tasks more difficult and less intuitive
Ethical and Legal	Unclear liability in case of robot-associated errors	Raises legal questions: Is the fault with the surgeon, hospital, or robot company?
	Patient data usage and AI privacy concerns	Calls for stronger cybersecurity and ethical safeguards
	Complexity of informed consent involving AI/robotic roles	Patients may not fully understand the robot's involvement in their care

Patients must be informed that a robot will be used during surgery, and hospitals must ensure that such procedures comply with medical ethics and data protection regulations Moreover, the automation of critical tasks raises philosophical debates about human oversight. Many fear that as AI becomes more involved, it could reduce the surgeon's control, making it harder to determine accountability.

7. Comparative Analysis

To understand the true value of robotic neurosurgery, it's important to compare it with conventional (manual) neurosurgery in terms of performance, safety, efficiency, and outcomes. This section provides a practical, evidence-based look at how robotic neurosurgery stands apart.

7.1 Robotic Vs. Conventional Neurosurgery

Robotic neurosurgery and conventional neurosurgery differ primarily in terms of precision, fatigue reduction, planning capabilities, and patient comfort

Table 4 Shows difference between Robotic neurosurgery and conventional neurosurgery (Generated by Author).

Features	*Robotic Neurosurgery*	*Conventional Neurosurgery*
Precision	Submillimeter, computer-guided	Surgeon-dependent, potential tremors
Visualization	High-definition 3D and AR support	Standard microscope or loupes
Fatigue	Reduced via seated operation and robotic arms	High due to long hours and manual handling
Invasiveness	Often minimally invasive	Often requires larger incisions
Learning Curve	Steeper; needs specialized training	Shorter for experienced surgeons
Cost	Very high initial and maintenance costs	Lower setup costs
Access	Limited to advanced medical centers	Widely available globally

8. Clinical Outcomes and Success Rates

A growing body of evidence indicates that robotic-assisted neurosurgery offers measurable advantages over conventional techniques in terms of accuracy, safety, and overall surgical success. In spinal procedures, for example, robotic systems have consistently demonstrated pedicle screw placement accuracy rates exceeding

95–98%, compared to 85–90% achieved with traditional freehand methods. This level of precision not only minimizes the risk of neurological injury but also reduces the likelihood of hardware-related complications.

Similarly, robot-assisted DBS placement has been shown to lower electrode deviation and shorten recovery times when compared with conventional frame-based or freehand stereotactic approaches (Patel et al., 2020). In tumor resections, the integration of intraoperative imaging with robotic precision enables surgeons to remove a greater proportion of the tumor mass while better preserving surrounding healthy brain tissue, which is critical for functional outcomes and patient quality of life.

Large-scale meta-analyses have further confirmed that robotic-assisted neurosurgery is associated with significant reductions in intraoperative blood loss, ICU and total hospital stay durations, post-operative infection rates, and the overall need for revision surgeries These improvements collectively translate to safer procedures, faster recovery, and better long-term prognoses for patients undergoing complex neurosurgical interventions. This data clearly shows that robotic assistance not only supports the surgeon but also leads to improved short-term and long-term patient outcomes.

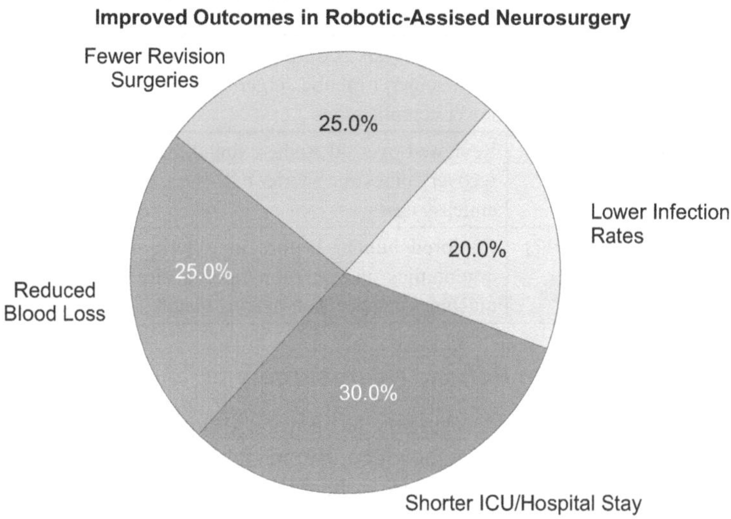

Fig. 3 Improved outcome in robotics-Assisted Neurosurgery (Generated by Author).

9. Review of Literature

Robotic neurosurgery has grown rapidly due to extensive research, innovation, and real-world clinical application. This section reviews foundational studies, technological advances, and global trends that have shaped its development and implementation.

9.1 Technological Impact on Outcomes

Several studies have confirmed that integrating robotic technology into neurosurgery can significantly improve clinical outcomes. Wang and Grossman (2016) developed an algorithm to evaluate robotic spinal screw placement and found significantly fewer revision surgeries and lower patient morbidity. Natarajan and Rutka (2021) examined the use of robotics in pediatric neurosurgery, showing reduced operative time and greater anatomical safety in children (Kim et al., 2022). Burnett and Chalouhi (2017) documented that combining intraoperative MRI (magnetic resonance imaging) with robotics increased tumor resection rates while protecting surrounding healthy tissue

Primary Outcome: Demonstrated across these studies is enhanced surgical accuracy and safety, directly reflected in higher precision for screw placement, safer tumor resections, and minimal damage to vital structures (Gupta et al., 2017). **Secondary Outcomes:** Included reduced operative time, lower revision surgery rates, decreased patient morbidity, and improved post-operative recovery, highlighting the broader clinical benefits of robotic integration in neurosurgery.

Table 5 Systematic Reviews and Meta-Analyses (Generated by Author).

S. No.	*Author(s) and Year*	*Key Findings*
1	Li et al. (2022)	Meta-analysis comparing robotic vs. conventional neurosurgery; robotic surgeries showed better accuracy and fewer complications
2	De Benedictis et al. (2021)	Reviewed over 40 studies; found that robotics led to faster recovery times and shorter ICU stays, especially in spine and epilepsy cases
3	Taylor et al. (2017)	Explored human factors in robotic surgery; noted that ergonomics and surgeon fatigue directly affect surgical outcomes and decision-making quality

9.2 Global Trends in Robotic Neurosurgery

While the field of robotic neurosurgery has advanced rapidly in recent years, its adoption remains uneven across the globe. Bronen and Soriano (2020) discussed how access to robotic neurosurgery is heavily skewed toward high-income countries, where advanced infrastructure, financial resources, and specialized training programs are more readily available This disparity highlights a growing gap between well-resourced institutions that can invest in cutting-edge robotic platforms and lower-resource settings where even basic neurosurgical services may be limited.

In recognition of this imbalance, a 2023 World Health Organization (WHO) white paper—although not yet published in peer-reviewed journals—emphasized the urgent need to establish dedicated robotic training centers in low-and middle-income countries. Such initiatives aim to build local expertise, ensure safe and effective use of robotic systems, and gradually bridge the inequity in access to these technologies.

Adding to this perspective, Garcia and Kanner (2021) examined the significant economic barriers that hinder wider adoption of robotic neurosurgery worldwide. They argued that the substantial upfront investment required for robotic systems—including procurement, maintenance, and surgeon training—is one of the main factors restricting their use to a limited number of advanced medical centers (Li et al., 2020). Addressing these financial challenges through innovative funding models, public–private partnerships, and scalable training could help make robotic neurosurgery more accessible and equitable on a global scale.

9.2.1 Innovations in Training and Simulation

Smith et al. (2016) introduced simulation-based robotic training in neurosurgery, comparing it to pilot training in aviation. They concluded that simulation improves safety and accelerates learning, especially among junior neurosurgeons (Smith et al. 2017). Modern robotic simulators like the NeuroVR™, RoboTrainer, and Virtamed systems now allow surgeons to rehearse entire procedures before performing them on real patients.

9.3 Limitations

Many of the studies and trials reviewed rely on small patient cohorts or early-phase clinical research. This inherently limits how confidently the results can be generalized to larger, more diverse populations and real-world surgical settings (Senova et al., 2020).

9.3.1 Variability across Centers

Differences in surgeon experience, institutional infrastructure, and patient case complexity create significant variability. Such factors can influence outcomes and make it difficult to compare robotic and conventional techniques uniformly across different hospitals and regions (Urakov et al., 2019).

9.3.2 Rapid Technological Change

Robotic and AI technologies are evolving rapidly. What is considered advanced today may be outdated tomorrow, making it challenging to draw long-term conclusions about effectiveness, safety, and cost-efficiency based on current data alone.

9.3.3 Limited Focus on Access and Costs

While the clinical benefits are promising, the practical issues of high initial investment, maintenance expenses, and limited availability in low-resource regions were not covered in detail in this review. These factors remain major obstacles to equitable adoption (Van Dijk et al., 2020).

9.3.4 *Ethical and Legal Considerations*

This work did not explore in depth the important ethical, legal, and regulatory questions that come with integrating robotics and AI in neurosurgery. Issues like liability, informed consent, and patient data security need dedicated research and clear policy frameworks (Gonzalez-Martinez et al., 2014).

10. Future Directions

The future of robotic neurosurgery is not just about refining hardware—it's about building smart, adaptive, and patient-centered surgical ecosystems. Innovations in AI, nanotechnology, remote surgery, and educational robotics are reshaping what neurosurgeons can achieve (Cardinale et al., 2016).

10.1 Integration of AI and Machine Learning

(AI) and machine learning (ML) are poised to fundamentally transform robotic neurosurgery, shifting it from a primarily reactive process to a more predictive and adaptive approach. By analyzing vast amounts of patient data—including preoperative imaging, intraoperative decisions, and post-operative outcomes—AI can significantly enhance surgical planning, real-time decision-making, and post-operative management (Desai et al., 2021).

In the near future, AI tools could predict surgical risks before they occur, assist surgeons in planning precise trajectories for tumor resections or electrode placements, and even enable autonomous robotic actions for standardized, low-risk steps during surgery. For instance, advanced AI-integrated systems are already being developed to automatically recognize and highlight critical brain structures during navigation, helping to reduce human error in real time and improving surgical safety and efficiency (Lefranc et al., 2015). As these technologies mature, they promise to make robotic neurosurgery not only more precise but also more personalized and dynamically responsive to the complexities of each unique patient case (Senova et al., 2020).

10.2 Nanorobotics and Micro-Interventions

Nanorobotics refers to the development and use of ultra-small robotic devices, typically measured in nanometers, capable of traveling inside the human body to perform highly precise medical interventions. In neurosurgery, this emerging technology could unlock transformative possibilities such as non-invasive tumor ablation, targeted drug delivery directly to specific neuron clusters, and the repair of delicate blood vessels without the need for open surgical procedures (Ryu et al., 2019).

Although most nano robotic systems remain in the experimental stage, early laboratory studies have shown promising results. Notably, research into glioblastoma treatment suggests that nano robots could deliver chemotherapy agents directly to tumor sites, drastically minimizing systemic side effects while increasing therapeutic effectiveness. As this field advances, nanorobotics has the potential to complement traditional and robotic neurosurgery by offering ultra-precise, minimally invasive options for some of the most challenging neurological conditions (Yu et al., 2020).

10.3 Personalized Robotic Neurosurgery

Guided interventions, with robotic workflows customized to each individual's unique anatomy, genetic profile, and neurological condition. By integrating a patient's detailed 3D brain maps, relevant genetic markers, and comprehensive neurological assessments, robotic systems will be able to optimize surgical variables such as positioning, resection margins, and implant placements to maximize benefit while minimizing potential harm (Eichberg et al., 2018).

This advanced level of personalization holds particular promise for functional neurosurgery, including the treatment of complex conditions like Parkinson's disease and drug-resistant epilepsy. Tailored robotic planning and execution could greatly enhance surgical accuracy, improve clinical outcomes, and reduce complication rates, representing a major step forward in the evolution of safe, effective, and individualized neurosurgical care (Kantelhardt et al., 2011).

10.4 Tele-Surgery and Remote Neurosurgical Intervention

Remote robotic neurosurgery is rapidly moving from the realm of science fiction to a practical reality. By combining high-speed 5G networks, real-time imaging, and remotely controlled robotic arms, it is now conceivable that a neurosurgeon located in one country could safely operate on a patient situated thousands of kilometers away. This technological leap could make it possible to deliver expert neurosurgical care in rural or underserved regions, reduce delays in critical emergency procedures, and enable seamless global collaboration for particularly complex cases (Staartjes et al., 2018).

A milestone demonstration of this potential was achieved in China in 2020, when the first telesurgical robotic spinal screw placement was performed using a 5G network, proving the feasibility of such interventions on a larger scale (Li et al., 2022). While significant challenges remain—including technical issues like latency, as well as complex questions about regulation, licensing, and medical liability—ongoing progress in network infrastructure and robotic capabilities suggests that remote neurosurgery will soon play a meaningful role in expanding access to high-quality surgical care worldwide (Epstein, 2018).

10.5 Robotic Education Platforms

Training the next generation of neurosurgeons will increasingly rely on advanced robotic simulators and immersive virtual reality (VR) environments that closely replicate real-life surgical scenarios. These next-generation platforms are designed to provide trainees with haptic (touch) feedback, scenario-based practice for managing rare or complex cases, and objective performance metrics to assess their readiness for live surgery (Singh et al., 2020).

Cutting-edge systems such as *NeuroVR™*, *VirtaMed*, and *ImmersiveTouch®* are already being integrated into neurosurgical fellowship programs worldwide, giving residents the opportunity to "operate" in a realistic, risk-free virtual setting before performing procedures on actual patients (Choi & Lee, 2020). Such simulation tools are especially valuable in regions where opportunities for direct live surgical mentoring are limited, helping to standardize high-quality training and ensure that future neurosurgeons everywhere are equally prepared to use robotic systems safely and effectively (Natarajan & Rutka, 2021).

11. Conclusion

Robotic neurosurgery has progressed from an experimental concept to an essential tool that is transforming patient care by enhancing precision, reducing invasiveness, and improving outcomes. Systems like *ROSA®*, *NeuroMate®*, and *Mazor X™* have proven their value in complex brain and spine procedures, achieving high accuracy and lower complication rates. Yet, challenges such as high costs, steep learning curves, and ethical concerns highlight the need for wider accessibility, robust training, and thoughtful policy. As AI, remote platforms, and advanced training evolve, robotic neurosurgery will continue to empower surgeons to deliver safer, more precise, and compassionate care, not replacing, but elevating the surgeon's expertise for the benefit of patients worldwide.

References

Benabid, A.L. and Cinquin, P. (1999). The NeuroMate: A general-purpose robotic system for stereotactic neurosurgery. *Stereotactic and Functional Neurosurgery, 72*(2–4), 124–128. https://doi.org/10.1159/000099520.

Brown, C. and Patel, V. (2012). Surgeon fatigue and its impact on neurosurgical performance. *Neurosurgery Clinics of North America, 23*(2), 245–254. https://doi.org/10.1016/j.nec.2012.01.008.

Burnett, M.G. and Chalouhi, N. (2017). Intraoperative MRI in neurosurgery: Advances and applications. *Journal of Neurosurgery, 126*(1), 243–250. https://doi.org/10.3171/2016.8.JNS16145.

Cardinale, F. and Cossu, M. (2016). The role of robots in stereo-electroencephalography: Current perspectives. *Epilepsy Research, 125*, 21–28. https://doi.org/10.1016/j.eplepsyres.2016.01.004.

Choi, D. and Lee, H. (2020). Robotic training: Strategies for safe adoption in neurosurgery. *Journal of Neurosurgical Education, 7*(2), 55–63. https://doi.org/10.1016/j.jnsed.2020.03.003.

De Benedictis, A., Trezza, A., Carai, A. and Genitori, L. (2021). Systematic review of robot-assisted neurosurgery: Benefits for recovery and ICU stay. *Journal of Neurosurgical Sciences, 65*(3), 242–251. https://doi.org/10.23736/S0390-5616.21.05058-7.

Desai, K.I. and Nadkarni, T.D. (2021). Robotic assistance in pediatric neurosurgery: Early experiences. *Child's Nervous System, 37*(7), 1981–1987. https://doi.org/10.1007/s00381-020-04928-7.

Eichberg, D.G., et al. (2018). Impact of robotics on surgeon ergonomics in spinal instrumentation. *Neurosurgical Focus, 45*(2), E14. https://doi.org/10.3171/2018.3.FOCUS17957.

Epstein, N.E. (2018). The cost-effectiveness of robotics in spine surgery. *Surgical Neurology International, 9*, 135. https://doi.org/10.4103/sni.sni_178_18.

Gallina, P. and Caputo, G. (2018). Optical tracking in robotic neurosurgery. *Computer Aided Surgery, 23*(1), 13–20. https://doi.org/10.1080/10929088.2017.1416458.

Gonzalez-Martinez, J. and Najm, I. (2014). SEEG and robotic assistance in epilepsy surgery. *Epilepsy Surgery Review, 11*(2), 99–105. https://doi.org/10.1016/j.epsur.2014.03.001.

Gonzalez-Martinez, J.A., Vadera, S., Mullin, J., Enatsu, R., Khalifa, M. and Najm, I. (2014). Robot-assisted stereotactic laser ablation in medically intractable epilepsy: Operative technique. *Neurosurgery, 10*(Suppl 2), 167–172. https://doi.org/10.1227/NEU.0000000000000170.

Gupta, R. and Suri, A. (2017). Nanorobotics in neurosurgery: A futuristic approach to brain tumor therapy. *Journal of Clinical Neuroscience, 38*, 1–6. https://doi.org/10.1016/j.jocn.2016.10.021.

Horgan, S. and Vanuno, D. (2001). Robots in laparoscopic surgery. *Journal of Laparoendoscopic and Advanced Surgical Techniques, 11*(6), 415–419. https://doi.org/10.1089/109264201753212930.

Integrated Surgical Systems. (1997). *NeuroMate®: The first FDA-approved Robot for Stereotactic Neurosurgery* [Company brochure]. [Brochure]

Jannin, P. and Meurice, L. (2018). Modus V™ robotic exoscope in modern neurosurgery. *Operative Neurosurgery, 14*(Suppl 4), 417–422. https://doi.org/10.1093/ons/opy221.

Jones, D.R. and Clark, R. (2013). The evolution of medical robotics: From orthopedics to soft tissue. *Surgical Innovation, 20*(6), 545–552. https://doi.org/10.1177/1553350613482447.

Kantelhardt, S.R., et al. (2011). Robot-assisted pedicle screw placement: Operative time and accuracy benefits. *Neurosurgical Review, 54*(1), 93–99. https://doi.org/10.1007/s10143-010-0284-2.

Kantelhardt, S.R., Martinez, R., Baerwinkel, S., Burger, R., Giese, A. and Rohde, V. (2011). Accuracy of screw positioning in conventional, open robotic-guided, and percutaneous robotic-guided pedicle screw placement. *Spine, 36*(6), 456–461. https://doi.org/10.1097/BRS.0b013e3181f4baa8.

Kim, Y. and Park, S. (2022). Real-time AI-guided navigation in neurosurgery: A systematic review. *Neurosurgical Review, 65*(1), 1–9. https://doi.org/10.1007/s10143-021-01650-7.

Kumar, P. and Singh, A. (2016). Robotics in neurosurgery: Improving accuracy and patient safety. *World Neurosurgery, 88*, 661–667. https://doi.org/10.1016/j.wneu.2016.01.054.

Kwoh, Y.S., Hou, J., Jonckheere, E.A. and Hayati, S. (1988). A robot with improved absolute positioning accuracy for CT-guided stereotactic brain surgery. *IEEE Transactions on Biomedical Engineering, 35*(2), 153–160. https://doi.org/10.1109/10.18802.

Lee, J. and Park, J. (2021). Learning curves in robotic neurosurgery: Challenges and solutions. *World Neurosurgery, 145*, 74–81. https://doi.org/10.1016/j.wneu.2020.09.179.

Lefranc, M., et al. (2015). Frameless robotic stereotactic biopsy: A prospective comparative study. *Neurosurgery, 76*(4), 353–361. https://doi.org/10.1227/NEU.0000000000000614.

Lefranc, M. and Capel, C. (2016). The ROSA robotic device: Current applications in neurosurgery. *International Journal of Medical Robotics and Computer Assisted Surgery, 12*(1), 134–142. https://doi.org/10.1002/rcs.1689.

Li, J., et al. (2022). Meta-analysis of robotic vs. freehand spine surgery: Outcomes and safety. *Spine, 47*(5), E185–E192. https://doi.org/10.1097/BRS.0000000000004107.

Li, X. and Chen, Y. (2020). First remote robotic spinal screw placement using 5G networks: A Chinese milestone. *Spine, 45*(21), E1351–E1356. https://doi.org/10.1097/BRS.0000000000003633.

Mazor Robotics Ltd. (2016). *Renaissance™ and Mazor X™: Advanced Spinal Robotic Guidance Systems* [Product overview].

Miller, K. and Lee, J. (2015). Robotics in soft tissue surgery: A review of the da Vinci system and its applications. *Journal of Robotic Surgery, 9*(1), 1–7. https://doi.org/10.1007/s11701-014-0471-3.

Natarajan, M. and Rutka, J. (2021). Technical failures and safety incidents in pediatric robotic neurosurgery. *Child's Nervous System, 37*(9), 2719–2724. https://doi.org/10.1007/s00381-021-05233-1.

Patel, A.P. and Thomas, A. (2020). Haptic feedback and skill acquisition in robotic neurosurgery. *Journal of Robotic Surgery, 14*(3), 451–458. https://doi.org/10.1007/s11701-020-01050-y.

Ryu, W.H. and Kam, J.K. (2019). Minimally invasive techniques using robotics in skull base surgery. *Journal of Clinical Neuroscience, 60*, 1–6. https://doi.org/10.1016/j.jocn.2019.08.012.

Schatlo, B., Molliqaj, G., Cuvinciuc, V., Schaller, K. and Tessitore, E. (2015). The role of robotic systems in spinal surgery: Current applications and future perspectives. *Expert Review of Medical Devices, 12*(6), 733–745. https://doi.org/10.1586/17434440.2015.1060144.

Senova, S., et al. (2020). Diagnostic yield and safety of robotic stereotactic biopsy: A large cohort study. *Stereotactic and Functional Neurosurgery, 98*(1), 31–39. https://doi.org/10.1159/000501112.

Senova, S. and Benabid, A.L. (2020). Robotic accuracy in stereotactic procedures: Review and perspectives. *Journal of Neurosurgical Sciences, 64*(1), 1–10. https://doi.org/10.23736/S0390-5616.20.04817-4.

Shin, D.H. and Lee, C.H. (2018). Hybrid operating rooms with AI-enhanced intraoperative imaging for complex neurosurgery. *Journal of Neurosurgical Imaging, 5*(2), 85–92. https://doi.org/10.1055/s-0043-123456.

Singh, R. and Agrawal, A. (2020). Accessibility of robotics in low-resource neurosurgical centers. *Journal of Neurosurgical Sciences, 64*(2), 123–130. https://doi.org/10.23736/S0390-5616.20.04698-6.

Smith, A.B. (2010). *Fundamentals of Neurosurgery: An Introduction to the Specialty*. Journal of *Neurosurgery, 112*(1), 1–7. https://doi.org/10.3171/2010.1.JNS09123.

Smith, R. and Patel, H. (2017). Virtual reality and simulation in robotic neurosurgical training. *Operative Neurosurgery, 13*(5), 567–572. https://doi.org/10.1093/ons/opx049.

Staartjes, V.E. and Schröder, M.L. (2018). Robotic guidance improves screw placement accuracy and clinical outcomes. *European Spine Journal, 27*(2), 245–255. https://doi.org/10.1007/s00586-017-5290-y.

Taylor, R.H. and Funda, J. (1993). Image-guided robotics: Stereotactic neurosurgery and beyond. *Proceedings of the IEEE, 81*(7), 1083–1097. https://doi.org/10.1109/5.235754.

Taylor, R.H. and Stoianovici, D. (2003). Medical robotics in computer-integrated surgery. *IEEE Transactions on Robotics and Automation, 19*(5), 765–781. https://doi.org/10.1109/TRO.2003.817453.

Urakov, T., et al. (2019). Accuracy of robotic-assisted spinal fusion: A meta-analysis. *European Spine Journal, 28*(8), 1785–1794. https://doi.org/10.1007/s00586-019-05902-6.

Van Dijk, J.D., et al. (2020). Accuracy of robot-guided spinal instrumentation: A prospective study. *The Spine Journal, 20*(3), 403–408. https://doi.org/10.1016/j.spinee.2019.09.015.

Watanabe, E. and Sato, T. (2000). Frameless stereotaxy with image-guided navigation. *Neurosurgery Clinics of North America, 11*(4), 593–605. https://doi.org/10.1016/S1042-3680(05)70085-9.

Yu, H. and Zuo, Z. (2020). Laser interstitial thermal therapy and robotic guidance for brain tumors. *World Neurosurgery, 133*, e52–e60. https://doi.org/10.1016/j.wneu.2019.09.125.

Zhang, Y. and Wang, H. (2018). Ergonomics in neurosurgery: The impact of robotic platforms. *Neurosurgery Review, 61*(4), 451–457. https://doi.org/10.1007/s10143-018-1017-2.

Zimmer Biomet. (2020). *ROSA® ONE Brain: Manufacturer's Technical White Paper*. Zimmer Biomet. [Link unavailable]

14 Robotics in Minimally Invasive Surgery

Dipika Rawat[1*], Rohit Ranjan[2] and Minakshi[3]

Performing procedures without causing the morbidity linked to conventional surgical incisions is the aim of limited access techniques. This was made feasible by a blend of three technological innovations: the Hopkins rod lens system and shrinking cameras for videos, which permit the surgeon to look within the body in a way similar to open surgery while keeping a normal posture. The controlled distension of bodily cavities is made possible by insufflation devices using gas, allowing the surgeon to work with more space. For many abdominal treatments, minimally invasive surgery is taking the place of the more conventional open surgical method. The benefits of less discomfort, quicker oral uptake recovery, reduced length of hospitalizations, and better esthetic results all add to the expanding popularity of the laparoscopic technique. However, this method has drawbacks, including a lengthier learning curve and more expenses because of disposable devices and specialized equipment. Surgical robotics, image guidance, NOTES, and SILS are just a few of the ongoing developments in MIS that have occurred since its inception in the early 1980s. Many surgical and non-surgical fields now employ MIS procedures. Through telepresence technologies, robotics in particular is transforming complicated surgeries, including heart surgery. These technologies improve safety, accuracy, and dexterity, but they are expensive and need a lot of training. The capabilities and accessibility of robotic-assisted MIS are expected to be significantly enhanced by upcoming advancements, such as enhanced haptic systems, AI-driven decision support, and 5G-enabled telesurgery.

1. Introduction

The goal of minimal access techniques is to perform surgeries without creating the morbidity associated with traditional surgical incisions. Three technological

[1, 2] Uttaranchal College of Health Sciences, Uttaranchal University, Dehradun-248007, Uttarakhand, India.

[3] College of Computer Science, King Khalid University, Saudi Arabia.
Email: rohitranjan@uumail.in[2]; msingh@kku.edu.sa[3]

* Corresponding author: dipikarawat1994@gmail.com

DOI: 10.1201/9781003655121-14

advancements came together to make this possible: the Hopkins rod lens system and the shrinking video cameras enable the surgeon to see into the body in a manner comparable to open surgery while maintaining a normal posture. In order to give the surgeon room to work, insufflation devices enable the controlled distension of bodily cavities with gas (Jaffray et al., 2005). For many abdominal treatments, minimally invasive surgery (MIS) is taking the place of the additional conventional open surgical method. The benefits of less pain, faster oral intake recovery, reduced length of hospital stays, and better esthetic results all add to the expanding popularity of the laparoscopic technique (Robinson & Stiegmann, 2004). The implementation of this new technique has resulted in two significant disadvantages: First, the learning curve is lengthier for the majority of surgeons in contrast to the learning process in open surgery; second, increased expenses because of the purchase of extended operating periods, the use of disposable devices, and the required equipment. Shorter hospital stays do not always offset these higher expenses in the various healthcare systems around the world (Fuchs, 2002). For the first few decades of the 20th century, laparoscopy was used to diagnose diseases of the abdomen (Antoniou & Granderath, 2015). Since MIS's inception in the early 1980s, numerous changes have been made to enhance it, although the fundamental ideas have remained mostly unchanged. These include advancements in laparoscopic instruments and sutures, as well as MIS-related technologies including image guidance systems, surgical robots, single-incision laparoscopic surgery (SILS), natural orifice transluminal endoscopic surgery (NOTES), and surgical robotics (Siddaiah & Nyandowe, 2017). All surgical subspecialties as well as a few nonsurgical specialties, including interventional radiology, cardiology, and gastroenterology are currently using minimally invasive technology (MIT). MIT has successfully managed the majority of known surgical procedures to date; the question now is not how to employ these techniques, but rather why, where, and when to use them (Darzi & Munz, 2004). Whether using a little or big incision, this technique has benefits over direct vision. This venture has been a small but developing experience. This is the upcoming task for cardiac surgeons, which calls for the development of video dexterity. Cardiac valve replacement or repair is being done endoscopically using a voice-activated robotically controlled camera. It is obvious that robotic manipulation has a role in the modern cardiac surgery age. These devices operate on the principle of telepresence surgery, in which the surgeon uses robotic operations that are controlled electronically rather than directly manipulating tissue (Ochsner, 2000). Various procedures in various surgical disciplines can now be performed endoscopically instead of openly, thanks to developments in video imaging, endoscope technology, and instruments. Through voice command over the developed relationships operating room, improved dexterity to enable microscale operations, and the creation of trainers for virtual simulators to improve learning new complex operations, the application of robotics and computers promises to make complex endoscopic procedures easier (Mack, 2001). A manipulator operated by a computer with artificial sense that is reprogrammable to move and relocate equipment to perform a variety of surgical operations would be the surgical robot according to Davies's strict definition of the term (Kuo & Dai, 2009). MIS's full potential has been achieved with increased accuracy, security, and consistency because of the use of robot assistance. As imaging and human-robot interface have advanced, so too has the creation of articulated, accurate tools to increase the surgeon's agility. With the ability to navigate via intricate anatomical pathways, this has enhanced hand-eye coordination and manual precision down to nano scales (Vitiello, & Yang, 2012). Both the patient and the surgeon benefit from the rapid advancements in robotic surgery that need the least amount of incision (Gomes, 2011). Better clinical results, reduced blood loss, and a shorter operating time are all linked to the minimally invasive approach (Staub & Sadrameli, 2019). To attain truly "non-invasive" surgery, more research is being done on minimally invasive surgery in the areas of diagnostic and therapeutic modalities. As a result, MIS has garnered attention lately and has been getting better with encouraging results (Rudiman, 2021).

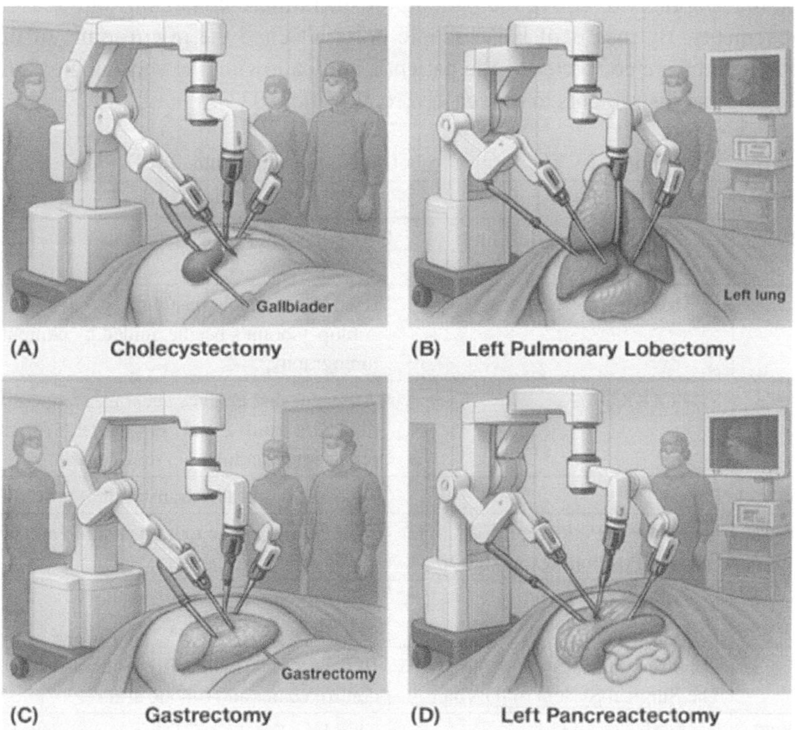

Fig. 1 The Robotic cart for cholecystectomy (A), left pulmonary lobectomy (B), gastrectomy (C), and left pancreatectomy (D) (Giulianotti & Caravaglios, 2003).

2. History, Background, and Milestones

Notable medical advancements involving the application of robotics for various tasks date back to the early 1980s, but in many circumstances today, robotic aided procedures stand as the benchmark for an ever-increasing variety of medical treatments (Vaida & Pisla, 2019). "Robot" is derived from the word "robota", which means "forced labor". In 1993, the first voice-controlled camera holder (AESOP) prototype robot was put into clinical use, and the US FDA marketed it as the first surgical robot ever in 1994, marking the start of the surgical robot era (Palep, 2009). The control gadgets and master console of the surgeon are the two primary parts of this system, which are connected to a computer via data cables. The principal surgeon is situated in the master console of the surgeon, which offers a using an endoscopic camera within the body of the patient to create a three-dimensional picture of the surgery field. The surgeon can control the camera from the console to feel as though they are actually in the surgical field. The surgeon makes surgical movements with control devices like handles or joysticks, and the robotic arms above the patient transform those commands into real-time movements. By means of laparoscopic ports attached the micro-joints of these robotic arms are connected to the patient's body allowing the endoscopic camera and surgical instruments to move (Rivero & Avila, 2023).

Table 1 The surgical robot's history (Ng & Tam, 2014).

Year	*Robot*	*Description*
1983	"Arthrobot", the world's first surgical robot	Support orthopaedic operations.
1985	PUMA 560	Used to accurately position A biopsy brain's needle guided by computed tomography.
1988	ROBODOC	A system that enables accurate preoperative planning and exact femur fits for hip replacement in total hip replacement.
1988	PROBOT	Research studies for transurethral procedure
1993	Autonomous Endoscopic System for Optimal Positioning, or AESOP	Arm that is robotic to help position and hold the laparoscopic camera.
1994	CyberKnife	Neurosurgery using stereotactic radiosurgery.
1998	Robotic Surgical System ZEUS and The Surgical System of da Vinci	Both systems included an operating room control center and robotic arms.
2000	the da Vinci robot	The US Food and Drug Administration (FDA) approved the da Vinci robot for use in laparoscopic procedures.

3. Pioneering Robotics Systems (EG Vinci Surgical System)

The sole gadget that is sold commercially that satisfies the fundamental principles of surgical robotics in the laparoscopic field is the da Vinci Surgical System (Douissard & Morel, 2019). It has four arms: three of them hold surgical instruments, while the fourth one contains a dual-lens endoscopic camera that gives the surgeon stereoscopic three-dimensional vision (Hussain & Ali, 2014). The da Vinci uses two cameras with a 5-mm wide angle inside an individual 12-mm laparoscope to create a three-dimensional image. Mobility is significantly increased with articulated tools at the ends of each surgical arm. The surgeon can feel inside the abdomen "wrist-like" because of the seven degrees of mobility freedom. Making use of both foot pedals and hand controllers, the surgeon controls the robot continuously from a remote panel. In addition to providing a grasping mechanism for centering and moving the hand controls, the foot pedals enable control over camera movement and focus. The instruments, which can be used for manipulation, dissection, coagulation, suturing, and camera movement, are controlled by hand controls. The robotic system lacks bipolar cautery but is capable of harmonics and monopolar cautery. Additionally, the system's computer offers graduated instrument grip, tremor reduction, and movement scaling. The da Vinci system's setup time, cost, and tactile/haptic feedback are its drawbacks (Ferguson & Daucher, 2004). The following are some of the primary elements that made da Vinci and its telerobotic concept so successful (Haidegger & Satava, 2022):

- Enhanced technological features, such as improved instrumentation and eyesight (Haidegger & Satava, 2022).
- Safety and ergonomics (Endo Wrist for better situation awareness, tremor filtering, and suturing) (Haidegger & Satava, 2022).
- Solid proof of better patient outcomes gathered over time (Haidegger & Satava, 2022).
- Focusing on operations that are capable of greatly improving life quality (benign hysterectomy, prostatectomy, etc. (Haidegger & Satava, 2022).

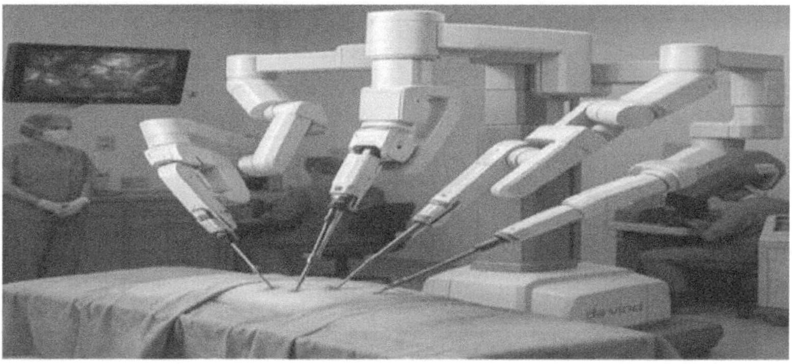

Fig. 2 The Da Vinci robot.

- A robust training program using simulators that has been proven over time (Haidegger & Satava, 2022).
- Since high-level autonomy was not introduced, and the surgeon continued to bear legal responsibility (Haidegger & Satava, 2022).
- Large-scale advertising and advertising (Haidegger & Satava, 2022).
- Solution selling (business model centered on services and consumption) (Haidegger & Satava, 2022).

An immersive operating environment with excellent stereo visualization is offered by the da Vinci system, and a direct contact between humans and machines links the surgeon's hand movements to the movement of the tip of the instrument within the patient (Freschi & Cuschieri, 2013).

4. Transition from Conventional Laparoscopy to Robotic Surgery

MIS implementation is no longer unjustified. A number of variables determine when open, laparoscopic, or robotic surgery should be performed. The surgery (cholecystectomy, hysterectomy, etc.), the surgical expertise, the severity of the indication (progression of the disease, low risk/high risk), and influence the technique that is employed (Williamson & Song, 2022). Robotic surgery has an impact on a wide range of medical specializations rather than being limited to just one. Beyond the limitations of conventional surgical techniques, the versatility of robotic systems has extended beyond general surgery to urology, gynaecology, and even heart surgery (Fairag & Alshehri, 2024).

Table 2 Robot-Assisted Surgery's Benefits and Drawbacks Compared to Traditional Surgery (Lanfranco & Meyers, 2004).

Human Capabilities	*Human Limits*	*Robot Capabilities*	*Robot Limits*
Excellent hand-eye coordination	Restricted agility beyond the natural scale	High geometric precision	No condemnation
Quick-witted	Prone to weariness and tremors	Consistent and persistent	Not being able to use qualitative data
Adequate and versatile	Inadequate geometric precision	Motion on a scale	Lack of tactile perception
Able to incorporate a wide range of information	Limited proficiency with quantitative data	Able to employ a variety of sensors for control	Pricey
Primitive haptic skills	Restricted sterility	It could be sterilized	A changing technological landscape
Capable of using qualitative data	Radiation and infection susceptibility	Radiation and insfection-resistant	More research is required.

5. Components of Robotics Surgical System

One way to conceptualize the robots is as data-driven surgical instruments that allow medical professionals to treat each patient safer, more efficiently, and with less morbidity than they otherwise could. Furthermore, computer-integrated surgery may become as crucial as Computer-assisted production in healthcare relates to the manufacturing of industrial products because of the information infrastructure and consistency of medical robotic technology systems for computer-assisted surgery (Taylor & Dario, 2016). Robots are categorized using functional categorization into three groups (Bann & Darzi, 2003).

- **Improvement in dexterity:** The surgeon controls the robot with an input device, but the robot and its software can enhance the surgeon's natural abilities, such as reducing tremor (Bann & Darzi, 2003).
- **Exact localization:** The surgical site's exact location can be determined with the assistance of preoperative investigations (Bann & Darzi, 2003).
- **Exact manipulation:** The robot can function in the designated area thanks to the creation of a preoperative plan (Bann & Darzi, 2003).
- Surgical robots can be divided into three main groups (Dwivedi & Mahgoub, 2012).

5.1 Supervisory Controlled System (SCS)

A lot of information is gathered by the surgeon in the first step, including mapping the body and the area of interest. In the second phase, known as registration, the surgeon links a connection in line with areas on the patient's image in real-time to the body image that was gathered. The exact procedure, in which the surgeon positions the robot in its initial position, is the third and last stage. The robot then completes its lesson while traveling along its preprogrammed route (Dwivedi & Mahgoub, 2012).

5.2 Tele Surgical

These devices are more commonly referred to as remote surgical systems. The surgeon controls the robot's arms in real- time when occupying a console. Although the robot technically performs the operation, the surgeon controls its movement during the process (Dwivedi & Mahgoub, 2012).

5.3 Shared Control System

The surgeon is mainly participating in the system of shared control. A robot assists the doctors in carrying out the process by offering consistent instrument manipulations. Neurosurgery and orthopaedic surgery frequently use the same control systems (Dwivedi & Mahgoub, 2012).

Three primary categories of robotic systems are currently employed in the surgical field: master-slave, semi-active, and active systems. In essence, Active systems perform pre programmed responsibilities and function on their own (but still under the operational surgeon's supervision). This is exemplified by the PROBOT and ROBODOC platforms that are discussed later. The part of these that is pre programmed robot systems can be enhanced by a surgeon-led component in semi-active systems. None of the autonomous or pre programmed parts of other systems are present in formal master-slave systems, of which the da Vinci® and ZEUS platforms were the precursors. They rely solely on the action of the surgeon. Laparoscopic surgical tools receive the surgeon's movements and the hands and faithfully replicate them, but intracorporeally (Lane, 2018). However, the primary barriers keeping current robotics from becoming the norm for MIS worldwide are its high lack of haptic feedback and expense. Thus, reducing costs, developing and testing simulators that are virtual and curricula, conducting clinical trials that are randomized to identify the most effective robotics applications, and launching new technologies and platforms are all essential components of robotic surgery's future (Bramhe & Pathak, 2022).

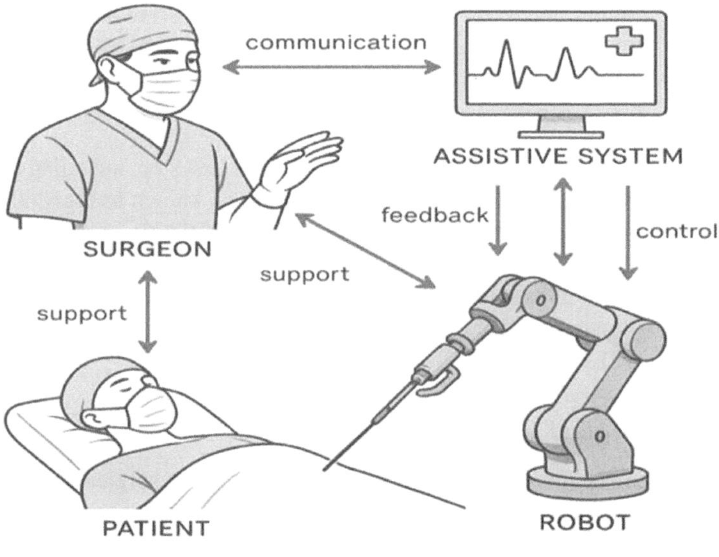

Fig. 3 The surgeon communicates with the robot, which then gives the doctor virtual fixtures or manual guidance. In this instance, the surgeon closes the control loop and maintains complete control over the machine throughout the process (Attanasio & Valdastri, 2021).

6. Surgeon Console and User Interface

It has been demonstrated that limitations in traditional MIS can be overcome by the development of teleoperated surgical robotic systems (TSRSs), which enable surgeons to perform surgeries across both short and long distances utilizing networks for wireless and/or wired communications. In fact, the use of teleoperated surgical robots has led to safer procedures, more accurate and efficient surgery, improved cosmetics, lower radiation exposure for surgeons, faster recovery times, and less postoperative discomfort for patients (Nguyen & Do, 2023). By reducing vibrations and translating precise movements, robotic systems improve camera scope performance. Robotic systems may now be controlled with intuitive user interfaces. These can be grouped according to the input method, which includes image-based monitoring of surgical instruments as well as control by foot, hand, voice, head, and eyes (Hamza & Navkar, 2023). There will soon be new robotic systems on stage. These can be categorized based on the kind of console, the configuration of the robotic arms, handles, and instruments, as well as other particular characteristics (such as eye tracking and haptic feedback). The first clinical studies of the Telelap ALF-X robot were published in 2016. It has an open console with eye-tracking, grips that resemble laparoscopies and have haptic feedback, and arms that are mounted on different carts. The Medtronic robot uses three arms and three-dimensional high-definition video technologies to provide an open console. The Avatera robot has four limbs on a single cart, a closed console with 6-degree-of-freedom 5-mm instruments and oculars that resemble microscopes (Rassweiler & Liatsikos, 2017).

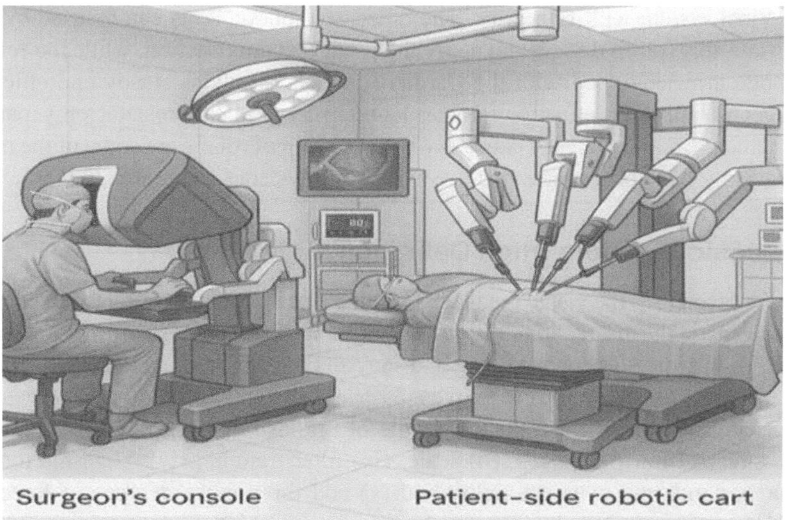

Fig. 4 The da Vinci surgical system (Murphy & Costello, 2008).

7. Patient-Side Robotic Arms

The effectiveness of assistant surgeons is crucial to robotic surgery, which requires a team effort. Interventions with the assistance of a skilled team are safer and

Table 3 An overview of the features of the robotic surgical systems that are currently approved (Koukourikis & Rha, 2020).

Robotic System	*Console*	*Camera Diameter (mm)*	*Features*
da Vinci Xi	Closed	8	Surgery in many quadrants Port-hopping dual console camera
da Vinci SP	Closed	12X10	360-degree spinning boom with a single port articulating camera
Senhance	Open/3D Glass	10	Eye-tracking apparatus Feedback that is haptic. No docking at the port
Revo-I	Closed	10	Warning signals about excessive force usage.
Versius	Open/3D Glass	10	Feedback that is haptic Arms that are independent and portable. Standing surgeon. No docking at the port
Avatera	Semi-Closed	10	Conserving space (2 units)
Hintori	Semi-Closed	NA	No docking at the port

quicker (Sgarbura & Vasilescu, 2010). The world's first report of a left-sided colorectal resection performed entirely with robotic assistance using a regular da Vinci system with four arms. The other two robotic arms can be used by the console surgeon to dissect and apply the proper countertraction, while the fourth robotic arm, equipped with the Cardiere forceps, provides steady and efficient surgeon-controlled retraction (Koh & Kim, 2011). Radical prostatectomy, partial nephrectomy, and radical cystectomy with the help of robots are some of the most frequently done procedures that use the robotic system (Zhu & Ye, 2025).

8. Vision System (High Definition 3D Imaging)

The surgeon uses the visual feedback from the laparoscopic imaging to teleoperate the robot via the master arms. By employing a high ratio of master to slave motion, this lessens the surgeon's fatigue and may improve motion accuracy (Krupa & Marescaux, 2003). With the help of da Vinci system, surgeons can: (i) easily translate the movement from the handle of the instrument to the tip, removing the effect of mirror images; (ii) scale; (iii) filter tremors; (iv) Align the tooltip image, hand, and eyes coaxially; and (v) add three more degrees of freedom with an internal articulated endoscopic wrist (Hashizume & Tsugawa, 2004). Augmented Reality (AR) technologies can raise awareness about surgery and give the surgeon a cozier and more productive environment during the intraoperative phase. This entails combining the intra-operative image of the surgical field with the pre-operative data and the surgical plan. Registration is the process of accurately modifying the virtual 3D model to correspond with the patient's actual anatomy. This is essential for developing intraoperative navigation tools and an

AR environment (Penza & Mattos, 2020). A robotic tool's position and orientation can be quickly and accurately measured and controlled using a variety of methods, such as: (a) electromagnetic (EM) tracking; (b) image-based tracking employing medical imaging modalities; (c) Robot kinematics for feed-forward, model-based control, and other less common techniques (Azizian & Patel, 2014).

9. Haptic Feedback in Robotic Surgery

A significant obstacle in teleoperated robotic surgery is the absence of haptic input. According to studies, a haptic feedback system can enhance skilled surgeons' competence and precision during robot-assisted surgery while lowering the amount of time new doctors need to learn robotic surgical procedures since they can find it hard to understand them just by looking at them (El Rassi, 2020). The term "haptics" encompasses both kinesthetics (force) and cutaneous (tactile) information. For the human hand to provide the usual sensations, both are required. This kind of input can be given by a haptic device like the PHANTOM from Sens Able Technologies (Woburn, MA). Since devices using tactile displays are not currently commercially accessible, it is unlikely that they will soon be able to fulfil the weight and size requirements for multi-degree-of-freedom systems (Okamura, 2004). In robotic knot tying, haptic feedback—an illustration of a Color bar scale—allows surgeons to be more accurate, constant, and use much higher tensions to delicate sutures without breaking them (Bethea & Yuh, 2004).

10. Innovation in Robotic Surgery

The advancement of high-fidelity sensors, akin to the improvements seen in 3D visualization, will facilitate sensations that extend beyond the conventional capabilities of human touch. Future surgical systems are poised to integrate all accessible data and imaging studies seamlessly, empowering surgeons to conduct microsurgical manipulations with unparalleled precision. Next-generation robots must enhance, not diminish, a surgeon's sense (Joseph & Patel, 2005). Surgeons are sought after by hospitals. Possessing a robotic surgical instrument boosts patient demand, helps recruit talent, and showcases a hospital's innovative program. The surgeon's learning curve or training to employ robots in surgery may be the cause of the elevated risk and slightly variable results. But how much time was spent in the operation room as well as the interval between opening and shutting also reduces as surgeons gain proficiency with new techniques (Vyas & Cronin, 2015).

11. Artificial Intelligent and Machine Learning in Robotic Surgery

Computers trained to solve problems by simulating human cognition are known as artificial intelligence (AI) systems. The AI subfields of machine learning (ML) and deep learning (DL) enable computers to generate predictions by analyzing underlying patterns in data. There is evidence that combining medical experts with ML algorithms enhances decision-making by lowering the mistake rate (Andras & Mottrie, 2020). Surgical competence is being objectively evaluated using AI in a number of ways. These consist of direct capture from the robot, force, and torque sensors connected to surgical equipment, hand-mounted eye trackers, and electromagnetic sensors linked to devices. The force with which the instruments are handled can be ascertained by measuring the robotic instruments' vibrations. With the use of this new technology, data may be gathered objectively, including how frequently an instrument encounters particular buildings (Egert & Sundaram, 2020). Policies should be put in place to address the serious ethical and legal concerns around patient data privacy and confidentiality, which range from intraoperative video utilized in predictive AI models to electronic health records (Moglia & Cuschieri, 2021).

12. Future Applications for Robotics

Two cutting-edge methods that could further lessen the intrusiveness and morbidity of surgery are laparoendoscopic single-site surgery (LESS) and natural orifice transluminal endoscopic surgery. However, the requirement for specific tools makes the process more technically challenging. With the creation of new robotic prototypes for single-port surgery and the quick advancement of robotic technology, robotic LESS is anticipated to advance with the aim of reducing problems and enhancing results (Ng & Tam, 2014). The present status of robotic surgery applications, discussing both their advantages and disadvantages. Future advancements are also covered, with special attention paid to how improved AI, ML, and sensory feedback will advance robotic surgery. Even though robotics possess the capacity to improve accessibility, lower problems, and improve patient outcomes, there are still technological, ethical, and financial issues that must be resolved. As robotic technologies develop further, they could change the way that necessary surgeries and treatments are performed (Rahman & Islam, 2025). It is anticipated that the use of 5G technology for remote surgery with robot assistance will advance contemporary surgical techniques and open up new avenues for the treatment of patients. The main benefit of 5G is its low-latency and fast network which enables almost instantaneous data transfer between the robotic system and the surgeon, even when they are located far apart. This allows for crucial real-time answers and modifications during surgery. Stereoscopic 3D and 4K high-definition video can be transmitted in real- time thanks to 5G technology's strong communication capabilities, which also make it easier to diagnose and treat patients using advanced imaging methods like examinations using magnetic resonance imaging (MRI), computed tomography (CT), and ultrasound exams (Xie & Chen, 2025). One extremely effective way to operate robots is by teleoperation. It makes it possible for people to travel to far-off places and engage with people and things there virtually (Lenz & Behnke, 2023).

13. Conclusion

By drastically lowering patient trauma, speeding up recovery, and enhancing clinical results, minimally invasive surgery, or MIS, has transformed surgical practice. Rapid technology improvements aimed at improving accuracy, safety, and surgeon ergonomics are reflected in the progression of open surgeries to laparoscopic and now robotic-assisted procedures. Superior dexterity, vision, and control have been demonstrated by robotic systems, especially the da Vinci Surgical System, which has made complex treatments more accessible and effective across a range of specialties. Nevertheless, obstacles including exorbitant expenses, the absence of tactile input, and challenging learning curves continue to prevent widespread use. New developments that promise to get around these obstacles and improve surgical accuracy include haptic feedback devices, augmented reality, and AI integration. MIS is well-positioned to advance toward a future of increasingly less intrusive, more sophisticated, and highly customized surgical care as long as research and development continue.

References

Andras, I., Mazzone, E., van Leeuwen, F.W., De Naeyer, G., van Oosterom, M.N., Beato, S., ... & Mottrie, A. (2020). Artificial intelligence and robotics: A combination that is changing the operating room. *World Journal of Urology*, *38*, 2359–2366.

Antoniou, S.A., Antoniou, G.A., Antoniou, A.I. and Granderath, F.A. (2015). Past, present, and future of minimally invasive abdominal surgery. *JSLS: Journal of the Society of Laparoendoscopic Surgeons*, *19*(3).

Attanasio, A., Scaglioni, B., De Momi, E., Fiorini, P. and Valdastri, P. (2021). Autonomy in surgical robotics. *Annual Review of Control, Robotics, and Autonomous Systems*, *4*(1), 651–679.

Azizian, M., Khoshnam, M., Najmaei, N. and Patel, R.V. (2014). Visual servoing in medical robotics: A survey. Part I: Endoscopic and direct vision imaging–techniques and applications. *The International Journal of Medical Robotics and Computer Assisted Surgery*, *10*(3), 263–274.

Bann, S., Khan, M., Hernandez, J., Munz, Y., Moorthy, K., Datta, V., ... & Darzi, A. (2003). Robotics in surgery. *Journal of the American College of Surgeons*, *196*(5), 784–795.

Bethea, B.T., Okamura, A.M., Kitagawa, M., Fitton, T.P., Cattaneo, S.M., Gott, V.L., ... & Yuh, D.D. (2004). Application of haptic feedback to robotic surgery. *Journal of Laparoendoscopic and Advanced Surgical Techniques*, *14*(3), 191–195.

Bramhe, S. and Pathak, S.S. (2022). Robotic surgery: A narrative review. *Cureus*, *14*(9).

Darzi, A. and Munz, Y. (2004). The impact of minimally invasive surgical techniques. *Annu. Rev. Med.*, *55*(1), 223–237.

Douissard, J., Hagen, M.E. and Morel, P. (2019). The da Vinci surgical system. In: *Bariatric Robotic Surgery: A Comprehensive Guide* (pp. 13–27). Springer Nature Link.

Dwivedi, J. and Mahgoub, I. (2012, May). Robotic surgery: A review on recent advances in surgical robotic systems. In: *Florida Conference on Recent Advances in Robotics* (pp. 10–11).

Egert, M., Steward, J.E. and Sundaram, C.P. (2020). Machine learning and artificial intelligence in surgical fields. *Indian Journal of Surgical Oncology*, *11*(4), 573–577.

El Rassi, I. and El Rassi, J.M. (2020). A review of haptic feedback in tele-operated robotic surgery. *Journal of Medical Engineering and Technology*, *44*(5), 247–254.

Fairag, M., Almahdi, R.H., Siddiqi, A.A., Alharthi, F.K., Alqurashi, B.S., Alzahrani, N.G., ... and Alshehri Sr, R. (2024). Robotic revolution in surgery: Diverse applications across specialties and future prospects review article. *Cureus*, *16*(1).

Ferguson, J.L., Beste, T.M., Nelson, K.H. and Daucher, J.A. (2004). Making the transition from standard gynecologic laparoscopy to robotic laparoscopy. *JSLS: Journal of the Society of Laparoendoscopic Surgeons*, *8*(4), 326.

Freschi, C., Ferrari, V., Melfi, F., Ferrari, M., Mosca, F. and Cuschieri, A. (2013). Technical review of the da Vinci surgical telemanipulator. *The International Journal of Medical Robotics and Computer Assisted Surgery*, *9*(4), 396–406.

Fuchs, K.H. (2002). Minimally invasive surgery. *Endoscopy*, *34*(02), 154–159.

Gomes, P. (2011). Surgical robotics: Reviewing the past, analysing the present, imagining the future. *Robotics and Computer-Integrated Manufacturing*, *27*(2), 261–266.

Giulianotti, P.C., Coratti, A., Angelini, M., Sbrana, F., Cecconi, S., Balestracci, T. and Caravaglios, G. (2003). Robotics in general surgery: Personal experience in a large community hospital. *Archives of Surgery*, *138*(7), 777–784.

Haidegger, T., Speidel, S., Stoyanov, D. and Satava, R.M. (2022). Robot-assisted minimally invasive surgery: Surgical robotics in the data age. *Proceedings of the IEEE*, *110*(7), 835–846.

Hamza, H., Baez, V.M., Al-Ansari, A., Becker, A.T. and Navkar, N.V. (2023). User interfaces for actuated scope maneuvering in surgical systems: A scoping review. *Surgical Endoscopy*, *37*(6), 4193–4223.

Hashizume, M. and Tsugawa, K. (2004). Robotic surgery and cancer: The present state, problems, and future vision. *Japanese Journal of Clinical Oncology*, *34*(5), 227–237.

Hussain, A., Malik, A., Halim, M.U. and Ali, A.M. (2014). The use of robotics in surgery: A review. *International Journal of Clinical Practice*, *68*(11), 1376–1382.

Jaffray, B. (2005). Minimally invasive surgery. *Archives of Disease in Childhood*, *90*(5), 537–542. Joseph, J.V., Arya, M. and Patel, H.R. (2005). Robotic surgery: The coming of a new era in surgical innovation. *Expert Review of Anticancer Therapy*, *5*(1), 7–9.

Koh, D.C.S., Tsang, C.B. and Kim, S.H. (2011). A new application of the four-arm standard da Vinci® surgical system: Totally robotic-assisted left-sided colon or rectal resection. *Surgical Endoscopy*, *25*, 1945–1952.

Koukourikis, P. and Rha, K.H. (2020). Robotic surgical systems in urology: What is currently available? *Investigative and Clinical Urology*, *62*(1), 14.

Krupa, A., Gangloff, J., Doignon, C., De Mathelin, M.F., Morel, G., Leroy, J., ... and Marescaux, J. (2003). Autonomous 3-D positioning of surgical instruments in robotized laparoscopic surgery using visual servoing. *IEEE Transactions on Robotics and Automation*, *19*(5), 842–853.

Kuo, C.H. and Dai, J.S. (2009). Robotics for minimally invasive surgery: a historical review from the perspective of kinematics. In: *International Symposium on History of Machines and Mechanisms: Proceedings of HMM 2008* (pp. 337–354). Springer Netherlands.

Lane, T. (2018). A short history of robotic surgery. *The Annals of the Royal College of Surgeons of England*, *100*(6_sup), 5–7.

Lanfranco, A.R., Castellanos, A.E., Desai, J.P. and Meyers, W.C. (2004). Robotic surgery: A current perspective. *Annals of Surgery*, *239*(1), 14–21.

Lenz, C. and Behnke, S. (2023). Bimanual telemanipulation with force and haptic feedback through an anthropomorphic avatar system. *Robotics and Autonomous Systems*, *161*, 104338.

Mack, M.J. (2001). Minimally invasive and robotic surgery. *Jama*, *285*(5), 568–572.

Moglia, A., Georgiou, K., Georgiou, E., Satava, R.M. and Cuschieri, A. (2021). A systematic review on artificial intelligence in robot-assisted surgery. *International Journal of Surgery*, *95*, 106151.

Murphy, D.G., Hall, R., Tong, R., Goel, R. and Costello, A.J. (2008). Robotic technology in surgery: Current status in 2008. *ANZ Journal of Surgery*, *78*(12), 1076–1081.

Ng, A.T. and Tam, P.C. (2014). Current status of robot-assisted surgery. *Hong Kong Medical Journal.*

Nguyen, C.C., Wong, S., Thai, M.T., Hoang, T.T., Phan, P.T., Davies, J., ... and Do, T.N. (2023). Advanced user interfaces for teleoperated surgical robotic systems. *Advanced Sensor Research, 2*(4), 2200036.

Ochsner, J.L. (2000). Minimally invasive surgical procedures. *The Ochsner Journal, 2*(3), 135.

Okamura, A.M. (2004). Methods for haptic feedback in teleoperated robot-assisted surgery. *Industrial Robot: An International Journal, 31*(6), 499–508.

Palep, J.H. (2009). Robotic assisted minimally invasive surgery. *Journal of Minimal Access Surgery,* 5(1), 1–7.

Penza, V., Moccia, S., De Momi, E. and Mattos, L.S. (2020). Enhanced vision to improve safety in robotic surgery. In: *Handbook of Robotic and Image-Guided Surgery* (pp. 223–237). Elsevier.

Rahman, M.A., Bristi, S.A., Yesmin, T. and Islam, M.T. (2025). Application of robotics in modern surgery and critical operations: Current status, challenges, and future directions. *INNOSC Theranostics and Pharmacological Sciences,* 4664.

Rassweiler, J.J., Autorino, R., Klein, J., Mottrie, A., Goezen, A.S., Stolzenburg, J.U., ... and Liatsikos, E. (2017). Future of robotic surgery in urology. *BJU International, 120*(6), 822–841.

Robinson, T. N. and Stiegmann, G.V. (2004). Minimally invasive surgery. *Endoscopy, 36*(01), 48–51.

Rivero-Moreno, Y., Echevarria, S., Vidal-Valderrama, C., Pianetti, L., Cordova-Guilarte, J., Navarro-Gonzalez, J., ... and Avila, G.L.D. (2023). Robotic surgery: A comprehensive review of the literature and current trends. *Cureus, 15*(7).

Rudiman, R. (2021). Minimally invasive gastrointestinal surgery: from past to the future. *Annals of Medicine and Surgery, 71,* 102922.

Sgarbura, O. and Vasilescu, C. (2010). The decisive role of the patient-side surgeon in robotic surgery. *Surgical Endoscopy, 24,* 3149–3155.

Siddaiah-Subramanya, M., Tiang, K.W. and Nyandowe, M. (2017). A new era of minimally invasive surgery: Progress and development of major technical innovations in general surgery over the last decade. *The Surgery Journal, 3*(04), e163–e166.

Staub, B.N. and Sadrameli, S.S. (2019). The use of robotics in minimally invasive spine surgery. *Journal of Spine Surgery, 5*(Suppl 1), S31.

Taylor, R.H., Menciassi, A., Fichtinger, G., Fiorini, P. and Dario, P. (2016). Medical robotics and computer-integrated surgery. In: *Springer Handbook of Robotics* (pp. 1657–1684).

The Da Vinci robot, the latest member of the CGHMC surgical team. (2022, September 30). CGHMC. https://cghmc.com.ph/the-da-vinci-robot-the-latest-member-of-the-cghmc-surgical-team/.

Vaida, C., Al Hajjar, N., Lazar, V., Graur, F., Burz, A., Elisei, R., ... and Pisla, D. (2019). Robotics in minimally invasive procedures: History, current trends, and future challenges. In: *6th International Conference on Advancements of Medicine and Health Care through Technology*; 17–20 October 2018, Cluj-Napoca, Romania: MEDITECH 2018 (pp. 267–273). Springer Singapore.

Vitiello, V., Lee, S.L., Cundy, T.P. and Yang, G.Z. (2012). Emerging robotic platforms for minimally invasive surgery. *IEEE Reviews in Biomedical Engineering, 6,* 111–126.

Vyas, D. and Cronin, S. (2015). Peer review and surgical innovation: Robotic surgery and its hurdles. *American Journal of Robotic Surgery, 2*(1), 39.

Williamson, T. and Song, S.E. (2022). Robotic surgery techniques to improve traditional laparoscopy. *JSLS: Journal of the Society of Laparoscopic and Robotic Surgeons, 26*(2).

Xie, X., Tian, Y., Huang, J., Luo, Q. and Chen, T. (2025). Surgery without distance: Will 5G-based robot-assisted telesurgery redefine modern surgery? *Translational Lung Cancer Research, 14*(5), 1821.

Zhu, L., Xia, D., Wang, S. and Ye, S. (2025). Optimizing Robotic Surgical Assistance: Shorten the Learning Curve for Urologic Oncology Cases. *JSLS: Journal of the Society of Laparoscopic and Robotic Surgeons, 29*(2).

15 Artificial Intelligence and Machine Learning in Robotic Surgery

Gaurav Mittal[1*] and Quazi Taif Sadat[2]

Artificial Intelligence (AI) and Machine Learning (ML) are fast changing the future of contemporary robotic surgery. This chapter examines how these technologies are being used to incorporate them into surgical robotics, outlining a detailed insight into their roots, applications, benefits, and ethics. Beginning with the evolutionary history of robotic systems, the chapter provides an overview of the basic concepts of AI and ML, including supervised, unsupervised, and reinforcement learning, deep learning, natural language processing, and computer vision. Finally, it is time to discuss the current three most common robot platforms, da Vinci, ROSA, and MAKO, and how they interact with the AI-based technologies in surgical planning, image-guided navigation, intraoperative decision-making support, and even autonomous actions. To give insight into these capabilities, the chapter offers a series of case studies in urology, neurosurgery, orthopedics, and also in laparoscopic surgery. The context is most obvious in terms of the advantages achieved in the case of AI: enhanced surgical precision, a decrease in postoperative complications, tailor-made procedures to the needs of an individual patient, and enhanced training experiences of surgical teams. There are, however, numerous problems left to be addressed, such as data privacy concerns, issues of trust and openness, regulation and equality of access issues. Following this description, the chapter tries to overview such future developments as autonomous surgery, AI-augmented reality, and distant telesurgery. All these trends together reflect a story of the future with the more intelligent, advanced mechanisms revolutionizing contemporary surgical practice. It is worth mentioning that this awkward material is worth the price for clinicians, researchers, and system developers who are involved in creating the next generation of AI-assisted robotic healthcare.

1. Introduction

Robotic surgery started as an experimental endeavor to expand the surgeon's capability to execute intricate procedures with more precision, flexibility, and

[1] Uttaranchal College of Health Sciences, Uttaranchal University, India.
[2] Director, Bangladesh University, Bangladesh.
Email: taif@bu.edu.bd[2]
* Corresponding author: gauravmittal@uumail.in

DOI: 10.1201/9781003655121-15

control than traditional methods. First created for remote-controlled military use in the 1980s, robotic systems made their way into general operating rooms gradually, particularly after the release of the da Vinci Surgical System in 2000. These systems enable surgeons to operate hand controls and foot pedals to move the robotic arm that holds instruments and a high-definition camera. With better visualization and minimal access, robotic-assisted surgery has demonstrated advantages such as less blood loss, fewer days in the hospital, and faster patient recovery (Herron & Marohn, 2008).

In our study, we can describe Artificial Intelligence (AI) as computer programs capable of performing tasks, normally requiring human intelligence. Within the medical field, AI has expanded significantly, from the original diagnostic systems and rule-based expert systems to the much more advanced machine learning (ML) algorithms that can work with large data sets, process medical images, and even perform a clinical decision support role. Since both have the same purpose of better accuracy, it is logical that AI and robotics merge; one of the contributions of the merge is the desire of better precision in surgery and decision-making. Discussing this phenomenon, Jiang et al. (2017) remark that AI has already started transforming all the significant fields in medicine, including radiology and pathology and surgery (Jiang et al., 2017).

Operative management involves sensitivity as well as instant judgment. Fatigue, variability, and human error affect even seasoned surgeons. Intelligent algorithms and ML are perfectly applicable to process the vast amount of surgical data, detect trends, and advise on decisions during an operation: they would be able to warn the surgeon about the developing complications, suggest the optimal direction of cuts, or help locate anatomical markers. This chapter centers on AI and ML in the process of transforming the field of robotic surgery. With the concepts on their back, the topic is broached regarding the actual deployment of these technologies in surgical robots, the practical application of robots, and how robotics can evolve in the future (Table 1).

1.1 Fundamentals of AI and Machine Learning

AI systems are computer programs that can carry out functions that require a human intellect. Such functions include image perception, understanding language, decision-making, and speech recognition. While traditional software limits itself to a set of rules, AI may be trained by as well as reprogrammed to deal with new information. In the medical field, AI assists the practitioners with diagnosis, prognosis, and prescribing regimes of treatment. It also enables a more accurate navigation of instruments during robotic surgery (Herron et al., 2008; Jiang et al., 2017).

ML is a branch in AI that empowers computers to learn without being specifically programmed. Unlike hard-coded programs, ML algorithms learn by observing patterns and they get better with experience. Applied in surgery, ML assists in identifying anatomical tissue types, monitoring of equipment, and estimating outcomes. The fact that it can be trained on "true patient and surgical data" makes ML especially strong in medical facilities and hospitals, where accuracy and constant learning are essential (Jiang et al., 2017; Hashimoto et al., 2018).

Supervised learning: Labeled data is trained as supervised learning. As an example, a system is shown thousands of surgical images, and each image has information associated with it, e.g., tissue type, or state of the disease. Through this training, the algorithm is capable of learning to trace new unseen pictures. Supervised learning in robotic surgery could help to identify relevant anatomy or predict the past cases complications (Hashimoto et al., 2018).

Unsupervised Learning: Unsupervised learning discovers latent patterns in unlabeled data. It clusters data points according to similarities without having prior knowledge of what these groups signify. It is applied in robotic surgery for image segmentation, anomaly detection, or revealing new procedural patterns that are not yet known. It's commonly applied in pre-operative planning or surgical performance metric analysis (Jiang et al., 2017). Reinforcement learning replicates how humans learn by trial and error. A robotic system is provided with feedback (reward or penalty) on its actions and learns to maximize the rewarding ones in the long run. To increase accuracy and autonomy, reinforcement learning has been used in surgery to teach robots to perform tasks like suturing and knot tying with minimal supervision (Topol et al., 2019).

Table 1 AI and ML Techniques in Robotic Surgery.

Technique	*Function*	*Application in Surgery*
Supervised Learning	Learn from labeled data	Classifies tissues, predicts complications
Unsupervised Learning	Finds patterns in unlabeled data	Image segmentation, anomaly detection
Reinforcement Learning	Learn via trial and error	Robotic suturing, skill acquisition
Deep Learning	Uses deep neural networks	Video analysis, instrument tracking
Natural Language Processing	Interprets human language	Reads surgical notes, voice commands
Computer Vision	Analyzes visual data	Recognizes organs/tools, tracks movements

1.2 Deep Learning and Neural Networks

Deep Learning is a branch of ML that employs artificial neural networks with numerous layers—deep neural networks—to process data. These devices are very good at identifying patterns in intricate sets of data such as surgical videos or medical images. Deep learning, during robotic surgery, allows real-time video processing, instrument detection, and even a surgeon's next action prediction. For example, convolutional neural networks (CNNs) are frequently used for image processing during minimally invasive surgical procedures (Hashimoto et al., 2018; Topol et al., 2019). Natural Language Processing (NLP) lets AI Programs break and interpret the language of human beings. In surgery, NLP can read electronic health records (EHRs), attend to surgical notes, or voice instructions in making clinical decisions. Computer Vision (CV), instead, is the ability of machines to see and process visual information like pictures, films. This is crucial in robotic surgery, whereby the system must recognize organs, instruments, and movement. NLP and CV should enhance the interaction between humans and machines, thereby making performing surgery safer and more effective (Jiang et al., 2017).

2. Overview of Robotic Surgery Systems

The field of robotic surgery systems began with a form of vision that enhanced human accuracy beyond conventional laparoscopic surgery. The early concepts were developed in the 1980s as NASA and the U.S. military studied the potential of remote surgery to operate on the battlefield or for space operations. PROBOT (United Kingdom) and ROBODOC (United States) were the first robotic systems for proactive and orthopedic surgeries (Davies et al., 2000). These initial robots showed the capabilities of robot assistance, but were not very autonomous and flexible. By the late 1990s, advances in technology and greater interest among engineers and surgeons opened the door to more advanced robotic systems. The turning point came with the FDA clearance of the Da Vinci Surgical System in 2000, which brought robot-assisted laparoscopic surgery into commercial reality and general acceptance (Lanfranco et al., 2004). Since then, the industry has exploded, incorporating AI tools, ML algorithms, and computer vision to further increase performance and results (Shademan et al., 2016).

2.1 Robotic Surgical Platforms

2.1.1 da Vinci Surgical System

The da Vinci Surgical System is created by Intuitive Surgical; it is the most popular and studied robotic unit worldwide. It has a surgeon console, a patient robotic cart, which has four interactive arms, and a vision system that gives a 3D high-definition view of the surgery site. The system permits movements of the instruments with a higher amount of freedom made by the wrist instead of the human hand with a reduction of tremor and the possibility of finesse manipulation. Newer models, like da Vinci Xi, can facilitate the surgical procedures in multiple quadrants and provide enhanced ergonomics, whereas a combination with AI algorithms has become possible to provide superior task identification and modeling (Shademan et al., 2016).

2.1.2 ROSA, MAKO

There have also been other robot platforms that have come up to meet the needs in the niche. Zimmer Biomet The ROSA (Robotic Surgical Assistant), to be used in neurosurgery to orthopedic procedures, includes image-guided navigation (Wang et al., 2013). In the same way, the MAKO System by Stryker specializes in the partial knee and total knee as well as in hip arthroplasty. It employs preoperative CT imaging, coupled with intraoperative kinematic data, to generate (Lonner et al., 2019).

Other similar developing systems are the VERSIUS (Cursorial) and Senhance (Asensus) systems, which propose to do modular, cost-competitive, and scalable systems with superior haptics and surgeon feedback systems (Ashton et al., 2020).

A robotic surgery system typically comprises three major components:

- **Surgeon Console:** This is where the surgeon sits and operates the robot via hand controllers and foot pedals. A stereoscopic monitor provides real-time, magnified 3D images of the surgical field.
- **Patient-Side Cart:** The robotic arms that hold the surgical instruments and endoscopic cameras are connected to this cart. The surgical instruments move according to the brilliant direction of the surgeon's hands.
- **Vision and the Software System:** This consists of high-resolution digital cameras, lighting, and an image acquisition area. The feedback is in real- time, with haptic feedback and motions based on scaling factors. This system has features utilizing AI, tracking instruments, skillset analysis, and predicting errors (Shademan et al., 2016; Ashton et al., 2020).

3. Role of AI in Robotic Surgery

AI has a revolutionary effect on robotic surgery, converting such systems from passive devices to smart surgical assistants. AI integration increases robotic accuracy, real-time decision-making, safety, and responsiveness.

The following are the major areas in which AI is having a very positive impact.

- Image-guided surgery employs real-time imaging with modalities such as MRI (magnetic resonance imaging), CT (computed tomography), and ultrasound to image the anatomy in real-time intraoperatively. AI and CV algorithms assist the robotic system in better interpreting images.
- Computer vision allows surgical robots to recognize tissue types, detect tumors, and distinguish between anatomical landmarks in real-time. Such systems can superimpose 3D models over the operative field so that the surgeon can work based on a virtual topography of the patient's anatomy (Figure 1).
- Deep learning algorithms such as CNNs are highly suitable for computer processing of medical images and have been utilized in robotic systems to enhance tool tracking and surgical navigation (Esteva et al., 2017).

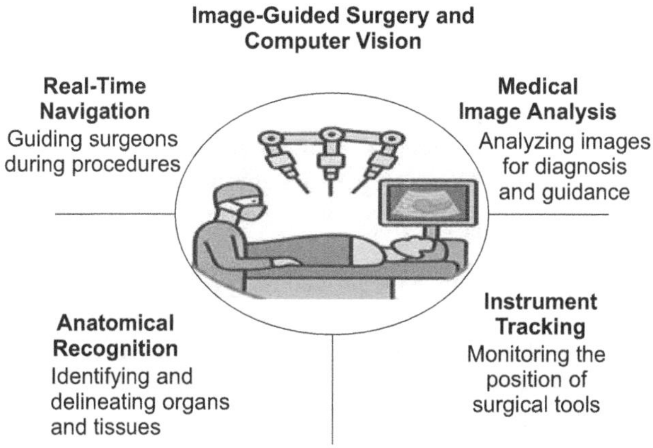

Fig. 1 Image-Guided Surgery and Computer Vision.

AI-enhanced vision also facilitates Augmented Reality (AR) in surgery, allowing critical information to be displayed directly on the surgical field, improving spatial orientation and reducing reliance on manual interpretation (Maier-Hein et al., 2017).

AI-planning minimizes variation among surgeons and rationalizes complicated operations, e.g., those of orthopedic surgery. AI assists, for instance, in the ideal placement of implants via scanning CT scans and estimating joint alignment (Figure 2). Robotic platforms make such plans generated by AI feasible to translate into accurate motion, enhancing results and reducing invasion (Chen et al., 2020).

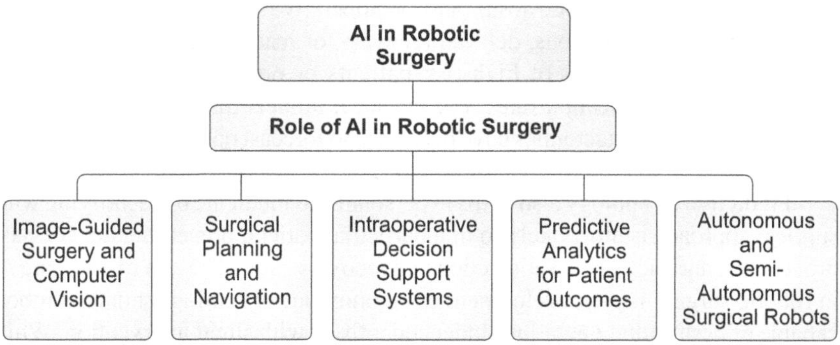

Fig. 2 Role of AI in Robotic Surgery.

Intraoperative decision support systems powered by AI serve as an adjunct to the surgeon. They consider concurrent data: video feed, vital signs of the patient, and movement of the instrument, and produce alerts, suggestions, or warnings in a timely fashion. They may measure active bleeding, unusual tissue characteristics, or intraoperative signs of surgical complications.

More advanced systems utilize ML models trained by multiple surgical videos to identify key phases of a surgery and predict the next steps based on what the surgeon has performed and provide alerting for violations of each surgical protocol (Twinanda et al., 2016). These system features may improve efficiency in the surgical field, reduce the likelihood of human error, and lessen the cognitive load on the surgeon.

Decision-support systems have proved their potential in the case of robotic-assisted laparoscopic surgery to offer alternative options when the robotic system detects restricted visibility or obstruction and thus improves intraoperative safety (Padoy et al., 2019) AU based gesture and motion sensing allow robots in surgery to recognize the surgeon's hand, eye, or instrument movement with high accuracy. The algorithms pick up on patterns of instrument use that assist in interpreting small hand movement into precise robot movement. Additionally, AI systems can recognize aberrant gestures signaling possible mistakes or complications. Aside from control, gesture recognition enables measurement of surgical skill. Through comparison with expert-level procedure databases, AI is able to provide an objective assessment to residents or practicing surgeons to optimize technique and enhance surgical training (Ahmidi et al., 2017). In cooperative settings, gesture recognition can enable the robot to predict the surgeon's next move and make the interaction more natural and intuitive. This will be especially beneficial in multi tasking settings where surgeons are communicating with assistants or frequently changing tools (Rivas-Blanco et al., 2020). AI-driven predictive analytics enable better predictability of surgical outcomes. These models screen preoperative information (e.g., vital signs, demographics, comorbidities), intraoperative factors (e.g., anesthetic time, blood loss), and postoperative measurements to forecast complications like infections, delayed recovery, or readmissions. ML algorithms can notify surgical teams of high-risk patients or procedure steps that would lead to higher complication rates. For instance, models trained on thousands of laparoscopic cholecystectomies have been used to forecast open surgery conversion from initial presentation.

Predictive technology also helps in personalized medicine by identifying what surgical approach is most likely to fit a particular patient, preventing unnecessary procedures, and increasing satisfaction and recovery rates. The aim of applying AI in robotic surgery is the development of autonomous or semi-autonomous robots capable of performing operations independently or with slight intervention. While full autonomy is not yet being developed, semi-autonomous systems already had the capability to execute subtasks such as suturing, cutting, or camera placement. One of the biggest highlights was the autonomous anastomosis of soft tissue performed by the Smart Tissue Autonomous Robot (STAR), which had better consistency than human surgeons under laboratory settings (Krieger et al., 2016). These robots can adapt to change during procedures using real-time feedback from force sensors, vision systems, and AI algorithms. As the systems age, ethical and regulatory paradigms will have to change to answer responsibility, accountability, and transparency of data (Hashimoto et al., 2020).

4. Machine Learning Applications in Surgical Robotics

ML is the force behind robotic surgery because robots can perceive, learn, and reason in complex surgical environments (Figure 3). Unlike current robotic systems running under known algorithms, robots with the potential of ML can process information in real-time, identify patterns, and infer conclusions based on experiences in the past. This section conveys the main applications of ML in surgical robotics, which range from analysis of training data to real-time notification and estimation of the findings at the postoperative period. Surgical video is one of the richest data sources for machine learning when talking about robotic surgery. Video cameras can capture high-definition intraoperative video, which can be utilized for deep learning model development with large video datasets. The training can allow models to identify important surgical phases, instrument actions, tissue reactions, and motions of the surgeon. For example, through CNNs, computers can be trained to autonomously annotate video by parsing video into discrete actions such as cutting, suturing, or cauterizing without the annotator being human. Not only would this speed up analysis of the data, but it would also allow for systematic scrutiny of surgeries and scale. With time, the models would become better at recognizing even slight differences between experts and novices or safe and unsafe responses (Madani et al., 2020). So far, labeled surgical videos are applied to procedural simulation in virtual reality (VR) or AR environments to produce immersive data-driven training spaces for residents and students (Jarc et al., 2017).

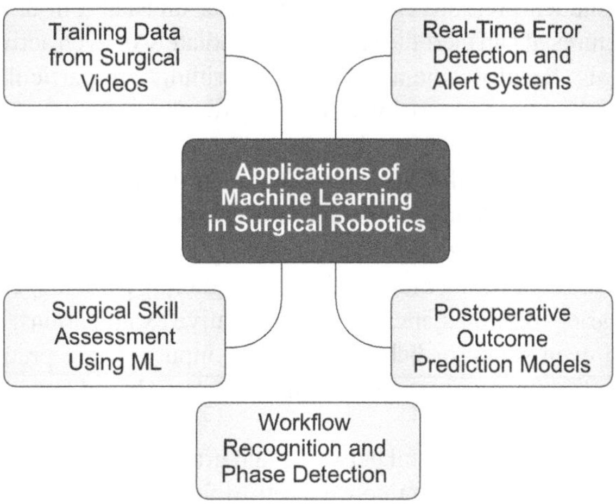

Fig. 3 Machine Learning in Surgical Robotics.

Objective, measurable metrics have been introduced by ML for evaluating surgical proficiency, which are based on kinematic data like instrument velocity, path length, and smoothness of motion. This is particularly important in robotically assisted surgery, where fine-grained tool tracking is already inherent in the system. ML can be used to differentiate between trainee and expert surgeons using support vector machines (SVMs) and random forests algorithms to train on. Characteristics of economy of motion, time to task completion, and tremor frequency are compared to benchmark datasets and yield precise skill-level classification. Such a data-driven strategy has helped create automated skill feedback tools that provide real-time recommendations, enabling continuous improvement within academic as well as clinical environments (Vedula et al., 2017).

Knowing how the procedure goes in real-time enables robots to aid intelligently. The surgical steps, including access, dissection, hemostasis, and closure, can be trained by ML models while examining the integration of videos, audio, and instrument movements. Temporal models, including long short-term memory (LSTM) deep learning networks, will perform well in modeling temporal data and identifying movement from one procedural step to another. After training, the models can be coupled with robotic devices to forecast surgeons' requirements for further action and indicate deviations from predicted workflows. It is also capable of dynamic control of the camera. For instance, during dissection, as dissection is carried out, the system will position the endoscope so that it remains focused on the target, enhancing visibility without the need for verbal command (Lea et al., 2016). One of the most widespread ML applications in robotic surgery is the detection of errors. Intraoperative accidents often occur as a result of minute errors that are not even noticed until they are too late. ML algorithms are able to detect such events by learning from thousands of previous operations and reporting deviation in force application, motion patterns, or instrument trajectories. For instance, whenever the robot detects sudden pressure changes in tools or unusual tool orientations near sensitive structures, it can alert the surgeon immediately or even activate automatic safety protocols. Reinforcement learning algorithms are particularly useful in learning optimal responses to risky scenarios through emulation of trial-and-error outcomes under simulated safe environments (Murali et al., 2019).

Besides, ML-based alarm systems enhance human-robot interaction by reducing the cognitive load on surgeons to enable them to focus on complex procedures and allow the robot to attend to safety in the background (Maier-Hein et al., 2022). ML is becoming more utilized in predicting patient-specific outcomes from a wide variety of inputs, including preoperative examinations, intraoperative variables, and even social or behavioral health inputs. These predictive models allow for complications such as surgical site infection, blood loss, or readmission need to be predicted.

ML methods like deep neural networks and gradient boosting are learned over big sets of clinical data to determine what sets of factors lead to adverse outcomes. They are then used to inform intraoperative decisions and customize care. For example, if the model indicates that the risk of postoperative infection is very high, the surgical team can carry out prophylactic action such as intensified antibiotic regimens or wound management plans (Rajkomar et al., 2019)

4.1 Impact of AI in Robotic Surgery

Through increased procedure accuracy, safety, and customization, surgical care is being reimagined by AI. AI improves many levels of surgical work flows through its implementation within robotic platforms, across preoperative planning and intraoperative guidance through postoperative recovery and education (Table 2). The following sections detail the key advantages and wider implications of the use of AI in robotic-assisted surgery (Table 2). One of the primary advantages of the use of AI in robot-assisted surgery is reduced human error. Hand tremors, tiredness, and restricted movement of joints are among the shortcomings of conventional surgery. The shortcomings can be remedied with the aid of AI-powered robotic platforms in providing motion scaling, tremor cancellation, and highly precise tool placement. AI algorithms continually track surgical progress, anatomical features, and instrument movement, with real-time feedback and corrective response. AI-enabled platforms, for example, can recognize unexpected tissue responses or movement away from predetermined norms and alert the surgeon in near real-time

Table 2 Benefits and Impact of AI in Robotic Surgery.

Benefit	*Description*	*Impact Area*
Enhanced Precision & Reduced Human Error	AI algorithms improve accuracy in identifying anatomy and guiding instruments.	Surgical outcomes, safety
Shortened Recovery Time & Hospital Stay	AI-guided procedures are less invasive, reducing trauma and accelerating healing.	Patient recovery, healthcare costs
Improved Surgical Training & Simulation	AI-based simulators provide real-time feedback and skill analysis for surgical trainees.	Education, performance improvement
Personalized & Patient-Specific Surgery	ML models tailor surgical plans based on patient anatomy and risk profiles.	Precision medicine, decision-making
Consistent Surgical Quality	Reduces variability between surgeons by standardizing critical decisions.	Equity in care delivery
Real-Time Intraoperative Support	AI systems assist with live image interpretation, alerts, and navigation.	Intraoperative decision-making
Outcome Prediction & Risk Assessment	Predictive analytics model complications and recovery likelihoods using patient data.	Postoperative care, resource planning

It can be fatal with a single millimeter error in cases of maximum risk surgeries like cardiac, neurosurgical, or urologic surgeries. The data-driven system provided by the AI improves standardization, reduces the intersurgeon variability, and maximizes the outcome of the surgery (Pangal et al., 2021)

Robot-assisted surgeries with the aid of AI are less invasive and involve less damage to tissues, less blood loss, and smaller incisions. They all contribute to shorter recovery times and shorter periods of hospital stay directly. Robot surgeries with the assistance of AI guidance have been found to have less risk of complications such as infection or incidental damage to organs and thus shorter periods of postoperative care and lower costs of care (Hung et al., 2018). Additionally, AI optimizes intraoperative efficiency with minimized operative time and resource usage. Computerized scheduling with the aid of AI improves the forecasting of surgery times better and optimizes better the management of the operating room (Zhang et al., 2021). To the patient, shorter recovery time equates to faster return to normal activity, less time away at work, and better quality of life. In surgeries such as robotic prostatectomy or hysterectomy, better visualization and guidance with the aid of AI increased marked postoperative satisfaction and diminished the pain and discomfort (Ebbing et al., 2020).

AI is changing surgical training by the vehicle of high-fidelity simulation and real-time feedback. ML algorithms built on huge stores of expert cases permit surgical trainees to practice virtual maneuvers that mimic the complexity of the real world.

AI simulators offer unbiased measures of trainee performance based on analysis of instrument motion, timing, and technique. They are used to select strengths and weaknesses and tailor the learning experience for everyone (Sethi et al., 2021). In addition, AI-based tools allow for curriculum adaptation automatically so that trainees are promoted to increasingly challenging cases only after having mastered previous levels. This data-driven, organized approach accelerates the acquisition of skills and enhances competency prior to clinical exposure (Mirchi et al., 2020). AI-powered virtual tutors and skill assessors are also being integrated into real-time robotic consoles, offering intraoperative suggestions and feedback just as flight simulators provide advice to pilots. This dual use in training and actual operations is one factor contributing to the development of safer and more skilled surgeons (Hashimoto et al., 2019).

Modern medicine is experiencing a transition to personalization, and surgeons will be able to make each procedure individualized to a patient's unique anatomy, pathology, and risk factors based on AI support. Preoperative imaging, laboratory and genomic results are being used by AI systems to identify the recommended surgical approach as well as determine likely complications. This individualization generates customized surgical plans for robotic surgery down to the angle of incision, best path of dissection, and optimal position of prosthetic components in the body. The robotic system will subsequently execute these customized surgical plans with sub-millimeter accuracy. Patient-specific information can also support intraoperative decision-making. For example, in robotic surgery, AI systems are able to identify real-time variations in tissue tension or vascularity and modify the robotic movements, in accordance with these predictive analyses, in order to minimize risk related to procedures, especially when treating orthopedic and oncologic requirements (Jayaraman et al., 2022). AI is allowing for transition from a value-based model of surgery to a precision surgery model, which will improve patient satisfaction outcomes, clinical success rates, and recovery patterns.

5. Challenges and Ethical Considerations of AI in Robotic Surgery

Robot-assisted surgery with AI would revolutionize the field, but it would also pose challenging problems and ethical concerns. Human-machine interaction, data privacy, autonomous system dependability, adherence to regulatory requirements, and worldwide availability are some of these challenges. To provide secure, equitable, and ethical application of AI in surgical interventions, the challenges must be met.

5.1 Patient Content and Data Privacy

Big data, preferably from intraoperative sensor data, images, EHRs, and surgery videos, are essential to AI models. Patient privacy, consent, and data ownership issues are raised through such sensitive data, especially where AI algorithms are trained on anonymized but substantial numbers of records (patients would not necessarily be aware of). Healthcare is used, stored, or transmitted (Price et al., 2019). Health care professionals need to employ robust data protection mechanisms according to the law like the Health Insurance Portability and Accountability Act (HIPAA) or the General Data Protection Regulation (GDPR). Anonymization could be insufficient, however, since re-identification risks occur when data sets are combined. Moreover, consent for the use of data in training AI systems is only achievable effectively through adequate explanation of secondary use of data, commercial opportunities, and long-term data storage (Mesko et al., 2020).

5.2 Legal and Regulatory Issues

The legal framework for surgical systems based on AI is under development. Traditional medical devices undergo rigorous FDA or CE clearance processes, but AI brings in a dynamic element: models shift over time as they receive more data. The issue of post-deployment verification, safety monitoring, and management for updates comes here (Topol et al., 2020). Further, it is not easy to determine who is liable in the case of an adverse event. If a surgical mistake is committed due to an AI-guided suggestion or autonomous robot movement, no one knows who should take the blame–manufacturer, software designer, hospital, or doctor. Legal systems are not yet set up to handle these sensitive situations, and new regulation and adjusting regulatory strategies are necessary (Gerke et al., 2020). Algorithmic bias is also threatened when training data are not diverse enough and can result in disproportionate outcomes by demographic groups. Fairness, accountability, and transparency of AI model development and deployment will need to be addressed through policies and regulations (Rajkomar et al., 2018).

Surgeons will be required to depend on AI recommendations to add them to judgment. Black-box algorithms, characterized by impenetrable internal processes, are an obstacle to faith. If an AI algorithm recommends a surgical action or detects an anomaly without specifying how it made that conclusion, clinicians would be abstaining from acting on that suggestion (Ghassemi et al., 2021). In order to be deemed reliable, AI models will need to be tested extensively against real clinical outcomes. Techniques such as explainable AI (XAI) are being developed to make algorithms transparent by giving understandable feedback. Breakdown of these safeguards can lead to automation bias when surgeons blindly follow AI output and violate safety (Tonekaboni et al., 2019). System robustness also impacts reliability. AI must work roughly the same way under countless different surgical configurations, bodies, and hardware combinations. Misfire or misread in these high-stakes situations can be deadly, so strict testing and human-in-the-loop safety measures are required (Yu et al., 2018).

Successful implementation of AI surgery requires surgeons to accept and collaborate with such intelligent systems. However, most professionals fear losing control, deskilling, or over-dependence on machines. Such resistance can be compounded by inadequate training, ambivalence about role definition, or fears of substitution (Coiera et al., 2021). To ensure integration results in acceptance, institutions of learning must integrate AI principles into training for surgical education. Surgeons must master how to create AI systems, interpret the outputs, and discuss bad ideas. This change in surgical culture—from lone operator to human-machine teaming—will require reengineering workflows, communication standards, and teaming dynamics (Shortliffe et al., 2018). Early involvement of clinicians in AI system design and testing can also improve usability, relevance, and trustworthiness, so that technology is an aid, not a disruptor.

5.3 Cost and Accessibility in Resource-Limited Settings

Even though AI-powered robotic surgery has many benefits, most health care systems do not have access to it, particularly in middle- and low-income countries. The major barriers are the high initial cost of robotic platforms, maintenance, training, and AI integration.

In addition, infrastructure for high-speed data processing, cloud access, and secure digital storage that are needed for AI-powered robotic surgery are typically nonexistent in resource-limited settings. Surgeries involving AI can worsen existing inequalities in access to care unless global policy actions towards technological democratization are taken (Duffy et al., 2022). Participatory models involving open-source platforms, public-private partnerships, and low-cost hardware options are central to narrowing this gap. Priority on equity so that AI serves many groups, and global surgical justice are all part of the ethical rollout.

6. Future Perspectives and Innovations

The use of AI in robotic surgery is still in its infancy. Revolutionary advancements that will change surgical practice all over the world are to be expected as the technology advances. Advances in the future will improve the interface between humans and machines, grant remote access to surgery, and enhance robotic system capabilities. The following section takes into consideration vital future advances.

6.1 *Fully Autonomous Surgery*

One of the most ambitious objectives of AI in surgery is to make fully independent surgical system robots that are able to carry out procedures independently without direct human involvement. Although present robotic systems are mostly "surgeon-in-the-loop", work is now trending towards automating individual tasks like suturing, tissue dissection, or hemostasis. One of the key milestones was the STAR, which carried out soft tissue suturing as accurately as human surgeons in clinical trials (Krieger et al., 2016). The next generation of autonomous systems will draw on reinforcement learning, real-time imaging, and sensor fusion to understand dynamic surgical environments and make autonomous choices (Ghassemi et al., 2021).

With the cost of overcoming ethical, regulatory, and reliability hurdles, surgeons will presumably transition from being explicit operators to overseers—operating automated procedures while monitoring and jumping in as needed (Yu et al., 2018). The integration of AI with AR and VR has transformative potential for surgery and training. AR can superimpose anatomical landmarks, surgical lines, and real-time warnings directly into the surgeon's line of sight for improved spatial awareness and accuracy. This is done by translating preoperative imaging and real-time information into precise, interactive 3D models specific to each patient. In intricate procedures such as neurosurgery or orthopedic surgery, AR-guided devices can navigate the surgeon's hand on optimal trajectories to minimize intraoperative complications (Sethi et al., 2021). AI-driven VR simulators are also transforming surgical training. Students can rehearse surgery in virtual environments from real-world surgical data with real-time feedback and progress monitoring being offered by AI algorithms (Mirchi et al., 2020). Cloud computing is transforming the storage, analysis, and sharing of surgical data.

Cloud-based robotic surgical systems enable constant updating, real-time monitoring, and distance collaboration among institutions. AI can be trained and deployed in the cloud, making scaling easier and systems optimization without explicit hardware modifications. Centralization of data is thus achievable, with anonymized data from surgeries in multiple hospitals pumping into better algorithm performance and accuracy improvements. These networks can then finally construct federated learning systems where models can learn and collaborate across institutions without revealing sensitive patient data (Price et al., 2019). Cloud robotics can also deliver real-time AI assistance during procedures based on massive databases to supply recommendations for best practices or alert to possible abnormalities. This would particularly help poorly resourced or rural locations where there is no specialist expertise (Duffy et al., 2022). AI is also accelerating the development of telesurgery, conducting long-distance surgeries via networked robot systems.

Where initial telesurgeries were limited by delay and communication constraints, AI overcomes these using predictive models, motion smoothing, and error-correction mechanisms. AI is able to anticipate delays in tool response as resulting from network latency and correct the robot trajectory in advance to produce smooth motion. Such developments set the stage for real-time remote surgery to be conducted in areas of disaster, conflict zones, or underdeveloped nations. Moreover, AI programs can also serve as a virtual assistant during remote operations, providing instantaneous alerts, anatomical identification, or procedural guidance. This human-computer hybrid approach to expertise can potentially make high-quality surgical care accessible to everyone (Coiera et al., 2021). Unlike completely autonomous robots, collaborative robots (cobots) are programmed to work alongside human surgeons.

Cobots merge human intelligence with the accuracy and efficiency of machines. Cobots are able to perform repetitive tasks like retraction or suction, allowing the surgeon to concentrate on high-level decision-making. AI allows real-time recognition of gestures, voice command, and anticipatory support, enhancing cobot interaction. As an example, depending on the procedure phase, the system may forecast what tool the surgeon would require next to use, or it may help move the camera based on tool movement (Maier-Hein et al., 2022). Cobots of the future will be able to calibrate responses as per user preference and surroundings. This shift is a compromise that optimizes robot support while keeping human control, finding the middle ground between full autonomy and human control (Tonekaboni et al., 2019).

7. Case Studies and Practical Uses of AI in Robotic Surgery

AI has evolved from conceptual models to actual operating rooms within robot-assisted procedures. Robotic platforms driven by AI are being used by hospitals and surgery centers around the world to aid various specialties such as general surgery, neurosurgery, orthopedics, and urology. Four case studies that illustrate the advantages and uses of AI in robotic surgery are presented in this section (Table 3).

7.1 AI-Assisted Prostatectomy

Robot-assisted radical prostatectomy (RARP) has been arguably the most productive application of AI in robot surgery.

To preserve sexual function and continence of urine following surgery, the da Vinci Surgical System often supplemented by AI-based technology enables precise dissection and nerve-sparing methods, assists in these procedures by reviewing preoperative MRI and biopsy data to help plan excisions and identify cancer margins. Intraoperative guidance systems with machine learning algorithms assist in preventing nerve injury and identifying anatomical landmarks (Ebbing et al., 2020). In addition, AI has been employed to analyze the performance of surgeons in RARP with instrument motion data. ML algorithms detect skill levels, predict outcomes, and give post-procedure feedback for improving future performance (Vedula et al., 2017). Outcomes from multi-institutional trials have shown that AI-assisted RARP results in fewer positive surgical margins, reduced operative time, and reduced complications, compared to operations without AI.

7.2 Neurosurgical Robots

Neurosurgery demands very high accuracy because of the extremely fine and intricate organization of the brain and spinal cord. AI has enormously improved the performance of neurosurgical robots such as ROSA (Medtech) and NeuroMate. In deep brain stimulation (DBS) and epilepsy surgery, AI planning tools apply machine learning algorithms to examine preoperative neuroimages, anticipating the best electrode paths and target areas. The tools account for anatomical variations, lessening their dependence on generalized atlases and boosting procedural precision (Bozkurt et al., 2021). Intraoperatively, AI-based systems assist in directing the robotic arm to accurate coordinates with sub-millimeter precision, enhancing results in tumor resections, biopsies, and cranial navigation. Moreover, AI systems interpret electrophysiological signals and brain mapping results and thus improve decision-making intraoperatively (Rughani et al., 2018). One of the main benefits of neurosurgical AI is that it can learn from high-resolution, multi-modal data sets and transform into patient-specific anatomy, which results in safer outcomes in high-risk settings.

7.3 Computer Vision in Laparoscopic Surgeries

CV is a machine intelligence that enables machines to interpret visual data, such as video from laparoscopic cameras in real-time. In minimally invasive surgery, e.g., laparoscopic cholecystectomy, CV has been used to recognize organs, stages of the surgery, and the use of instruments while performing surgery. These models, which have been trained on hundreds of videos of surgeries, can recognize individual steps such as gallbladder exposure, dissection of the cystic duct, and clipping. This can aid in real-time workflow analysis and can alert the surgeon if a step is omitted or performed in the wrong order (Madani et al., 2020).

Healthcare facilities that utilize CV-based systems like Touch Surgery Enterprise have reported improved surgical quality and safety. The platforms have postoperative video review and peer review, and help in continuous skill improvement (Hashimoto et al., 2021). AI solutions based on computer vision assist with camera control, reducing the number of assistants utilized and improving focus on the operating field, which is particularly beneficial in solo-surgeon or teaching settings (Lea et al., 2016).

Table 3 Application of AI/ML in Robotic Surgery.

Surgical Specialty	*AI/ML Application*	*Impact/Benefit*
Urology	AI in robotic prostatectomy (da Vinci system)	Enhanced precision, reduced complications, better outcomes
Neurosurgery	ML-guided planning in epilepsy/DBS surgeries (ROSA)	Accurate targeting, reduced intraoperative risk
Laparoscopic Surgery	Computer vision for phase detection and tool tracking	Workflow recognition, real-time error alerts
Orthopedic Surgery	AI-assisted implant planning (MAKO, NAVIO systems)	Personalized joint replacement, improved recovery
General Surgery	NLP on surgical notes and EHR integration	Better clinical decisions, pre- and post-operative planning
Training & Simulation	Deep learning and VR in surgical training platforms	Skill assessment, performance feedback, and simulation practice

7.4 AI-Supported Orthopedic Robotic Procedures

Orthopedic surgeries, such as joint replacements and spinal fusions, demand mechanical accuracy in bone preparation and implant positioning. AI supports robotic-assisted systems like MAKO and NAVIO by improving preoperative planning, intraoperative navigation, and postoperative alignment verification. AI programs scan CT or MRI for a patient-specific 3D bone model that simulates ideal implant size, alignment, and orientation. Surgeons can practice any surgical scenario and choose the optimal option for a given patient (Jayaraman et al., 2022). During surgery, AI-powered robotics navigators watched saw blades and drills with millimeter accuracy, saving bone stock and soft tissue. In real-time feedback, overcutting is avoided and consistency from one operation to another is achieved (Tewari et al., 2018). AI-based postoperative assessment can also measure joint function and detect early implant malalignment. Research has established that AI-assisted robotic orthopedic surgery leads to faster recovery, greater mobility and fewer complications (Domb et al., 2021).

8. Conclusion

This chapter discusses the underlying principles, technological developments, functional implementations, and ethics of incorporating AI in surgical robots. The greatest achievement in modern surgical history is our shift from conventional surgery to AI-augmented robotic platforms.

We subsequently followed the evolution of robot-assisted surgery over time, and the growth of AI in medicine; AI became a necessity to increase accuracy, decrease variability, and improve patient outcomes as surgery grew more complex and data-driven. Robotic platforms have already demonstrated usefulness across specialties with systems such as the da Vinci Surgical System, ROSA, and MAKO. Apart from that, sophisticated robotic platforms are currently able to process voluminous data, interpret the same, make decisions in real-time, and provide predictive results that guide surgery planning and performance when integrated with AI. Contrary to perceiving AI as a single problem, it is established to be an intersection of computation methods that include, for instance, CV, ML, deep learning, and NLP. These are employed for numerous applications during surgery, from predicting risk factors after surgery to visual interpretation in carrying out laparoscopic surgery. The convergence of these technologies is driving the shift towards more data-intensive and personalized surgery, where personal needs and anatomy of each patient are considered.

Real-world examples demonstrate how AI is having an impact in a range of medical disciplines. AI has taught various surgical procedures such as neurosurgery, laparoscopic surgery, orthopedics, and prostatectomies the capability to enhance accuracy, reduce complications, and even offer improved recovery time. The case studies present tangible proof of the disruption caused by AI when used in surgical procedures.

References

Ahmidi, N., Tao, L. and Sefati, S. et al. (2017). A dataset and benchmarks for segmentation and recognition of gestures in robotic surgery. *IEEE Transactions on Biomedical Engineering*, *64*(9), 2025–2041. https://doi.org/10.1109/TBME.2016.2637334.

Ashton, R.C. and Murff, R. (2020). Versius robotic surgical system: A next-generation surgical platform. *Annals of Medicine and Surgery*, *56*, 70–74. https://doi.org/10.1016/j.amsu.2020.05.035.

Bozkurt, M., Ozdemir, B. and Ince, N.F. (2021). Robotic neurosurgery and AI. *Frontiers in Robotics and AI*, *8*, 714130. https://doi.org/10.3389/frobt.2021.714130.

Chen, J., Su, Y. and Tai, B.L. (2020). AI-based preoperative planning in joint replacement surgery. *Journal of Orthopaedic Research*, *38*(5), 1055–1062. https://doi.org/10.1002/jor.24567.

Coiera, E. and Braithwaite, J. (2021). The interaction between clinical and artificial intelligence decision-making. *The Lancet Digital Health*, *3*(10), e582–e583. https://doi.org/10.1016/S2589-7500(21)00154-1.

Davies, B.L. (2000). A review of robotics in surgery. *Proceedings of the Institution of Mechanical Engineers, Part H: Journal of Engineering in Medicine*, *214*(1), 129–140. https://doi.org/10.1243/0954411001535117.

Domb, B.G., Redmond, J.M. and Gui, C. (2021). AI-enhanced robotic hip arthroplasty. *The Journal of Arthroplasty*, *36*(1), 115–123. https://doi.org/10.1016/j.arth.2020.07.056.

Duffy, M.C., Johnston, D.B. and Allanson, E.R. (2022). Artificial intelligence in surgery: Implications for global health equity. *BMJ Global Health*, *7*(3), e007780. https://doi.org/10.1136/bmjgh-2021-007780.

Ebbing, J., Gehrig, L.M., Zerwekh, J.E. (2020). Patient-reported outcomes after AI-assisted robotic gynecologic surgeries. *International Urogynecology Journal*, *31*(6), 1231–1240. https://doi.org/10.1007/s00192-020-04261-3.

Esteva, A., Kuprel, B., Novoa, R.A., Ko, J., Swetter, S.M., Blau, H.M. and Thrun, S. (2017). Dermatologist-level classification of skin cancer with deep neural networks. *Nature*, *542*(7639), 115–118. https://doi.org/10.1038/nature21056.

Gerke, S., Minssen, T. and Cohen, I.G. (2020). Ethical and legal challenges of artificial intelligence-driven healthcare. *The Hastings Center Report*, *50*(3), 38–45. https://doi.org/10.1002/hast.1111.

Ghassemi, M., Oakden-Rayner, L. and Beam, A.L. (2021). The false hope of current approaches to explainable artificial intelligence in health care. *The Lancet Digital Health*, *3*(11), e745–e750. https://doi.org/10.1016/S2589-7500(21)00208-9.

Hashimoto, D.A., Meireles, O.R. and Rosman, G. (2020). Artificial intelligence in surgery: Promises and perils. *Annals of Surgery*, *272*(1), 70–76. https://doi.org/10.1097/SLA.0000000000003611.

Hashimoto, D.A., Meireles, O.R. and Rosman, G. (2021). Surgical data science and AI platforms. *NPJ Digital Medicine*, *4*(1), 1–7. https://doi.org/10.1038/s41746-020-00342-6.

Hashimoto, D.A., Rosman, G., Rus, D. and Meireles, O.R. (2018). Artificial intelligence in surgery: Promises and perils. *Annals of Surgery*, *268*(1), 70–76. https://doi.org/10.1097/SLA.0000000000002693.

Hashimoto, D.A., Sirimanna, P., Gomez, E.D., et al. (2019). Artificial intelligence in surgery: Promises and limitations. *Annals of Surgery*, *270*(1), 70–76. https://doi.org/10.1097/SLA.0000000000003083.

Hashimoto, D.A., Ward, T.M., Meireles, O.R. (2020). The role of artificial intelligence in surgery: Decision support and beyond. *Surgical Clinics of North America*, *100*(4), 757–770. https://doi.org/10.1016/j.suc.2020.04.007.

Herron, D.M. and Marohn, M. (2008). A consensus document on robotic surgery. *Surgical Endoscopy*, *22*(2), 313–325. https://doi.org/10.1007/s00464-007-9724-x.

Hung, A.J., Chen, J., Shah, A.Y., et al. (2018). Integrating AI into surgical practice: Workflow efficiencies and clinical outcomes. *The Journal of Urology*, *199*(4), 937–944. https://doi.org/10.1016/j.juro.2017.10.009.

Jarc, A.M. and Curet, M.J. (2017). Constructing data-driven virtual reality surgical simulators using real-world video. *Journal of Biomedical Informatics*, *74*, 114–121. https://doi.org/10.1016/j.jbi.2017.09.004.

Jayaraman, S., Wright, A.S., Sudhir, K., et al. (2022). Personalized surgical planning using AI and 3D modeling. *Surgical Innovation*, *29*(1), 35–45. https://doi.org/10.1177/15533506211048945.

Jiang, F., Jiang, Y., Zhi, H., Dong, Y., Li, H., Ma, S., ... and Wang, Y. (2017). Artificial intelligence in healthcare: Past, present, and future. *Stroke and Vascular Neurology*, *2*(4), 230–243. https://doi.org/10.1136/svn-2017-000101.

Khatri, A., Ravi, S. and Fong, Y. (2021). Machine learning-based prediction models in surgery: A review. *Surgical Innovation*, *28*(5), 585–595. https://doi.org/10.1177/15533506211029037.

Krieger, A., Kim, P.C. and Shademan, A. (2016). Smart Tissue Autonomous Robot (STAR) system for autonomous soft tissue surgery. *Science Translational Medicine*, *8*(337), 337ra64. https://doi.org/10.1126/scitranslmed.aad9398.

Lanfranco, A.R., Castellanos, A.E., Desai, J.P. and Meyers, W.C. (2004). Robotic surgery: A current perspective. *Annals of Surgery*, *239*(1), 14–21. https://doi.org/10.1097/01.sla.0000103020.19595.7d.

Lea, C., Reiter, A., Vidal, R. and Hager, G.D. (2016). Segmental spatiotemporal CNNs for action segmentation in fine-grained activities. In: *European Conference on Computer Vision* (*ECCV*) (pp. 36–52). https://doi.org/10.1007/978-3-319-46487-9_3.

Lonner, J.H. (2019). Robotics in orthopedic surgery: MAKO and the future. *Journal of Arthroplasty*, *34*(7S), S41–S43. https://doi.org/10.1016/j.arth.2019.01.034.

Madani, A., Namazi, B., Altieri, M.S., et al. (2020). Artificial intelligence for intraoperative guidance: Using semantic segmentation to identify surgical anatomy during laparoscopic cholecystectomy. *Annals of Surgery*, *272*(6), 1110–1116. https://doi.org/10.1097/SLA.0000000000003974.

Maier-Hein, L., Eisenmann, M., Sarikaya, D., et al. (2022). Surgical scene understanding: A review of deep learning approaches and datasets. *Nature Biomedical Engineering*, *6*(8), 820–840. https://doi.org/10.1038/s41551-021-00827-8.

Maier-Hein, L., Vedula, S.S., Speidel, S., et al. (2017). Surgical data science for next-generation interventions. *Nature Biomedical Engineering*, *1*, 691–696. https://doi.org/10.1038/s41551-017-0132-7.

Meskó, B. and Görög, M. (2020). A short guide for medical professionals in the era of AI. *NPJ Digital Medicine*, *3*(1), 1–5. https://doi.org/10.1038/s41746-020-0252-7.

Mirchi, N., Ledwos, N., Szasz, P., et al. (2020). The future of surgical simulation: AI and adaptive learning systems. *Journal of Surgical Education*, *77*(6), 1434–1442. https://doi.org/10.1016/j.jsurg.2020.05.027.

Murali, A., Sen, S., Lan, X., et al. (2019). Learning by hallucinating: Generative adversarial networks for robotic surgical data simulation. *Medical Image Analysis*, *57*, 196–203. https://doi.org/10.1016/j.media.2019.06.002.

Padoy, N. (2019). Machine and deep learning for workflow recognition during surgery. *The British Journal of Surgery*, *106*(2), e93–e96. https://doi.org/10.1002/bjs.11147.

Pangal, D.J., Pitt, H.A., Hogg, M.E. (2021). Artificial intelligence in surgery: Emerging trends and challenges. *Annals of Surgery Open*, *2*(2), e060. https://doi.org/10.1097/AS9.0000000000000060.

Price, W.N. and Cohen, I.G. (2019). Privacy in the age of medical big data. *Nature Medicine*, *25*(1), 37–43. https://doi.org/10.1038/s41591-018-0272-7.

Rajkomar, A., Dean, J. and Kohane, I. (2019). Machine learning in medicine. *The New England Journal of Medicine*, *380*(14), 1347–1358. https://doi.org/10.1056/NEJMra1814259.

Rajkomar, A., Hardt, M., Howell, M.D., Corrado, G. and Chin, M.H. (2018). Ensuring fairness in machine learning to advance health equity. *Annals of Internal Medicine*, *169*(12), 866–872. https://doi.org/10.7326/M18-1990.

Rivas-Blanco, I., Sánchez-Margallo, J.A., Sánchez-Peralta, L.F., et al. (2020). AI-assisted robotic camera control using gesture recognition. *Journal of Healthcare Engineering*, *2020*, Article ID 8429753. https://doi.org/10.1155/2020/8429753.

Rughani, A.I., Dumont, T.M., Penar, P.L., et al. (2018). AI in neurosurgery: Real-time applications. *World Neurosurgery*, *114*, 417–423. https://doi.org/10.1016/j.wneu.2018.03.228.

Senders, J.T., Staples, P.C., Karhade, A.V., et al. (2018). Machine learning and neurosurgical outcome prediction: A systematic review. *World Neurosurgery*, *109*, 476–486. https://doi.org/10.1016/j.wneu.2017.09.149.

Sethi, M., Emam, T.A., Broek, R.P., et al. (2021). Artificial intelligence in surgical training: Current landscape and future directions. *Surgical Endoscopy*, *35*(12), 6709–6720. https://doi.org/10.1007/s00464-021-08502-y.

Shademan, A., Decker, R.S., Opfermann, J.D., Leonard, S., Krieger, A. and Kim, P.C. (2016). Supervised autonomous robotic soft tissue surgery. *Science Translational Medicine*, *8*(337), 337ra64. https://doi.org/10.1126/scitranslmed.aad9398.

Shortliffe, E.H. and Sepúlveda, M.J. (2018). Clinical decision support in the era of artificial intelligence. *JAMA*, *320*(21), 2199–2200. https://doi.org/10.1001/jama.2018.17163.

Tewari, A., Srivastava, A. and Sooriakumaran, P., et al. (2018). Precision surgery: Navigating anatomical variability with AI-enhanced robotic systems. *Nature Reviews Urology*, *15*(7), 417–430. https://doi.org/10.1038/s41585-018-0016-2.

Tomašev, N., Glorot, X. and Rae, J.W., et al. (2019). A clinically applicable approach to continuous prediction of future acute kidney injury. *Nature*, *572*(7767), 116–119. https://doi.org/10.1038/s41586-019-1390-1.

Tonekaboni, S., Joshi, S., McCradden, M.D. and Goldenberg, A. (2019). What clinicians want: Contextualizing explainable machine learning for clinical end use. *Proceedings of Machine Learning Research*, *106*, 359–380. https://proceedings.mlr.press/v106/tonekaboni19a.html.

Topol, E.J. (2019). High-performance medicine: The convergence of human and artificial intelligence. *Nature Medicine*, *25*, 44–56. https://doi.org/10.1038/s41591-018-0300-7.

Topol, E. J. (2020). A framework for the regulation of AI in healthcare. *Nature*, *586*(7831), E16–E17. https://doi.org/10.1038/s41586-020-2793-0.

Twinanda, A.P., Shehata, S., Mutter, D., Marescaux, J., Padoy, N. (2016). Endonet: A deep architecture for recognition tasks in laparoscopic videos. In: *IEEE Conference on Computer Vision and Pattern Recognition* (*CVPR*) (pp. 5849–5857). https://doi.org/10.1109/CVPR.2016.632.

Vannabouathong, C., Duong, A., Al Dhaheri, B., et al. (2021). Machine learning in neurosurgical outcomes. *Neurosurgical Review*, *44*(1), 29–44. https://doi.org/10.1007/s10143-020-01241-0.

Vedula, S.S., Ishii, M., Hager, G.D. (2017). Objective assessment of surgical technical skill and competency in the operating room. *Annual Review of Biomedical Engineering*, *19*, 301–325. https://doi.org/10.1146/annurev-bioeng-071516-044549.

Wang, M.Y., Green, B.A. and Shahlaie, K. (2013). ROSA: Robotic technology for neurosurgery. *Surgical Neurology International*, *4*(Suppl 6), S398–S403. https://doi.org/10.4103/2152-7806.119479.

Yu, K.H., Beam, A.L. and Kohane, I.S. (2018). Artificial intelligence in healthcare. *Nature Biomedical Engineering*, *2*, 719–731. https://doi.org/10.1038/s41551-018-0305-z.

Zhang, X., Kim, J., Patriciu, A. (2021). Predictive analytics in surgical scheduling using artificial intelligence. *Journal of Biomedical Informatics*, *117*, 103758. https://doi.org/10.1016/j.jbi.2021.103758.

16 The Role of Artificial Intelligence in Next-Generation Surgical Robotics

Kapil Kumar Sharma[1*], Dr. Tripti Choudhary[2], Nidal Al Said[3] and Nidhi Sharma[4]

By using artificial intelligence within surgical robotics, healthcare is experiencing a radical shift in the way surgery is planned and performed and how surgical outcomes are qualitatively measured. The first robots created in surgery were only extensions of the surgeon's dexterity (the ability to move with precision). These early systems aided the surgeon by allowing for better visualization of the surgical field and a more expansive range of motion. The availability of AI technologies (e.g., machine learning, computer vision, natural language processing, and predictive analytics) has allowed surgical robots to become "intelligent" assistants to surgeons: They can provide real-time decision-support and perform some tasks on their own while offering tailored solutions for each individual patient. This chapter provides a framework for the application of AI in surgical robotics by emphasizing that the foundation for precision, flexibility, and learning over time lies in having accurate data and valid algorithms. The chapter reviews the applications of AI to surgical robots for pre-operative imaging; intraoperative navigation; and robotic-assisted surgery. The chapter also discusses machine learning-based algorithms to improve surgical success, adaptive learning capabilities, and intelligent error detection and reporting. The chapter reviews the da Vinci, Senhance, Versius, and STAR surgical robotics systems, and compares their measurable improvements in safety, efficiency, and recovery when compared to traditional methods of surgical intervention. This chapter evaluates several critical aspects of current technical hurdles, ethical and legal issues, and the need for popular support among both the surgical team and patient groups, while examining future potential avenues in the development of new surgical techniques through the use of AI-based autonomous surgical robotic

1 Department of Computer Science and Engineering, Accurate Institute of Engineering and Technology, Greater Noida.
2 Department of Computer Science and Engineering, Hi-Tech Institute of Engineering and Technology, Ghaziabad.
3 College of Mass Communication, Ajman University, Ajman, UAE.
4 Department of Computer Science and Engineering & Hi-Tech Institute of Engineering and Technology, Ghaziabad.
Email: triptichoudhary06@gmail.com[2]; n.alsaid@ajman.ac.ae[3]; nidhisharma5496@gmail.com[4]
* Corresponding author: k.kapil.s@gmail.com

DOI: 10.1201/9781003655121-16

systems, AI-powered training simulators, and human-AI collaborative procedures. Throughout this chapter, the reader is shown how AI-surgical robotic systems should not simply be viewed as substitutes for surgeons; instead, these systems represent a large step forward in the collaboration and development of the future of precision medicine and patient-centered care.

1. Introduction

One of the most substantial strides in modern medicine is the application of robotics to surgical practice. The intended purpose of surgical robotics was to improve a surgeon's precision, decrease invasiveness, and better patient outcomes. Early robotic systems illustrated the ability of an advanced machine to provide additional dexterity, visualization, and stability to the human surgeon, but the robot would again be at the command of the surgeon. Robotics systems were dependent on the intuition and decision-making of the surgeon.

As AI (artificial intelligence) has rapidly accelerated, particularly with machine learning (ML), computer vision (CV), and advanced data analytics, there is now an opportunity for transformative change in surgical robotics (Adegbesan et al., 2024). The synergy of AI and robotics represents the start of the next generation of surgical robotics. Robots, or machines, will not only serve as a device for precision surgical instruments, but will also be intelligent collaborators able to leverage the machine's data, intuition, decision-making, and perform on behalf of the surgeon independently or in a collaborative effort.

1.1 Evolution of Surgical Robotics

The journey of surgical robotics can be broadly divided into three distinct phases:

1. First Generation: Foundational Stage (1980s–1990s)

In its earliest phases, surgical robotics was experimental and primarily focused on demonstrating feasibility. That is, these systems depended heavily on a human operator for strict guidance and were limited in their operational capabilities beyond the manipulation of motion (Ghimire et al., 2025).

2. Second Generation: Advanced Assistance (2000s)

The da Vinci Surgical System exemplifies the commercialization of robotic platforms in the beginning of the 21st century and how significantly the da Vinci System changed the current world of surgical practice with the ability to perform laparoscopic appendectomy surgery these days using the da Vinci Surgical Robot. The da Vinci surgical robot features a 3D View of the inside of the patient's abdominal area, as well as motion scaling and wristed instruments which provide for a much higher level of dexterity than the human hand. The da Vinci surgical robot cannot perform surgery on its own and as such, the surgeon is still the ultimate decision-maker as the da Vinci is simply an extension of human experience and knowledge (Probst, 2023).

3. Third Generation: Intelligent Systems (Present)

Surgical robotics is currently evolving into a new era through the addition of AI- and ML- powered systems used in robotic surgery. Surgical robots are no longer a mechanical arm operated by humans; they are now more like AI-based systems of algorithms, CV, and data analytics utilization in the process of surgical procedures. Current research is exploring the development of robots that can independently perform surgical steps in the surgical workflow, assist in making surgical decisions in real-time, and tailor the robot to the unique anatomical variations of patients. This is a movement from robot-assisted surgery to AI-enabled robot surgery, preparing the ground for eventual full autonomous surgical robots.

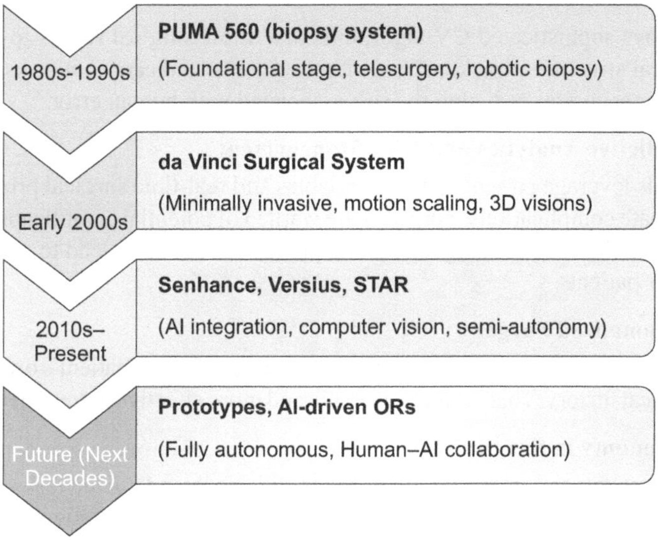

Fig. 1 Evolution of Surgical Robotics.

4. Fourth Generation: Prototypes, AI-driven Ors (Future)

Prototypes and AI-enabled Operating Rooms (ORs) characterize the future of surgical robotics, where fully autonomous systems conduct complex tasks with minimal supervision. Human-AI collaboration ensures surgeons supply their expertise and judgment to give a human touch to the precision, data-driven insight, and workflow orchestration of the AI, with the goal to create safer, more efficient, and patient-centered surgical environments (Riad et al., 2025).

This timeline, represented in Figure 1 the four generations of surgical robotics: the primitive stage in the 1980s–1990s (the PUMA 560), advanced assistance of the 2000s (the da Vinci system), intelligent systems in the 2010s and beyond (Senhance, Versius, STAR), and the future of fully autonomous AI-driven operating rooms.

1.2 Why AI is Transforming Surgery

AI has emerged as the driving force behind the next phase of surgical innovation. Its transformative impact can be understood through several dimensions:

- **Enhanced Decision-Making**

AI technology analyses large amounts of data throughout the course of the operation to provide surgeons with recommendations based on historical evidence and perform similar analysis of what they could expect for their patient, while significantly reducing uncertainty and bolstering the surgeon's confidence during stressful times in the OR.

- **Precision and Accuracy**

AI employs sophisticated CV algorithms that allow surgical robots to recognize anatomical structures, track instrument movements, and carry out tasks with sub-millimeter accuracy, reducing the risk associated with human error.

- **Predictive Analytics and Risk Management**

AI models leverage patient-specific variables and real-time surgical progress data to anticipate complications. Surgeons are warned of potential complications before they occur, allowing the surgeon to take preventive action to lead to an improved safety for patients.

- **Personalized Surgery**

AI can use patient data to develop surgical techniques for that patient's own anatomy and medical history. This is patient specific and more effective in treatment options.

- **Autonomy in Surgical Tasks**

AI allows robots to perform many of the repetitive or standardized tasks in surgery, such as suturing or tissue dissection, which can help alleviate fatigue and shorten procedure time. While robots are still under development for full autonomy, they are currently in use semi-autonomously.

- **Training and Simulation**

Additionally, robotic systems powered by AI serve as teaching platforms and offer simulations based on immersive virtual reality (VR) environments, allowing young surgeons to practice when the context is safe and controlled. These systems will evaluate performance and provide feedback for accelerated learning.

2. Foundations of AI in Surgical Robotics

The move to intelligent systems in surgical robotics entails utilizing Artificial Intelligent (A.I.) technologies. Traditional robots use precision through mechanics, and the surgeon, motioning to move safely inside the body. Modern surgical robots possess hardware that integrates "smarter" A.I. models, allowing robots to perceive, reason, learn, and adapt during a procedure. All of these changes directly come from the key A.I. technologies themselves, and in how we collect data, and develop the algorithms.

2.1 Core AI Technologies in Surgical Robotics

Transitioning to intelligent systems in robotics for surgical procedures means "more and more" using A.I. technologies. Once, robots utilized precision through mechanics and the surgeon chose motional actions and motioning to make sure they maneuvered safely inside the body. Today, surgical robots can be designed to incorporate "smarter" A.I. modalities allowing the robots to perceive, reason, learn, and adapt during a surgical procedure. All these advancements are happening because the A.I. technology itself is changing, and then accordingly, the ways we are collecting data, and developing algorithms. The advancements in the next generation of surgical robotics are based on advancing and integrating core AI technologies that offer unique capabilities to improve surgical practice. ML allows the robot to learn from large surgical data sets and operate more effectively over time. It also enables predictive analysis of the patient outcomes and provides adaptive control during surgery. In turn, Deep Learning (DL) utilizes multi layered neural networks to analyze complex and unstructured data sets (e.g., medical images and videos of procedures), thereby enhancing the robot's image recognition capabilities (Liu et al., 2024a). For example, the robot learns to differentiate between tissue, instruments, and anatomy with greater precision. Natural Language Processing (NLP) takes use of AI to give surgical robots the ability to interact in and with natural spoken language; for example, a surgeon may control a robotic system with voice commands or could use voice to help seamlessly document procedures. And lastly, CV allows robots to be intelligent in how they interpret visual information to visualize and analyze aspects of the surgical anatomy; for example, creating 3D models of the patient anatomy, tracking surgical instruments in real- time, and improving intraoperative safety by alerting the surgeon to the presence of potential risks. Collectively, these components—ML, DL, NLP, and CV—represent the technological foundation of AI-enabled surgical robotics that converts a mechanical tool into an intelligent partner in surgery.

2.2 Importance of Data and Algorithms in Surgery

AI is the source of intelligence behind surgical robots; however, the true value of surgical robots comes from using the combination of multiple forms of both algorithmic and patient-related data. Like most modern surgical robots, which utilize many different forms of data in addition to that entered by surgeons, these types of data include (but are not limited to) comprehensive patient data, medical imaging, such as MRIs (magnetic resonance images) and CT (computed tomography) scans, video feeds gathered by endoscopes, and sensor input gathered by instruments during surgery. By combining these different forms of information, surgical robots create a more thorough and better understanding of the surgical environment than previous generations of robots. Thus, through the robot's ability to process the gathered information from various sources, the robot adjusts for each patient's unique anatomical and clinical situation, allowing a surgeon to provide tailored, individualized surgical care. The algorithms (i.e., computer programs) that process the data collected are also important for the robot. These algorithms represent how computers will convert raw gathered data into real-time, useful, and relevant information at the time of surgery by using the previously identified data. For example, some advanced algorithms might help the surgeon to make the most effective surgical decision, to identify and predict complications that might occur during surgery, and/or help the robot perform movements in a manner that is precise and safe (Hashimoto et al., 2018). Additionally, the use of feedback mechanisms within these algorithms allows for robotic surgical systems to continuously develop and advance based upon the increased number of procedures that they are utilized for. The combination of high-quality data along with advanced algorithm technology creates AI-based robotic surgical systems which will provide greater levels of accuracy, adaptability, and improvement in performance with time and use which in turn will generate superior surgical results and enhance patient safety.

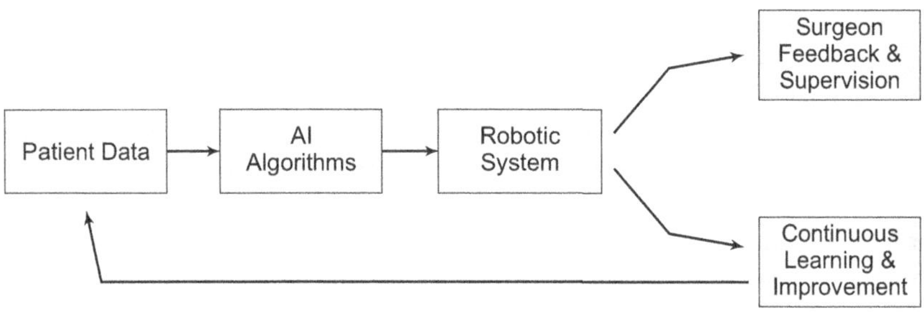

Fig. 2 Data Flow in AI-Supported Surgery.

Figure 2 shows how patient data such as electronic medical records, images, and intraoperative information from sensors are input into AI algorithms. The Robot performs the surgical maneuvers prescribed by the AI algorithm based on the patient's data. The surgeon observes the procedure and provides feedback to the robot. The robot uses this feedback to continually learn from its experience and become more proficient during each surgical procedure.

3. Applications of AI in Surgical Robotics

AI has transformed robotic surgery from a high level of mechanical accuracy to one where AI teaches a robot how to make intelligent decisions while adapting to situations. AI's strength in the surgical space is its ability to process vast amounts of complex medical data, support the surgical team when things go wrong, and in many instances, even perform surgical procedures independently. In this chapter, we will summarize some of the more interesting applications of AI found in various robotic systems used in the surgical field, such as the imaging process (preoperatively), navigation during surgery and the ability to make real-time decisions as well as increased capability for either fully autonomous or semi-autonomous surgical executions (Habuza et al., 2021) (Table 1).

Table 1 Applications of AI in Surgical Robotics.

Application	*Purpose*	*AI Techniques Used*
Preoperative Image Analysis	3D models, risk assessment, and surgical planning	Deep Learning (CNNs), ML-based prediction
Intraoperative Guidance	Real-time navigation, tissue recognition	Computer Vision, Reinforcement Learning
Autonomous Procedures	Execution of repetitive tasks	Reinforcement Learning, Robotics Control
Error Detection	Prevent damage, improve safety	CNNs, Anomaly Detection, Autoencoders
Personalized Surgery	Patient-specific strategies	Predictive Analytics, Adaptive ML Algorithms

3.1 Preoperative Image Analysis and Surgical Planning

AI can assist in the preoperative planning of surgical robot operations. There is extensive research on how AI can analyze CT scans, MRI scans and ultrasound images more quickly and accurately than a human being. The first step in using AI to improve surgical efficiencies is through the construction of three-dimensional models of the anatomy of the patient, along with visual representations of areas of concern. AI can also help the surgeon visualize and evaluate how well multiple approaches to the same site can be used to treat a patient, thereby allowing for a decision as to which surgical strategy presents the best chance of success. AI helps to make the surgical process more individualized by providing specific and relevant surgical steps based on the circumstances of the specific patient ("Use of AI in Diagnostic Imaging and Future Prospects," 2025). Additionally, by utilizing data from previous surgical procedures performed on those patients, AI can generate predictions of the outcomes and consequently develop preoperative plans to ensure safety and effectiveness.

3.2 Intraoperative Guidance and Real-Time Decision-making

Operating rooms are often very busy environments where things can change often, therefore any type of decision support that is needed for the operating room must be provided in real-time, and with the introduction of AI, decision support will be greatly changed through the ability to analyse live streaming of data collected from cameras, sensors, and robotic surgical instruments. Computer vision will enable robotic surgical instruments to be able to identify anatomical structures, identify the position of tools, and detect changes in tissue during the surgical procedure. The ability to identify critical anatomical structures (i.e., blood vessels and nerves) will help avoid injury to these important structures. In addition, AI will allow algorithms to assess all intraoperative signals, including vital signs and other signals that may alert the surgical team to issues before they develop. Access to real-time statistics and decision support enables surgeons to make more informed decisions based on data while in the operating room. The combination of real-time analytics and decision support increases precision through augmentation and decreases the occurrence of human errors. Ultimately, AI will create a robotic surgery tool that will continuously be scanning and directing the surgeon during the execution of the surgical procedure (Park et al., 2025).

3.3 Autonomous and Semi-Autonomous Surgical Procedures

AI in robotic surgery is now making surgical procedures more independent. AI-assisted robotic systems can execute a restricted number of surgical tasks automatically, whereas prior robotic systems had to rely entirely on human interaction to perform every task. A robot can repeat standardized procedures during surgery, such as suturing, cutting, or drilling, with unrivalled consistency. Semi-autonomous systems provide for a division of discretion between the robot and the surgeon in which the AI can autonomously perform discrete actions while providing the surgeon the ability to supervise and intervene as necessary. Research is underway examining even fully autonomous systems executing complex operations with minimal supervision. However, even with these systems, the AI is fully dependent on learning from a dataset of past surgical procedures to improve autonomous activity over time (Gode et al., 2025). The use of surgical robotics raises implications related to ethics, legal accountability, and especially trust-based decision-making or judgment. Autonomous care is close to being realized and is already increasing surgical efficiencies and decreasing fatigue in semi-autonomous surgery. In the long term, enabled by improvements in autonomy, humans and intelligent surgical robots will partner to allow the human to utilize their judgement and sophistication with the precision and reliability of a machine.

4. Machine Learning in Surgical Robotics

Cantered in the realm of AI as it applies to next-gen surgical robotics, ML offers the opportunity for robotic systems to not be programmed in the traditional sense, but rather learn from data, adapt to changing circumstances, and become more effective as they learn. In a surgical setting, this would permit patients to have their outcomes predicted, to have the surgical technique adjusted at the time of surgery, and to have errors (if errors were committed) detected in real time. The benefits that would be gleaned would come from synoptically applying data-driven models, adaptive algorithms, and state-of-the-art (often DL-based) ML techniques to transform surgical robots into smart surgical assistants.

4.1 Predictive Models for Patient Outcomes

One strong application of ML in surgical robotics is the development of predictive models that can aid in anticipating patient outcomes. These models would use plentiful historical patient data, imaging data, and surgical outcomes to find correlations that may not be noticeable in the moment by a human surgeon. Using predictive insights, these models can estimate the risk for post-surgical complications, estimate time to recover, and, in some cases, suggest the best surgical approach for a patient. There are tools and techniques to suddenly support predictive models: for example, Scikit-learn can be used to build traditional models like logistic regression, decision trees, and support vector machines; DL models can be trained using TensorFlow and PyTorch to analyze complicated data such as CT or MRI imaging; and traditionally, for structured, large-volume clinical datasets predictive models, XGBoost, and LightGBM are used (Eloranta & Boman, 2022). For example, a predictive ML model that has been trained on thousands of heart surgery cases could predict the risk of complications based on person-specific aspects such as age, number of comorbidities, and imaging results, giving surgeons a more thoughtful method to plan surgical interventions with the best outcomes and safety.

4.2 Adaptive Learning from Surgical Data

Surgery is a constantly changing setting in which each patient presents different anatomical and clinical characteristics, and this variability requires systems capable of adapting in real-time. Adaptive learning allows surgical robots to improve performance in real time by learning from real surgical data, which allows them to evolve much like human surgeons. In order to drive changes to the robot's surgical actions, ML algorithms will derive actions from sensor data, robotic motion data, and intraoperative images. These algorithms automatically learn to adapt the robotic surgical actions to enhance accuracy, minimize forces to delicate tissues, and lower the risk of error. The adaptive capability of a robotic surgical system can be improved through training with simulations, where according to (Wu et al., 2024) advanced methods like Reinforcement Learning (RL) allow the development of a model where the system will perform certain actions on an object based on either positive (reward) or negative (punishment) feedback. The RL algorithms used in robotic systems can be more sophisticated than the early algorithms using Q-learning; in addition to the use of RL to train the robot's movements and actions, more sophisticated methods like Deep Q Networks (DQN) and Policy Gradient Methods can be incorporated for the purposes of controlling the robot in an uncertain environment and to prevent degradation of the robot's performance as the complexity of the surgical task increases. Additionally, platforms for training robotic systems, such as OpenAI Gym and robotic simulators designed for surgical applications, provide the appropriate environment for the robots to conduct millions of simulated surgical procedures before performing actual surgical procedures on live patients to hone their skills through trial and error. For instance, the Robotic Suturing System described above, which incorporates an RL algorithm, is able to progressively adapt to improve the accuracy of stitch placement.

4.3 Intelligent Error Detection Systems

Errors during procedures, including unintentional alterations of tissue or misplacement of an instrument, may result in the development of harmful consequences; thus, error detection remains a salient aspect of intelligent surgical robotics. Error detection systems that operate based on ML methods have emerged to assist with this challenge by methodically monitoring surgical environments in real- time through video feeds, sensor inputs, and robotic kinematics, with the intent to detect potential errors and alert the surgical team. Specifically, error detection systems identify deviations from known patterns of normal surgical activity and are capable of detecting potential threats prior to an error increasing in risk level and resulting in an adverse event (Hamilton, 2024). For example, advanced methods employing CV with convolutional neural network (CNN) practices are capable of detecting unusual instrument movement or atypical tissue response with substantial accuracy. Furthermore, methods of anomaly detection, for example, Isolation Forest or Autoencoders, in the ML space, have performed well on pre-clinical studies identifying abnormal characteristics of streaming surgical data in excess of substantial variation that may indicate a developing harmful error. Furthermore, each of these approaches requires real-time data processing programs, such as Apache Kafka and Spark Streaming, for managing health goals and streaming data in the operating room, especially given the noteworthy scale of intraoperative data, including possible raised alerts during surgeries as soon as feasible. For instance, an intelligent robotic system may identify an unusual pattern of force being utilized during the dissection of tissue and notify the surgeon accordingly (Table 2).

Table 2 Machine Learning Applications in Surgical Robotics.

Application	*Purpose in Surgical Robotics*	*Tools / Techniques Used*
Predictive Models for Patient Outcomes	Forecast surgical risks, recovery time, and outcomes based on patient data.	Scikit-learn (logistic regression, decision trees), TensorFlow & PyTorch (deep learning), XGBoost/LightGBM
Adaptive Learning from Surgical Data	Continuous improvement of robotic performance using surgical experience.	Reinforcement Learning (RL), Deep Q-Networks (DQN), Policy Gradient Methods, OpenAI Gym, Surgical Simulators
Intelligent Error Detection Systems	Detect abnormal actions, prevent tissue damage, and alert surgeons in real time.	Computer Vision (CNNs), Anomaly Detection (Isolation Forest, Autoencoders), Real-Time Processing (Apache Kafka, Spark Streaming)

5. Improving Precision, Safety, and Efficiency

AI may represent one of the most important opportunities for next-generation robotic surgery in terms of precision, safety, and efficiency of the procedure. Robotic systems exhibit greater dexterity and stability than humans do. While robotic systems have improved a surgeon's capabilities through enhanced dexterity and stability, they have only excelled to a certain stage when using AI; AI has provided an entirely different level of benefit. AI provides intelligent error avoidance, utilizes visual feedback with augmented reality (AR), and allows for customizing surgical procedures for an individual patient through computer programs. The combination of all of these technologies is producing a drastic transformation to robotic surgical systems that now provide feedback and optimization to robotic technologies along with assistance rather than relying solely on robotic surgical technology for assistance.

5.1 Minimizing Surgical Errors with AI

Errors that occur during surgical procedures can be fatal; they can be caused by physician fatigue, poor vision, and, to a lesser extent, the difficulty of the human anatomical structure. A robotic surgical system that incorporates AI can use a real-time safety protocol, along with predictive analytics and detection systems, to help mitigate surgical errors. The robotic surgical systems use CV and multiple sensors to monitor the surgeon's use of surgical instruments with a level of accuracy that has never been available in surgical environments. This enables them to provide an alert to the surgeon when their instruments are getting too close to an unsafe configuration. Furthermore, the thousands of surgical procedures that ML algorithms are trained on will allow the robotic surgical systems to detect changes in surgical instrumentation that could indicate an impending complication, allowing the surgeon to take action before a complication occurs.

An example is that an AI-enabled robotic surgical system can detect an abnormal amount of force when the surgeon is dissecting tissue and alert the surgeon to avoid possible damage. As robotic surgical systems accumulate new learnings of thousands of surgical procedures through AI technology, they will further minimize risks and lessen the chances of human errors in surgery. This will promote safer and more consistent surgical processes.

5.2 Enhanced Visualization and Augmented Reality (AR)

The use of traditional surgery relies heavily on 2D imaging for visualization, which can be misleading and therefore, restrict a surgeon's ability to comprehend how three-dimensional structures in the body relate to each other, especially when trying to visualize complex spatial relationships. The advent of surgical robots with AI, in contrast, allows for completely different visualization options through AR/VR technologies, whereby clinical imaging/video data is incorporated with AI algorithms to develop 3D models of the patient's anatomy that provide enhanced visualization capabilities to the surgeon during the procedure. Moreover, AR, by integrating the data from the AR model with the real-world view of the surgical site, in addition to highlighting specific structures such as blood vessels and tumors in the surgeon's field of view can support a reduction of inadvertent errors during surgical dissection (Cotsoglou et al., 2024). Additionally, through the use of AI algorithms and AR technology, AR can provide the necessary information for surgical navigation to guide robotic devices with a high degree of precision to their respective target anatomical structures, thereby reducing uncertainty associated with even the most challenging or minimally invasive surgical procedures. Ultimately, the use of AR technology is significantly impacting the surgical environment in which surgeons work; therefore, allowing them greater levels of visualization and knowledge to deliver optimal outcomes for their patients.

The integration of AI, with AR, for Surgical Visualization, is demonstrated in Figure 3. 3-Dimensional Anatomical Models,Tumor /Blood Vessel Overlays, and Real- Time Navigation, provide urgeons with enhanced Precision, Lower Risk, and Improved Decision-Making, while performing complex surgeries.

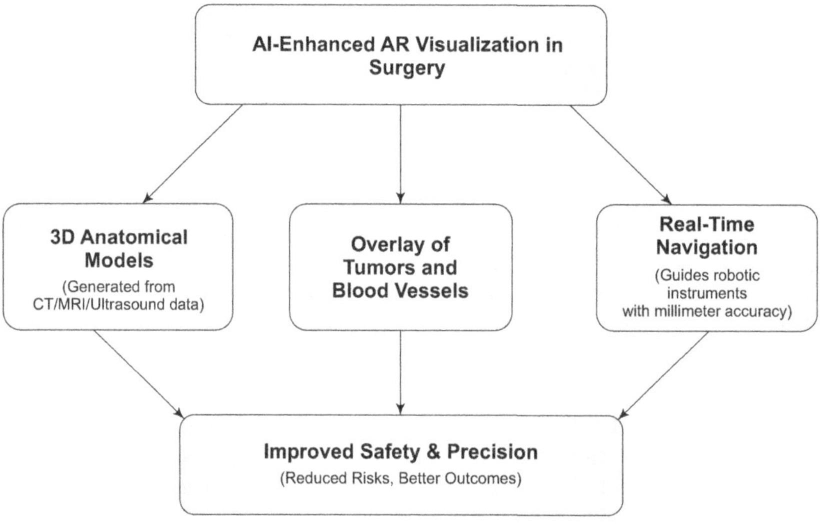

Fig. 3 AI-Enhanced Visualization and Augmented Reality in Surgery.

5.3 Personalized Robotic Surgical Procedures

Because every patient has different anatomies and different medical histories, the surgical experience for virtually everyone is a unique experience. Therefore the use of AI allows the development of a customized robotic surgical procedure for each patient utilizing analysis of data related to the individual (i.e., imaging data, genetics, and clinical information). The application of ML models will develop algorithms that will allow for prediction of the type of surgical procedure that is most appropriate for each patient, while the adaptive robotic control will allow for any changes made to the surgical instrument during the procedure to be made to fit the patient's anatomy (Neri et al., 2025). For instance, a robotic system may alter the angle of the incision or alter the amount of force applied to tissue based upon real-time feedback, enabling real-time tailoring of the surgical procedure to provide improved safety and effectiveness. The development of personalized surgical robotics will not only produce an improved outcome for patients, but also may decrease recovery time and incidence of postoperative complications.

6. Integration of AI with Healthcare Data

Because every patient has different anatomies and different medical histories, the surgical experience for virtually everyone is a unique experience. Therefore the use of AI allows the development of a customized robotic surgical procedure for each patient utilizing analysis of data related to the individual (i.e., imaging data, genetics, and clinical information). The application of ML models will develop algorithms that will allow for prediction of the type of surgical procedure that is most appropriate for each patient, while the adaptive robotic control will allow for any changes made to the surgical instrument during the procedure to be made to fit the patient's anatomy (Neri et al., 2025). For instance, a robotic system may alter the angle of the incision or alter the amount of force applied to tissue based upon real-time feedback, enabling real-time tailoring of the surgical procedure to provide improved safety and effectiveness. The development of personalized surgical robotics will not only produce an improved outcome for patients, but also may decrease recovery time and incidence of postoperative complications.

6.1 Minimizing Surgical Errors with AI

There are many potential causes of errors in surgery—human fatigue, limited visibility, complicated anatomy, and unexpected intraoperative events. These issues are resolved through the use of AI within surgical robotics through the real-time monitoring of surgical activity; the ability to predict surgical outcomes; and the detection of complications. The application of CV to identify the position of surgical instruments and the ability to accurately track the movement of the surgical instruments allows for the ability to ensure the precise placement of instruments with respect to the vulnerable structures of the body. Additionally, the application of AI on large volumes of surgical cases allows for AI to be trained to recognize patterns of complications that are associated with surgical procedures (i.e., small bleeds) and/or unusual tissue responses (i.e., excessive bleeding). Therefore, AI can be effectively applied as a tool to support surgeons in making better surgical decisions (e.g., identifying when they are about to cause a significant amount of unnecessary trauma to the patient) and ultimately leading to less trauma to the patient.

The advanced AI-Enabled frameworks that identify errors can use CNNs to identify sudden changes in the motion of surgical instruments and Anomaly Detection to detect anomalies in the motion or movements of surgical instruments. To capture the data used in these AI models in real-time, we can use Real-Time Processing Software Tools such as Apache Kafka and Spark Streaming to calculate and monitor surgical-related data nearly instantaneously, allowing for the immediate identification of errors (Liu et al., 2023a). This is critical in reducing unnecessary surgical trauma to patients and improving surgical accuracy and success rates. There are robotic platforms that can measure the abnormal force or force discernments during dissection or closure and halt action to alert the surgeon or instigate a course of action. AI, in conjunction with a prediction algorithm and continuous learning, can yield good results.

6.2 Enhanced Visualization and Augmented Reality (AR)

Visualization is an essential element in surgery, and AI technology has drastically changed the way that surgeons see and interact with the operative field. The original robotic systems enhanced magnification and stereoscopic visualization, but AI-enhanced robotic systems utilize AR, CV, and real-time imaging to deliver a truly immersive surgical environment. By integrating pre-operative imaging (i.e., CT or MRI scans) and intra-operative video feeds, AI-based algorithms can reconstruct precise, complex, patient-specific anatomy from highly detailed 3D models and display the models as overlays on the surgeon's field of vision, while instructing instruments to navigate to locations in the operative field with high fidelity (Amin et al., 2024).

AR utilization in robotic surgery is especially applicable to oncological and neurosurgical procedures that require strict and highly defined surgical precision. For example, AR can instantly identify tumor borders, blood vessel paths, or nerve waypoints in real- or near-real time, circumventing the usually disastrous accidental injury to critical anatomical structures. AI-enhanced visualization can many times determine the best next steps intra-operatively, allowing surgeons to follow the best and safest path to a tissue target area. In minimally invasive surgery or cases where visualization is limited, AI-enhanced visualization compensates for limited visualization by utilizing identification and characterization of hidden anatomical features, providing clues and insights that even highly skilled and experienced surgeons may miss or cannot see. The overall benefits to patients are improved surgeon precision, reduced time in surgery, and improved surgical outcomes.

6.3 Personalized Robotic Surgical Procedures

Every patient has their own unique characteristics; therefore, personalization represents the greatest potential for changing the future of Surgical Robotics through AI technology. Traditional surgical techniques often reside around pre-established

Standard Treatment Protocols; whereas, AI allows Surgical Personalized Planning and Surgical Implementation based upon Data Collected from Individual Patients. Based on an analysis of many different Data Sources (Genetic Data, Medical History Data, Imaging Data), AI will generate a recommended Surgical Plan for an Individualised Patient (Liu et al., 2024c). AI allows for the Robotic System to be modified according to Anatomy, Physiological State, and Risk Factors associated with the patient.

ML models can provide an AI recommended Surgical Technique and by using Real-Time Adaptive Feedback, Adaptive Robotic Systems can modify or alter their activities as dictated by User Input to provide the best outcomes. As an example, in Orthopaedic Surgery, AI may change Robotic Cutting Trajectories to consider Bone Density, which enables them to produce the most consistent results possible.

7. Challenges and Barriers

Although AI has the potential to evolve surgical robotics into highly sophisticated, adaptive, and efficient systems, the implementation of AI in surgery has multiple challenges to be addressed before it gains acceptance in the public domain (Table 3). Integration of AI in surgery raises a series of technical, ethical, legal, and social issues that must be addressed before achieving public acceptance of these systems. The aim of the chapter is to discuss the technical barriers, ethical and legal issues, and acceptance by surgeons and patients of AI-enabled robotics, which determine the pace and extent of AI adoption in surgery.

7.1 Technical Limitations of AI in Surgery

Although significant progress has been made, AI-supported surgical robotics still faces technological limits that inhibit reliability and adoption as a standard of care. Accuracy is heavily reliant on large, high-quality datasets to train algorithms, and when it comes to healthcare, data are rarely high-quality, standardized, fragmented, repeatable, and are biased toward specific populations. Without stronger datasets, generalizability across patient populations is limited. Another limitation is the interpretation of AI systems; DL models are mainly black boxes, and their output can be difficult for a surgeon to interpret and understand how a decision or prediction was made. In a high-stakes procedure like surgery, ambiguity raises the issue of accountability and trust (Shin et al., 2025).

Another obstacle to overcome is creating an environment for real-time performance. The surgical environment requires real-time analysis and visualization of video and sensor data and the use of AI based on temporal reasoning that has algorithmic complexity. The use of robotic systems includes limitations imposed by the amount of power available from the hardware, the dexterity of the robotic systems, and the ability to integrate multiple types of data from different modalities. Although robots may execute repeated or structured tasks better than people, they remain incapable of adapting to unexpected variations or surprises during surgery in the same way that people are. To achieve greater levels of accomplishment in these areas, it is necessary to use advanced algorithms and hardware, sophisticated sensor technologies, and multiple sources of integrated data beyond those used in constructing datasets in a conventional manner (Levendovics et al., 2024).

Table 3 Challenges and Possible Solutions in AI- driven Surgical Robotics.

Challenge	*Description*	*Possible Solutions*
Technical Limitations	Lack of large, diverse datasets; limited interpretability; real-time performance issues.	Federated learning for multi-institutional data; Explainable AI; High-performance computing and optimized hardware.
Ethical and Legal Concerns	Unclear accountability in case of errors; algorithmic bias; data security issues.	Clear legal frameworks; ethical guidelines; strict data governance (HIPAA, GDPR compliance).
Privacy of Patient Data	Need for large volumes of imaging and clinical data for training AI models.	Data anonymization, blockchain for secure medical data sharing, and federated training.
Acceptance Among Surgeons	Resistance due to fear of losing control, lack of trust in AI decisions.	Continuous medical education (CME), AI-assisted training, and human-in-the-loop design.
Patient Trust and Consent	Patients may hesitate to accept robot-assisted or autonomous procedures.	Transparent communication, informed consent, and public awareness campaigns.
Cost and Accessibility	High installation and maintenance costs; limited availability in low-resource settings.	Scalable modular systems; cloud-based AI platforms; government/ industry collaborations.

7.2 Ethical, Legal, and Privacy Concerns

The ethical and legal implications associated with the implementation of AI within surgical robotics are highly controversial. A significant concern is that of accountability. Who will be held accountable when AI-operated surgical robots make mistakes resulting in harm to the patient? Is it the surgeon, the hospital, the manufacturer of the robotic system, or the developer of the AI-based algorithm? The uncertainty surrounding these issues has complicated malpractice laws and may delay the utilization of these technologies until appropriate legal frameworks are developed.

Protecting patient privacy also presents major challenges. To effectively train AI systems, a vast quantity of information regarding each patient must be used. This includes imaging studies, electronic health records (EHRs), and intraoperative or surgical video. In order to comply with regulations set forth by civil rights authorities such as the Health Insurance Portability Act, or HIPAA (United States), and the General Data Protection Regulation, or GDPR (the European Union), security and de-identification of this sensitive information pose unique hurdles to implementation. In addition, AI systems can potentially introduce algorithmic bias against patients who belong to subpopulations that have historically not had adequate representation in the training datasets. This could result in inequitable surgical results among these populations (Alonso & Siracuse, 2023). The introduction of autonomous surgery raises many ethical concerns regarding how far AI machines should be allowed to go in making critical life decisions. Autonomous surgery will enable patients to access surgical procedures using AI technologies. However, the lack of human oversight presents ethical challenges, particularly with respect to the ethical principles of autonomy, beneficence, and non-maleficence. Therefore, it is essential for medical professionals to develop appropriate ethical guidelines, regulatory frameworks and strong data governance systems to ensure that AI supports patient safety without undermining patient rights, safety, or equity (Khan et al., 2024).

7.3 Acceptance among Surgeons and Patients

If the technical and legal obstacles are overcome, the success of AI in surgical robots will ultimately depend on the acceptance of surgeons and patients. Surgeons are likely to have some resistance to using AI-enabled robots because they fear that they will lose control, develop an over-reliance on machines, and/or be replaced by machines in the future. There are also many surgeons who are skeptical about how reliable the use of AI will be, especially in the case of scenarios that are unpredictable. For example, these scenarios rely on human judgment and experience, which cannot be replicated by machines. Therefore, in order to train surgeons to effectively collaborate with AI-driven robots, one must also build trust in the AI system's reliability (O'Sullivan et al., 2019).

Patient acceptance of AI-enhanced surgery will depend on their perceptions of safety, trust, and eventual outcomes. Some patients will likely see the value of an AI-enhanced surgery due to the precision and speed of recovery time, while other patients will probably have concerns about having robots make decisions during a potentially life-threatening situation. In addition to perceptions of safety, the public perception of AI has been influenced by both positive and negative media portrayals of AI, which in turn can influence patient willingness to consent to AI-assisted surgeries. Developing trust in AI-enhanced surgeries will require increased transparency regarding the operation of AI systems, rigorous clinical validation, and communication between surgeons and patients about AI (Awuah et al., 2024).

8. Future Prospects and Innovations

The impact of AI on surgical robots has only begun to be felt in terms of changing how surgical robots are being used. Developments in technology will allow for the improvement of surgical robots as tools to co-operation (to learn, adapt and finally to work with full autonomy). There will be three main advancements as a result of future developments in AI-based surgical robots. The first is the introduction of fully autonomous surgical robots. The second is the introduction of AI-enabled training simulators for surgery. Thirdly, there will be an integration of human and AI support in surgery. The benefits of these advances will provide for safer, more reliable, and greater individualized surgical care.

8.1 Fully Autonomous Surgical Robots

One of the most anticipated developments in surgical robotics is the emergence of fully autonomous systems. In contrast to today's systems, which operate exclusively in direct surgeon control or semi-autonomous modes, future robots could conduct an entire procedure independently. Leveraging recent developments in ML, CV, and RL models, autonomous surgical robots will analyze patient data, devise a surgical plan, and take action almost entirely autonomously (Moustris et al., 2011).

The Smart Tissue Autonomous Robot (STAR), for example, has already shown during controlled experiments that it can perform suturing tasks with greater consistency than human surgeons. Building on this type of prototype, the next generation of autonomous robots will perform not just rote procedures but reliably manage complicated decisions. However, a uniquely autonomous solution necessitates addressing some challenges, like making the algorithms more explainable, who would be accountable if something goes wrong, and gaining the trust of patients. Although the global implementation of these types of robots may still be many years away, fully autonomous robots may be the future where surgical robots will extend surgical care to areas with no care, in emergencies, and with accuracy and precision we simply cannot replicate The STAR, for example, has already shown during controlled experiments that it can perform suturing tasks with greater consistency than human surgeons (Ostrander et al., 2024)

8.2 AI-Enhanced Surgical Training Simulators

Surgeons have always been trained by mentors and trained using either models, cadavers, or live patients. However, the emergence of advanced AI simulators will change this educational process forever by creating extremely realistic, adaptive, and individualized training experiences that will allow trainees to practice within frameworks that incorporate VR, AR, and performance metrics driven by AI. Such training simulators place the trainee in a realistic environment, similar to what is often needed in terms of training, that has not been easily replicated.

Unlike training with traditional modalities, such as models, cadavers, and live patients, the AI-enhanced simulator will constantly orchestrate assessments of the surgeon's performance, providing real-time feedback on how accurate, efficient, and error-prone surgery is being performed during that experience. The AI system can use the assessment to modify the difficulty of a simulation by using AI systems to monitor the trainee's experience and personalize it by adjusting the difficulty of a simulation to suit the trainee's skill level. For example, if a trainee is having trouble with laparoscopic suturing, the augmented intelligence simulator can continually produce exercises that replicate more advanced and progressively more challenging practice scenarios while providing corrective instructions. Additionally, AI can connect the trainee's performance to the performance of expert surgeon aggregates and provide performance gap assessments and recommendations for specific areas requiring deliberate practice to bridge those gaps. As the speed and adaptability of technology develop, the burden placed on patients will be decreased by enabling newly graduated surgeons to successfully complete key milestones of a surgical procedure prior to entering the OR with a decreased likelihood of complications for their patients. The educational environment for surgical training will also be improved because of innovative and significant educational platforms intended to enhance the overall education provided in surgical training programs from preclinical through beyond residency and advanced surgical practice.

8.3 Human–AI Collaboration in Operating Rooms

The future of surgery doesn't involve machines replacing the skills of surgeons. Rather than acting separately from AI-driven robots, surgeons will work together with them and have a symbiotic connection. In this new surgical climate, the OR will become a hybrid intelligent environment. Surgeons provide experience, intuition, and ethical judgement; robots provide computational strength, accuracy, and endurance.

By using AI systems, robotic systems will serve as a co-pilot, helping surgeons analyze data in real-time and identify previously hidden anatomical structures while helping them predict potential surgical risks. Further, robots will perform repetitive and boring tasks while allowing surgeons to focus on critical decision- making and complex patient-specific issues. Furthermore, there is no limitation on how many surgeons can work together and collaborate through AI between robots and skilled practitioners, allowing task completion as efficiently as possible. Surgeons and patients benefit from such collaborations by experiencing improved surgery and fewer post-operative complications due to tailored surgical experiences.

The OR of the future will utilize AI-assisted systems, surgical orchestration, AI-coordinated robotic actions, the surgical team's work process flow as well as the anaesthesia systems and available resources. These Cooperations will be a major advancement in the progress of surgery with Human Understanding and Intelligence combined.

9. Case Studies and Practical Insights

We will discuss how AI is changing the way we think about surgical robots by comparing the results of many different systems and providing examples to show the progress of AI technology in the area of surgical robotics. There are some new developments in AI technology and associated prototypes, as well as existing platforms that are already using AI to assist with medical procedures. These platforms demonstrate how surgery is currently being changed through the interaction of AI and technology through features such as CV motion tracking, and performance analytics. Also, comparative studies between traditional surgery and conventional robotic surgery augmented with AI provide tangible insight into the measurable improvements that AI can bring to the OR.

9.1 Existing AI-driven Robotic Surgery Platforms

Over the past two decades, robotic surgery has evolved from purely mechanical assistance toward intelligent, data-driven systems. Several AI-enabled platforms are already operational in hospitals worldwide, while others are under active development and clinical testing.

- **da Vinci Surgical System (Intuitive Surgical)**

The da Vinci system is still the leading robotic surgical device in use around the world. Originally developed for the purpose of minimally invasive surgery, it has expanded its range of applications to include AI features. The latest generation of da Vinci robots combines the existing robotic features of amplifying motion, removing shake, and improving presentation accuracy along with the inclusion of an enhanced level of AI analytic tools that will supply the surgeon with performance data following the surgery. They will also offer the surgeon some level of CV assistance in tracking instruments, distinguishing between tissue types, and recognizing tissue patterns.

- **Senhance Surgical System (Asensus Surgical)**

Senhance's Augmented Intelligence (AI) mechanism delivers real-time digital information during an operation. This intelligent technology provides haptic feedback, eye-tracking camera control, and performance analytics to assist surgeons with decision-making in the surgical field. In contrast to da Vinci, which focuses on enhancing surgical instrument performance through AI-assisted guidance, Senhance emphasizes increased training and skill development opportunities for surgeons via the use of embedded AI into the platform itself.

- **Versius Robotic Surgical System (CMR Surgical)**

The Versius automation system, which combines the modular and portable characteristics of robotics with AI-backed data collection and cloud analytics capabilities, helps to streamline surgical workflow and increase surgeon performance. Additionally, Versius's flexible design also gives hospitals that do not have adequate infrastructure the ability to incorporate robotic technology into their surgical practices, while using the data collected for the purpose of establishing training programs and continually improving.

- **Smart Tissue Autonomous Robot (STAR)**

The surgical device named STAR is among the most progressive AI-based systems currently available. It uses ML and computer vision technologies to perform sutures autonomously with consistency that exceeds many human surgical procedures. Experimental studies have demonstrated an ability to adjust to the dynamics of tissue movement instantaneously. The results of these studies suggest that the development of a completely autonomous surgical robot should soon be achievable.

9.2 Comparative Analysis of Outcomes

AI has been able to make great strides in surgery through advancements in robotic surgery. Studies that compared conventional surgical methods with conventional robotic-assisted techniques and AI-enhanced techniques have shown many distinct differences in quality of outcomes (Table 4).

1. **Precision and Accuracy**

The traditional surgical method allows for significant variations in the outcomes obtained based on the level of competence and skills of the surgeon performing the procedure. Traditional robotic systems use enhanced dexterity and motion scaling to increase the level of accuracy and precision for each surgical process. The AI- driven surgical systems provide the added benefit of real-time recognition of tissues within the patient's body, predictive modeling, and adaptive control—thus, providing sub-millimeter levels of accuracy within a procedure. For example, STAR demonstrated a consistency level in performing suturing procedures that far surpassed that of an expert surgeon.

2. **Safety and Error Reduction**

Risk of accidental injury to the tissue is greater with traditional methodologies. While modern robotic surgery has cut down on risks, the surgeon's input is still required. With predictive monitoring and abnormalities prevention built into AI-assisted systems, errors made during surgery can be reduced due to proactive risk flags when they begin to rise.

3. **Efficiency and Workflow Optimization**

Traditionally performed surgical procedures usually require extensive recovery time, taking much longer to operate than with robotics, however robotics offer improved workflow efficiency but are still limited to their capabilities. The majority of AI- enabled platforms utilize Predictive Analytic techniques through Automated Assistance offering decreased operating times, and total anesthesia requirements, as well as superior creation/management of hospital resources to eliminate the waste inherent in conventional ORs.

4. **Recovery and Patient Outcomes**

Traditional surgery has a longer recovery and higher complication rate than Robotics as performed with traditional means. When there are fewer areas to cut into during surgery, less trauma occurs to the body, resulting in faster healing times. By utilizing Robotics and AI to perform surgery using less invasive techniques with the application of personalized surgical plans, AI Robotics provide the best possible surgical outcome, resulting in quicker recovery rates and fewer surgical complications.

5. Surgeon Training and Performance Feedback

Conventional training methods follow an "apprenticeship model ", providing little quantitative information about what was learned or developed by the trainee. In contrast to traditional robotic training, which relies on simulation, AI-platforms provide adaptive support during skill acquisition. Technologies such as the Senhance and Versius robotic systems offer both real-time analytical feedback along with cloud-based benchmarking of individual clinician's skills. As a result, skill development and training time are dramatically improved.

Table 4 Comparative Outcomes in Surgery.

Parameter	*Traditional Surgery*	*Conventional Robotic Surgery*	*AI-Driven Robotic Surgery*
Precision	Variable, surgeon-dependent	High (mechanical assistance)	Very High (AI vision + learning)
Safety	Higher risk of errors	Reduced risk	Lowest risk (predictive monitoring)
Efficiency	Longer operation times	Moderate efficiency	Optimized with an AI workflow
Recovery Time	Longer hospital stays	Reduced compared to traditional	Shortest, personalized recovery
Training Support	Mentor-apprentice model	Simulators, limited feedback	AI analytics, adaptive simulators

10. Conclusion

10.1 Key Takeaways

AI in surgical robotics is a significant development in the evolution of medicine. This book has shown the capabilities of AI Technologies like ML, CV, NLP, and RL to modernize surgical practices to make them safer, more accurate, and more effective for patients. Current-use examples of da Vinci, Senhance, Versius, and STAR, demonstrate that the applications of AI are not confined to research laboratories, but are now routinely being utilized in surgical suites around the globe.

The main takeaways from this are:

- **Higher Precision/Safety:** AI will provide sub millimeter accuracies, near real-time error feedback and predictive risk assessment that will greatly reduce the likelihood of surgical complications.
- **Fast Training/Efficiency:** AI technology can be utilized to increase the efficiency of surgical workflow and create intelligent simulators that provide

opportunities for continued development of individual surgeon skill and knowledge after graduation from surgical school.

- **Individualized Patient Care:** AI will create individualized surgeries through predictive algorithms and adaptive models, which will lead to better outcomes and more rapid recovery of patients.
- **Collaboration not Replacement:** AI is designed to support the human surgeon's progression in surgery by providing a means of working together rather than taking over the human part of the surgical process. AI will help support decision-making, perform repetitive tasks, and collect, track, and analyze quantitative data continuously.

Each one of these observations provide evidence that AI is not an adjunct to robotic surgery, but a foundational necessity.

10.2 Future Outlook for AI in Surgical Robots

In the not too distant future, we expect the continued advancement of AI to lead to the development of more advanced and sophisticated autonomous surgical robots, which will be able to perform increasingly complex surgical procedures with minimal or no input from human operators. This will be particularly useful in areas of limited resources, where there is often little access to adequately trained surgeons. Furthermore, using adaptive simulations in surgical education and training will drastically change the way we learn and prepare for surgical practice. In addition to providing a completely immersive virtual environment for surgical education, adaptive simulation will also create a new and unique type of surgeon, who has been trained to work collaboratively with machines that possess, or are being imbued with, AI capabilities.

When we envision the operating room of the future, we foresee a collaborative ecosystem, in which humans and AI function as intelligent and strategic partners, in addition to functioning as partners. AI will facilitate the analysis of multimodal data sets and create augmented reality or overlay technology to assist surgical teams, while also improving the quality and consistency of surgical workflows. At the same time, humans will continue to provide critical aspects of surgical judgement, including ethical decision-making, imagination, and compassion, all unique attributes of the human condition that machines cannot duplicate.

In addition to improving access to surgical care for individuals who live in rural or underserved areas, the application of robotics and AI to surgery will revolutionize the delivery of surgical services and ultimately help to achieve global health equity. While the above represents some visions regarding what the future OR may look like, it is important to identify the many ongoing issues/challenges faced by healthcare providers that will affect future OR designs and functionalities (technical limitations, legal/ethical issues regarding security and privacy, patients' ability to trust the doctors performing surgery, costs associated with creating these new types of ORs). Continued research, clear regulations, collaborative innovations (incremental, evolutionary, etc.), and ultimately continued growth in the surgical field will lead to a safer, smarter, fairer, and more efficient surgery environment moving forward into the future.

References

Adegbesan, A., Akingbola, A., Aremu, O., Adewole, O., Amamdikwa, J.C. and Shagaya, U. (2024). From Scalpels to Algorithms: The Risk of Dependence on Artificial Intelligence in Surgery. *Journal of Medicine, Surgery, and Public Health, 3*, 100140.h ttps://doi.org/10.1016/J.GLMEDI.2024.100140.

Agius, S., Magri, C. and Cassar, V. (2025). A Cognitive Task Analysis for Developing a Clinical Decision Support System for Emergency Triage. *Journal of Emergency Nursing*. https://doi.org/10.1016/J.JEN.2025.05.013.

Alonso, A. and Siracuse, J.J. (2023). Protecting patient safety and privacy in the era of artificial intelligence. *Seminars in Vascular Surgery, 36*(3), 426–429. https://doi.org/10.1053/J.SEMVASCSURG.2023.06.002.

Amin, A., Cardoso, S.A., Suyambu, J., Saboor, H.A., Cardoso, R.P., Husnain, A., Isaac, N.V., Backing, H., Mehmood, D., Mehmood, M. and Maslamani, A.N.J. (2024). Future of Artificial Intelligence in Surgery: A Narrative Review. *Cureus, 16*(1), e51631. https://doi.org/10.7759/CUREUS.51631.

Awuah, W.A., Aderinto, N., Poornaselvan, J., Tan, J.K., Shah, M.H., Ashinze, P., Pujari, A.G., Bharadwaj, H.R., Abdul-Rahman, T. and Atallah, O. (2024). Empowering health care consumers & understanding patients' perspectives on AI integration in oncology and surgery: A perspective. *Health Science Reports, 7*(7), e2268. https://doi.org/10.1002/HSR2.2268.

Cotsoglou, C., Granieri, S., Bassetto, S., Bagnardi, V., Pugliese, R., Grazi, G.L., Guglielmi, A., Ruzzenente, A., Aldrighetti, L., Ratti, F., De Carlis, L., De Carlis, R., Centonze, L., De Angelis, N., Memeo, R., Delvecchio, A., Felli, E., Izzo, F., Belli, A., … Pugliese, G. (2024). Dynamic surgical anatomy using 3D reconstruction technology in complex hepato-biliary surgery with vascular involvement: Results from an international multicentric survey. *HPB, 26*(1), 83–90. https://doi.org/10.1016/J.HPB.2023.10.003.

Eloranta, S. and Boman, M. (2022). Predictive models for clinical decision making: Deep dives in practical machine learning. *Journal of Internal Medicine, 292*(2), 278. https://doi.org/10.1111/JOIM.13483.

Ghimire, S., Shrestha, S., Shrestha, D. and Awal, S. (2025). Robotics in neurosurgery: The past, present, and the future. *Egyptian Journal of Neurosurgery*, 40(1), 1–12. https://doi.org/10.1186/S41984-025-00395-9.

Gode, C., Kakkeri, R.B., Thoutam, N., Bagade, J.V., Deore, M.P. and Birari, D.R. (2025). Autonomous Suturing in Robotic Surgery Using Reinforcement Learning and 3D Visual Feedback. *Journal of Neonatal Surgery, 14*(10S), 24–35. https://doi.org/10.52783/jns.v14.2754.

Habuza, T., Navaz, A.N., Hashim, F., Alnajjar, F., Zaki, N., Serhani, M.A. and Statsenko, Y. (2021). AI applications in robotics, diagnostic image analysis and precision medicine: Current limitations, future trends, guidelines on CAD systems for medicine. *Informatics in Medicine Unlocked, 24*, 100596. https://doi.org/10.1016/J.IMU.2021.100596

Hamilton, A. (2024). The Future of Artificial Intelligence in Surgery. *Cureus, 16*(7), e63699. https://doi.org/10.7759/CUREUS.63699.

Hashimoto, D.A., Rosman, G., Rus, D. and Meireles, O.R. (2018). Artificial Intelligence in Surgery: Promises and Perils. *Annals of Surgery, 268*(1), 70. https://doi.org/10.1097/SLA.0000000000002693.

Khan, M.A., Researcher, J. and Khan, A. (2024). *Ethical Implications of AI (artificial intelligence) in Healthcare Mainly Focus on Surgical Procedures: Identification of Ethical Issues of AI in*

Surgical Procedures and Ranking of Ethical Issues Based on Criticality. (Master Thesis LUT University). https://lutpub.lut.fi/handle/10024/167840.

Levendovics, R., Levendovics, T., Kronreif, G. and Haidegger, T. (2024). *Surgical Data Science: Emerging Trends and Future Pathways*. 65–84. https://doi.org/10.1007/978-3-031-58257-8_5.

Liu, Y., Wu, X., Sang, Y., Zhao, C., Wang, Y., Shi, B. and Fan, Y. (2024a). Evolution of Surgical Robot Systems Enhanced by Artificial Intelligence: A Review. *Advanced Intelligent Systems*, *6*(5), 2300268. https://doi.org/10.1002/AISY.202300268

Liu, Y., Wu, X., Sang, Y., Zhao, C., Wang, Y., Shi, B. and Fan, Y. (2024c). Evolution of Surgical Robot Systems Enhanced by Artificial Intelligence: A Review. *Advanced Intelligent Systems*, *6*(5), 2300268. https://doi.org/10.1002/AISY.202300268.

Lu, T., Wang, L. and Zhao, X. (2023). Review of Anomaly Detection Algorithms for Data Streams. *Applied Sciences*, *13*(10), 6353. https://doi.org/10.3390/APP13106353.

Moustris, G.P., Hiridis, S.C., Deliparaschos, K.M. and Konstantinidis, K.M. (2011). Evolution of autonomous and semi-autonomous robotic surgical systems: A review of the literature. *The International Journal of Medical Robotics and Computer Assisted Surgery*, *7*(4), 375–392. https://doi.org/10.1002/RCS.408.

Neri, A., Penza, V., Baldini, C. and Mattos, L.S. (2025). Surgical augmented reality registration methods: A review from traditional to deep learning approaches. *Computerized Medical Imaging and Graphics*, *124*, 102616. https://doi.org/10.1016/J.COMPMEDIMAG.2025.102616.

Ostrander, B.T., Massillon, D., Meller, L., Chiu, Z.Y., Yip, M. and Orosco, R.K. (2024). The current state of autonomous suturing: a systematic review. *Surgical Endoscopy*, *38*(5), 2383–2397. https://doi.org/10.1007/S00464-024-10788-W/METRICS.

O'Sullivan, S., Nevejans, N., Allen, C., Blyth, A., Leonard, S., Pagallo, U., Holzinger, K., Holzinger, A., Sajid, M.I. and Ashrafian, H. (2019). Legal, regulatory, and ethical frameworks for development of standards in artificial intelligence (AI) and autonomous robotic surgery. *The International Journal of Medical Robotics and Computer Assisted Surgery*, *15*(1), e1968. https://doi.org/10.1002/RCS.1968.

Park, S., Chung, S., Kim, Y., Yang, S.A., Kwon, S., Cho, J.M., Lee, M.J., Cho, E., Ryu, J., Kim, S., Lee, J., Yoon, H.J., Choi, E., Kim, K. and Lee, H. (2025). A deep-learning algorithm using real-time collected intraoperative vital sign signals for predicting acute kidney injury after major non-cardiac surgeries: A modelling study. *PLOS Medicine*, *22*(4), e1004566. https://doi.org/10.1371/JOURNAL.PMED.1004566.

Probst, P. (2023). A Review of the Role of Robotics in Surgery: To DaVinci and Beyond! *Missouri Medicine*, *120*(5), 389. https://pmc.ncbi.nlm.nih.gov/articles/PMC10569391/.

Riad, A., Hadid, M., Elomri, A., Al-Ansari, A., Rejeb, M.A., Qaraqe, M., Dakua, S.P., Jaber, A.R., Al-Ansari, A., Aboumarzouk, O. M. and EL Omri, A. (2025). Advancements and challenges in robotic surgery: A holistic examination of operational dynamics and future directions. *Surgery in Practice and Science*, *22*, 100294. https://doi.org/10.1016/J.SIPAS.2025.100294.

Shin, Y., Lee, M., Lee, Y., Kim, K. and Kim, T. (2025). Artificial Intelligence-Powered Quality Assurance: Transforming Diagnostics, Surgery, and Patient Care—Innovations, Limitations, and Future Directions. *Life*, *15*(4), 654. https://doi.org/10.3390/LIFE15040654.

Wu, D., Zhang, R., Pore, A., Dall'Alba, D., Ha, X.T., Li, Z., Zhang, Y., Herrera, F., Ourak, M., Kowalczyk, W., De Momi, E., Casals, A., Dankelman, J., Kober, J., Menciassi, A., Fiorini, P. and Vander Poorten, E. (2024). A review on machine learning in flexible surgical and interventional robots: Where we are and where we are going. *Biomedical Signal Processing and Control*, *93*, 106179. https://doi.org/10.1016/J.BSPC.2024.106179.

17 Kinematics, Workflow Integration, and Clinical Applications

Archika Jain[1*], Kapil Joshi[2] and Nidal Al Said[3]

In modern surgical we integrate the surgical robotics and computer-assisted surgery (CAS) for using robotics. It improves the precision of computational power and patient outcomes. It also decreases intrusiveness. In this computer-assisted task, perform the kinematic structures, control methods, and interactions. To learn about surgical robotics, we study a large number of research articles that were published from 2020 to 2025. It gives detailed descriptions and workflow of CAS processes. In the experiment setup, we compare the robotic-assisted surgery with manual one. Robotic surgical procedure gives greater precision and less tissue damage.

1. Introduction

Modern surgical processes require precision, minimal intrusive, and fast patient recovery. Traditional surgical techniques are very effective techniques, but fundamentally they are less in human skill, and fatigue level. Surgical robots and CAS (computer-assisted surgery) provide the better solution for emerging the built-in restrictions. Surgical robots deliver the stability, precision in motor control, and the capacity to handle the highly specialized equipment. CAS significantly enhances the accuracy by combining preoperative imaging, with real-time guidance and assessment. These advanced systems are transforming standard practices including urology, cardiology, neurology, and orthopaedics. Figure 1 presents the robotic arm's kinematic structure which includes joints, linkages, and workspace. It also compares planned and actual instrument placement against AR (augmented reality) guidance to improve precision.

[1] Swami Keshvanand Institute of Technology, Management and Gramothan (SKIT) Jaipur, India.
[2] Department of Computer Science, Uttaranchal Institute of Technology, Uttaranchal University, Dehradun, India.
[3] College of Mass Communication, Ajman University, Ajman, UAE.
Email: kapilengg0509@gmail.com[2]; n.alsaid@ajman.ac.ae[3]
* Corresponding author: archikaagarwal@gmail.com

DOI: 10.1201/9781003655121-17

Evolution of Surgical Robotics

Early Systems

- The PUMA 560 Robot (1980s) is used in stereotactic neurosurgery for precision needle placement.
- PROBOT: An early prototype for transurethral prostatectomy.

Modern Systems

- The da Vinci Surgical System features a master-slave setup with 3-4 robotic arms, endoscopic imaging, and haptic feedback.
- ZEUS Robotic System: Telemanipulation for distant surgeries.
- MiroSurge: A modular robotic platform for minimally invasive procedures.

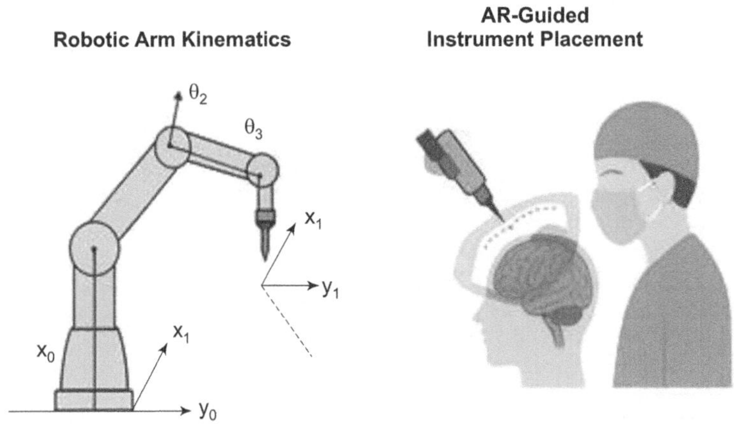

Fig. 1 Robotic Arm Kinematics Vs AR-Guided Instrument Placement (Shao, et al., 2025).

Table 1 Comparison Table of Key Robotic Systems.

Robotic System	*Application*	*Arms*	*Imaging Integration*	*Haptic Feedback*
PUMA 560	Neurosurgery	1	CT Guidance	No
PROBOT	Prostatectomy	1–2	MRI Guidance	No
Da Vinci	Multiple specialties	3–4	Endoscopic Video	Yes
ZEUS	Remote Surgery	3	Endoscopic Video	Yes
MiroSurge	Minimally invasive	2–4	Multi modal	Yes

Table 1 compares significant robotic surgical systems based on their application, number of arms, imaging integration, and haptic feedback capabilities. It contrasts single-arm, image-guided platforms like the PUMA 560 with multi-arm, haptics-enabled systems like the Da Vinci and ZEUS.

Kinematics of Surgical Robots

Forward Kinematics

- Determines the position and orientation of the end-effector given joint parameters.
- Essential for planning instrument movement in surgical workspace.

Inverse Kinematics

- Calculates joint angles needed to achieve a desired end-effector position.
- Critical for trajectory planning in constrained anatomical spaces.

Figure 2 shows a 3-DOF robotic arm with labeled joints, end-effector, and workspace coordinates. The diagram depicts the kinematic configuration of the arm, with its coordinate axes and joint angles θ_1, θ_2, and θ_3.

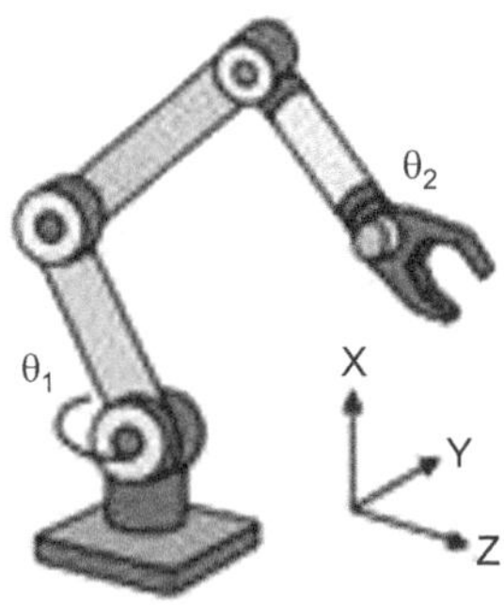

Fig. 2 3-DOF robotic arm showing joints, end-effector, and workspace coordinates. (Include axes and joint angles θ_1, θ_2, θ_3.) (Saeedi-Hosseiny, et al., 2021).

Differential Kinematics

- Velocity and force transmission from joints to end-effector.
- Important for smooth, precise instrument motion.

Control Systems

1. **Position Control:** Maintains desired end-effector position.
2. **Force Control:** Ensures safe interaction with tissues.
3. **Hybrid Control:** Combines position and force for delicate procedures.
4. **Haptic Feedback:** Provides tactile sensation to the surgeon for safer manipulation.

4. Literature Review

I. Tamadon et al. (2021) proposed a robot that is called a ValveTech for invasive surgery. It contains the flexible arm and control unit. The surgeons give the faster result by using this robot in their trials (Tamadon et al., 2021).

Peine and Stoyanov et al. (2025) explore the surgical technologies that combined the robotics hands, medical image, and AI-driven ecosystem. The integration of these technologies, robotics will increase the technical skills, imaging will boost clarity and AI will help in tough decision-making (Peine & Stoyanov et al., 2025).

Colleoni et al. (2022) integrate the attention modules that focus on the generation process like robotic instrument structure. It interacts with the surgical scene. The study evaluated segmentation accuracy and image quality. This validation demonstrates that the synthetic images can successfully train the binary and semantic segmentation models (Colleoni et al., 2022).

Tran et al. (2024) inferences and utilize a multi-modal model. This model is based on a transformer-like structure for output accuracy. It also describes a multi modal, transformer-based model to incorporate both spatial and temporal features. It validates the advantages of utilizing the ResNeSt model (Tran et al., 2024).

Min et al. (2023) developed the algorithm for handling deformation of soft tissue and maintaining the accuracy. It creates authentic, quick, and intra-operative metrics to access and register without interspersed surgical workflow (Min et al., 2023).

Jeon et al. (2024) provides the design, forging, and a one-time configuring and verifying technique for dual sensors. It gives the accuracy standards for the intended applications (Jeon et al., 2024).

Min et al. (2021) introduced a CAOS and PSR method. By using this, the authors can bring out and employ the normal and tangent vector, so that they can improve the registration accuracy and robustness (Min et al., 2021).

Tamadon et al. (2023) focused on the ValveTech platform that is a robotic platform. It is a safe and semi-autonomous navigation platform. It demonstrates the autonomous valve position for hybrid forward with endoscoping visual serving (Tamadon et al., 2023).

Lim et al. (2021) focused on an AR-based navigation unit. It created a CT image that is a 3D path for the epidural needle. The physician uses this path and determines the insertion point. It maintains the accuracy and it is confirmed by the phantom studies. It also reduced the process time X-ray utilization (Lim et al., 2021).

Hussain et al. (2022) reveals the RNN in RAS architecture when it was using JIGSAWS dataset. It improves the accuracy and precision while using gesture and trajectory segmentation tasks (Hussain et al., 2022).

Kim et al. (2023) proposed a supermicrosurgical robot that supports multi-surgeon teleportation. In the early stages, the robots can assist only primary surgeons. But now a days robots assist multiple surgeons and they also avoid dynamic collision avoidance. Authors used a post tracking algorithm that is effective in line tracing experiments (Kim et al., 2023).

Kennedy-Metz et al. (2020) demonstrate how heart rate variability (HRV) can detect emotional stress and surgical flow interruptions during cardiac surgery. In a near-miss pharmaceutical error, the anesthesiologist's sympathetic activity matched the reported stresses (Kennedy-Metz et al., 2020).

Shao et al. (2025) established SH-YOLO that incorporated a star operation and HAM. They are used for efficient feature extraction and adaptive feature fusion (Shao et al., 2025).

Martin-Gomez et al. (2024) utilized built-in cameras of AR and HMDs. By using these, the authors achieved accurate tracking without integration of additional electronics. They track multiple surgical tools simultaneously (Martin-Gomez et al., 2024).

Saeedi-Hosseiny et al. (2021) used an image processing algorithm to identify 2D pixel coordinates of radio reflective markers (Saeedi-Hosseiny et al., 2021).

5. Work-Flow of Computer-Assisted Surgery (CAS)

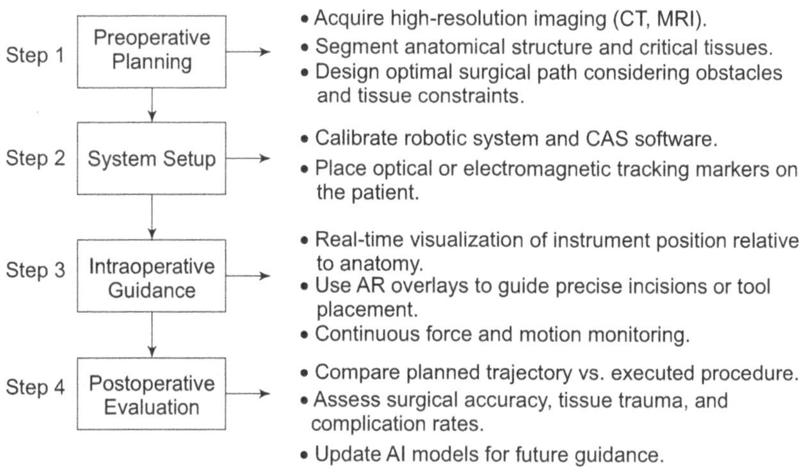

Fig. 3 CAS Workflow Diagram.

Figure 3 illustrates synergistic integration of imaging, planning, and robotic guidance.

6. Methodology

Robotic System Ex

Setup

Objective: Evaluate the system's comprehensive performance and dependability.

Equipment:

- 4-DOF robotic arm with haptic feedback.
- Phantom anatomical models.
- Optical tracking system (infrared cameras).
- CAS software for trajectory planning.

Table 2 Advantages, Limitations, and Clinical Examples of Surgical Robotics and CAS.

Section	*Key Points*	*Details/Examples*
Advantages of Surgical Robotics and CAS	Increased precision	< 1 mm in some systems
	Reduced invasiveness and trauma	Minimizes tissue damage
	Shorter operation times & faster recovery	Improved patient outcomes
	Enhanced surgeon ergonomics	Reduces fatigue during long procedures
	Remote/telesurgery capabilities	Enables surgery from distant locations
Limitations	High cost	Acquisition and maintenance expenses
	Steep learning curve	Requires extensive surgeon training
	Dependence on calibration/software	Accuracy relies on system reliability
	Ethical concerns	Autonomous decision-making risks
Clinical Examples	Robotic Prostatectomy	20–30% reduction in complication rates vs. open surgery
	Cardiac Bypass Surgery	Robotic assistance reduces blood loss by 40%
	Neurosurgical Biopsy	Robotic guidance improves targeting accuracy to <1 mm

Procedure:

1. Perform calibration routines.
2. Import pre operative imaging data.
3. By using a robotic system, execute the surgical path.
4. Simultaneously record critical data streams.
5. Track the position, time, data, and force.

Figure 4 illustrates the experimental setup, showing a robotic arm that integrated with CAS.

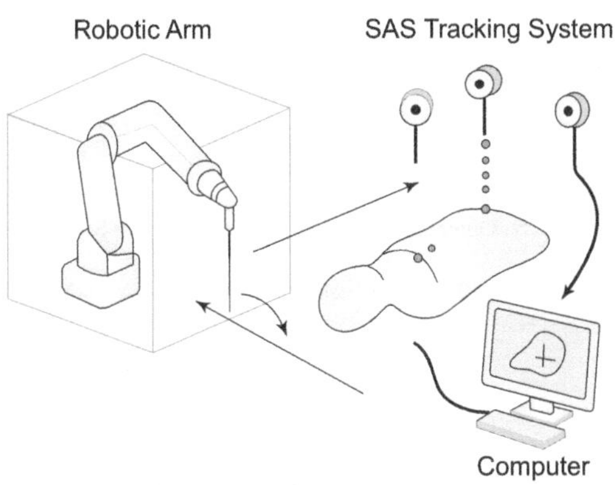

Fig. 4 Experimental layout. (Lim et al., 2021).

Table 3 provides an overview of key parameters defining robotic surgery.

Table 3 Metrics and Evaluation.

Metric	*Definition*	*Measurement Tool*
Precision (mm)	Distance from planned vs. actual position	Optical tracking
Tissue Trauma Score	Qualitative scale 1–10	Phantom evaluation
Operation Time (min)	Time from incision to completion	Stopwatch
Success Rate (%)	Number of successful procedures / total	Visual & software

7. Experiments and Results

Phantom Model Surgery

10 robotic-assisted procedures vs. 10 manual procedures.

Table 4 illustrates the significant improvements including precision, tissue safety, procedure time, and success rates.

Table 4 Comparison of manual versus robotic-assisted surgery.

Metric	*Manual Surgery*	*Robotic-Assisted*	*Improvement (%)*
Precision (mm)	2.4	0.6	75%
Operation Time (min)	120	95	21%
Tissue Trauma Score	8	3	62%
Success Rate (%)	88	98	10%

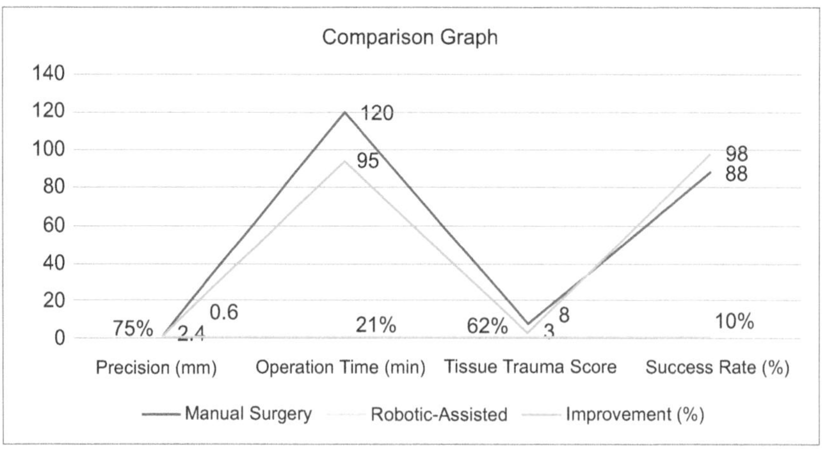

Fig. 5 Comparison graph.

Figure 5 demonstrates the clinical benefits of robotic-assisted procedures that provide high precision and low tissue injury.

8. Conclusion and Future Scope

Surgical robots and CAS are fundamentally changing modern surgery by enhancing precision, efficiency and patient safety. They enable minimally invasive treatments, and significantly reduce surgeon fatigue. Although many challenges faced like high cost, training, and workflow integration persist. The study examines a large number of research articles published between 2020–2025. They investigate the surgical robots. It also provides the workflow of CAS. In the experimental section we compare robotic assisted surgery with manual procedure. It gives greater precision and less tissue.

References

Colleoni, D. Psychogyios, B. Van Amsterdam, F. Vasconcelos and D. Stoyanov. (2022, Nov.). SSIS-Seg: Simulation-Supervised Image Synthesis for Surgical Instrument Segmentation. *IEEE Transactions on Medical Imaging, 41*(11), 3074–3086. doi: 10.1109/TMI.2022.3178549.

Jeon, S., K.T. Hnin, Y.G. Jung and S. Lim. (2024). Design and Calibration of Dual Sensor: Towards Simultaneous Instrument Tracking and Deformable Shape Sensing in Computer-Integrated Surgery. In: *2024 46th Annual International Conference of the IEEE Engineering in Medicine and Biology Society (EMBC)*, Orlando, FL, USA (pp. 1–4). doi: 10.1109/EMBC53108.2024.10781652.

Hussain, S.M., A. Brunetti, G. Lucarelli, R. Memeo, V. Bevilacqua and D. Buongiorno. (2022). Deep Learning Based Image Processing for Robot Assisted Surgery: A Systematic Literature Survey. *IEEE Access, 10*, 122627–122657. doi: 10.1109/ACCESS.2022.3223704.

Kennedy-Metz, L.R., A. Bizzego, R.D. Dias, C. Furlanello, G. Esposito and M.A. Zenati.(2020). Autonomic Activity and Surgical Flow Disruptions in Healthcare Providers during Cardiac Surgery. In: *2020 IEEE Conference on Cognitive and Computational Aspects of Situation Management (CogSIMA)*, Victoria, BC, Canada (pp. 200–204). doi: 10.1109/CogSIMA49017.2020.9216076.

Kim, G., J. Lee, R. Delgado, S.R. Oh and Y.S. Ihn. (2023). "Pose Tracking of Supermicrosurgical Robot Towards Multi-User Teleoperation. In: *2023 45th Annual International Conference of the IEEE Engineering in Medicine and Biology Society (EMBC)*, Sydney, Australia (pp. 1–4). doi: 10.1109/EMBC40787.2023.10339969.

Lim, S., et al. (2021). Augmented Reality Assisted Surgical Navigation System for Epidural Needle Intervention. In: *2021 43rd Annual International Conference of the IEEE Engineering in Medicine and Biology Society (EMBC)*, Mexico (pp. 4705–4708). doi: 10.1109/EMBC46164.2021.9629804.

Martin-Gomez, A., et al. (2024, July). STTAR: Surgical Tool Tracking Using Off-the-Shelf Augmented Reality Head-Mounted Displays, *IEEE Transactions on Visualization and Computer Graphics, 30*(7), 3578–3593. doi: 10.1109/TVCG.2023.3238309.

Min, Z., D. Zhu, J. Liu, H. Ren and M.Q.H. Meng. (2021, May). Aligning 3D Curve With Surface Using Tangent and Normal Vectors for Computer-Assisted Orthopedic Surgery. *IEEE Transactions on Medical Robotics and Bionics, 3*(2), 372–383. doi: 10.1109/TMRB.2021.3075784.

Min, Z., et al. (2023, May). 3-D Rigid Point Set Registration for Computer-Assisted Orthopedic Surgery (CAOS): A Review From the Algorithmic Perspective, *IEEE Transactions on Medical Robotics and Bionics*, 5, (2), 156–169. doi: 10.1109/TMRB.2023.3265708.

Peine and D. Stoyanov. (2025, Jan.–Feb.). Industry Perspective: The Future of Surgical Robotics—Augmenting a Surgeon's Hands, Eyes, and Brain. *IEEE Pulse, 16*(1), 8–11, Jan.–Feb. 2025, doi: 10.1109/MPULS.2025.3526482.

Saeedi-Hosseiny, M.S., F. Alruwaili, A.S. Patel, S. McMillan, I.I. Iordachita, & M.H. Abedin-Nasab. (2021). Spatial Detection of the Shafts of Fractured Femur for Image-Guided Robotic Surgery.

In: *2021 43rd Annual International Conference of the IEEE Engineering in Medicine and Biology Society* (*EMBC*), Mexico (pp. 3301–3304), doi: 10.1109/EMBC46164.2021.9630866.

Shao, Y., Z. Xu and Q. Zhu. (2025). SH-YOLO: Enhanced Real-Time Detection of Laparoscopic Surgical Instruments in Computer-Aided Surgery Based on Star Operation and Hybrid Attention Mechanisms. In: *IEEE Access*, *13*, pp. 135179–135195. doi: 10.1109/ACCESS.2025.3593635.

Tamadon, I., et al. (2021, Apr.). ValveTech: A Novel Robotic Approach for Minimally Invasive Aortic Valve Replacement. In: *IEEE Transactions on Biomedical Engineering*, *68* (4), 1238–1249. 1 doi: 10.1109/TBME.2020.3024184.

Tamadon, I., S.M.H. Sadati, V. Mamone, V. Ferrari, C. Bergeles and A. Menciassi. (2023, Dec.). "Semiautonomous Robotic Manipulator for Minimally Invasive Aortic Valve Replacement," in *IEEE Transactions on Robotics*, *39*(6), 4500–4519. doi: 10.1109/TRO.2023.3315966.

B. Tran, D. Kulić, S.M. Harrison, C. Pilgrim and E. Abdi. (2024). PCNet: Accurate Surgical Workflow Recognition with Phase Consistency. In: *2024 46th Annual International Conference of the IEEE Engineering in Medicine and Biology Society* (*EMBC*), Orlando, FL, USA (pp. 1–4). doi: 10.1109/EMBC53108.2024.10782329.

Index

A

Advanced Learning 47, 48, 56
AI-Based Personalized Learning 152
AI-Driven Neurorehabilitation 1, 2
AI-Supported Surgical Automation 168
Artificial Intelligence 1-4 65, 67, 131-133, 250, 251, 271, 272
Artificial Intelligence in Cardiology 133
Artificial Neural Network 142, 143
Autonomous Surgery 278, 287
Autonomous Surgical Robots 273, 288, 293

B

Bone Scanning 48
Brain Anomaly 26, 27
Brain–Computer Interfaces (BCI) 1, 12
Breaks 44, 46, 52, 54, 56

C

Cancer Detection 102, 103, 105, 112, 113, 115
Cardiac Magnetic Resonance 135
Cardiology 131-133, 136, 137
CAS 296, 300, 301, 303
Clinical Application 35, 40, 58, 59, 69, 171, 214, 227, 296
Clinical outcomes 218, 228, 231
Computer Vision 250, 252, 253, 255, 265, 266, 271, 272, 277, 280, 290
Computer-Assisted Surgery (CAS) 296, 300
Convolutional Neural Networks (CNNs) 48
Cosmetic Chemicals 145
CTG classification 26

D

Data Fusion 171, 177-180
Deep Brain Stimulation (DBS) 216, 230
Deep Learning (DL) 23, 24, 34, 35, 65, 68, 70, 72, 74-77, 79, 250, 252, 254, 257, 258, 266, 267
Dermatology 140, 141, 143, 147, 148
Disease Prediction 68-71
Domain Adaptation 97

E

Electrocardiograms 132, 135
Electrophysiology 135, 136, 137

F

Fetal health 23, 24, 25, 26, 29, 31, 32, 34, 38, 39, 40
Fetal Health Prediction 23, 25, 26, 32
Fetal MRI Segmentation 34
Few-Shot and Zero-Shot Learning 84, 97, 98
Fracture Detection 45, 47

H

Haptic Feedback Systems 154
Haptic Systems 177, 179, 180, 235
Healthcare 65-81
Human-AI Collaboration 273, 289
Human-Machine Interface 191, 194, 201

I

Image Fusion 102-106, 108-111, 113, 115
Image-Guided Surgery 254, 255
Intraoperative Decision Support Systems 255
Intraoperative Neuromonitoring 1

L

Laparoscopic Surgery 236
Laparoscopy 236, 240

M

Machine Learning (ML) 65, 68-71, 73, 77, 80, 267, 271, 272, 278, 280
Medical Image Analysis 67, 69-71, 74
Medical Image Segmentation 84, 92, 93, 94

Medical Imaging 44, 48, 55, 57, 60, 65, 66, 69, 70, 72, 80, 81, 84, 85, 88-90, 92, 93, 95-99
Melanoma 143, 146
Minimally Invasive Robotic Surgery 2
Minimally Invasive Surgery (MIS) 175, 195, 196, 199, 207, 236, 265
MRI 23, 24, 25, 26, 29, 34, 35, 36, 37, 38, 39, 40

N

Natural Language Processing 66, 72, 76, 79
Natural Orifice Transluminal Endoscopic Surgery (NOTES) 236
Neurosurgery 1-3, 5-9, 13, 16-19

P

Patient Care 65-68, 73-77, 80, 81
Personalized Medicine 256
Predictive Analytics 69, 70, 75, 76
Preoperative Planning and Intraoperative Guidance 259
Psoriasis 140, 143, 144, 145

R

Rehabilitation 1, 4, 5, 6, 9-19
Robotic Neurosurgery 214, 216, 217, 222-224, 226-232
Robotic Surgery 169, 171, 173, 177, 179, 185-187, 237, 240, 242, 243, 245, 246, 250-264, 266
Robotic-Aided Plastic Surgery 146
Robotic-Assisted Neurosurgery 1, 2, 5
Robotic-Assisted Surgery 197
Robotics 1-3, 5, 6, 9, 12-15, 17-19, 296, 297, 299, 301

S

Segmentation 23-26, 29, 34-36, 39, 40
Semi-Supervised Learning 85, 87, 89, 94
Sensor Integration 168, 171, 183
Single-Incision Laparoscopic Surgery (SILS) 236
Skin Cancer Detection 105
Smart Surgical Tools 171, 173, 183, 185
Surgeon Training 229
Surgery 131, 136
Surgical Innovation 223, 274
Surgical Robotics 118-121, 124-127, 129, 168, 178, 192, 193, 195, 197-202, 206, 208, 209, 214, 216, 250, 257, 271-280, 283-286, 288, 289, 292, 296, 297, 301, 302

T

Tactile Feedback 168, 179, 182, 185
Technological advancement 197

About the Editors

Dr. Kapil Joshi is an Associate Professor in the Department of Computer Science & Engineering at the Uttaranchal Institute of Technology (UIT), Uttaranchal University, Dehradun, India. He holds a Ph.D. in Computer Science & Engineering, with his doctoral research focused on image quality enhancement using fusion techniques. He has over a decade of experience in academia, industry, and research, and his teaching interests include Operating Systems, Database Management Systems, Web Development, and Machine Learning.

Dr. Joshi's research interests span image processing, computer vision, pattern recognition, deep learning, and intelligent systems. He is currently pursuing postdoctoral research (remote) at the Singapore Institute of Technology (SIT), Singapore, under international academic supervision. He has published extensively in reputed international journals and conferences and has contributed to several edited books and book chapters with leading publishers. Dr. Joshi is a Senior Member of IEEE and actively serves as an editor, reviewer, and technical committee member for various international journals and conferences. He has received multiple awards for excellence in research and academic contributions.

Dr. Kiruthigha R is an Assistant Professor in the Department of Information Technology at SRM Institute of Science and Technology (SRMIST), Ramapuram, India. She holds a Ph.D. from Anna University, Chennai, an M.Tech. from Anna University, and a B.Tech. from Bharathiar University. With over 12 years of teaching experience, Dr. Kiruthigha specializes in Machine Learning and Medical Image Processing. Her research contributions focus on applying intelligent computational techniques to healthcare-related image analysis, aiming to enhance diagnostic accuracy and medical decision-making. She is actively involved in both academic instruction and research supervision at the undergraduate and postgraduate levels.

Dr. Gopal Krishna is an Assistant Professor in the Department of Computer Science and Engineering at the Uttaranchal Institute of Technology, Uttaranchal University, Dehradun, India. He completed his Ph.D. on the design and implementation of an Artificial Intelligence-assisted predictive framework aimed at enhancing the efficiency and reliability of Battery Management Systems. Dr. Krishna is a prolific researcher with keen interests in Artificial Intelligence, the Internet of Things (IoT), and their applications in green energy and sustainability. He has authored textbooks and published numerous research papers in reputed journals. His academic pursuits and research contributions extend into the realm of advanced computational intelligence, focusing on cutting-edge developments for transformative solutions in renewable energy and sustainable technologies.

Dr. Prabhishek Singh (Senior IEEE Member) is an Associate Professor in the School of Computer Science Engineering and Technology at Bennett University (The Times Group), Greater Noida, India, and also serves as Honorary Adjunct Faculty at Maryam Abacha American University of Nigeria. He received his Ph.D. from Babasaheb Bhimrao Ambedkar University (Central University), Lucknow, in 2018. Dr. Singh has authored over 300 peer-reviewed publications in SCI, SCIE, ESCI, and Scopus venues. His research interests include multimodal medical image fusion, computer vision, deep learning, and AI-enabed healthcare analytics, and he actively contributes as journal editor and reviewer. He is listed among the World's Top 2% Scientists.

Dr. Manoj Diwakar is working as Professor in the Department of Computer Science and Engineering at Graphic Era Deemed to be University, Dehradun. His research interests include image processing, information security and medical imaging. He has published more than 200+ research papers in peer-reviewed journals, conferences, books and book chapters with national and international publishers of repute such as IEEE, Springer and Elsevier. He has also served as guest editor/associate editor/editorial member of many reputable journals and organized many international conferences. Dr. Diwakar's editorial expertise is evidenced by his role as an Associate Editor, Academic Editor, and Guest Editor for prominent journals published by Elsevier, SPIE, and Bentham Science, among others. He has also served as a book editor for leading international publishers such as Springer, Elsevier, CRC Press, and Bentham Science. Furthermore, he regularly serves as a reviewer for renowned journals, including IEEE Transactions, Elsevier, Springer, and Inderscience publications.